The Worried Student's Guide to Medical Ethics and Law

Thriving, not just surviving

Deborah Bowman
Professor of Bioethics, Clinical Ethics and Medical Law
at St George's, University of London

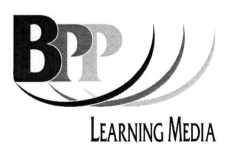

LEARNING MEDIA

First edition October 2011

ISBN 9781 4453 7949 4
e-ISBN 9781 4453 8572 3

British Library Cataloguing-in-Publication Data
A catalogue record for this book is available from
the British Library

Published by
BPP Learning Media Ltd
BPP House, Aldine Place
London W12 8AA

www.bpp.com/health

Typeset by Replika Press Pvt Ltd, India
Printed in the United Kingdom

Your learning materials, published by BPP
Learning Media Ltd, are printed on paper
sourced from sustainable, managed forests.

Contents

About the Publisher   ix
Free Companion Material   x
Abbreviations   xi
About the Author   xiii
Dedications   xiii
Acknowledgements   xiv
Introduction   xv

Chapter 1   **Entering the Medical Moral Maze**   **1**

Introduction: what is the subject of medical
ethics?   2
How is ethics learned and taught?   2
Why do students worry about ethics and
law?   3
What does this book offer the worried
student?   7
Ethical theories and frameworks   7
Methods for analysing an ethical problem
or case   8
The law   12
Reading about ethics and law   14
Professional codes and guidance   15
The student moral maze   16
Assessments: the Ethical Examination   17
The OSCE: ten top tips   23
Activities: Ethics in practice   25
Conclusion   26

Chapter 2   **Morality Tales: Ethics and Medical
             Education**   **27**

On being a medical student   28
Ethical erosion and how to avoid it   29
A student experience – taken from an
educational incident form   31
Conflicts of interest in education   31
Role models and cautionary tales   32
Chaperones and medical students   33

	Professional behaviour, the General Medical Council and medical students	34
	The six domains of professionalism	35
	An ethical education in practice	36
	Maintaining professional relationships	39
	Conclusion: the 'anti-Nike' approach to medical training: don't 'just do it'	41

Chapter 3	**It's My Life: Capacity and Consent**	**43**
3.1	Capacity: introduction	44
	The law	44
	Patients who lack capacity	46
	Lasting Power of Attorney	46
	Advance decisions	47
	Determination of best interests	50
	Capacity and medical students	51
	Core Concepts: Capacity	53
	Assessments: Capacity in practice	54
3.2	Consent: introduction	62
	Seeking consent	62
	Consent in medical education and training	64
	Core Concepts: Consent	65
	Assessment: Consent in practice	66

Chapter 4	**Trust Me, I'm A Medical Student: Confidentiality**	**73**
	Introduction	74
	The duty of confidence: extent and qualification	74
	Consent to share confidential information	75
	Confidential information and the patient's best interests	77
	Disclosure of confidential information in the public interest	78
	Confidentiality and defining the public interest	78
	Is there a duty to warn?	79
	Specific statutory provisions on disclosure of information	80
	Confidentiality and police requests	81
	Particular problems of confidentiality	82
	Patient access to medical information	84
	Confidentiality and death	85

Confidentiality and medical students 85
Core Concepts: Confidentiality 87
Assessments: Confidentiality in practice 88

Chapter 5 New Beginnings: Reproductive Ethics 95

Introduction 96
Personhood and slippery slopes 96
Ways of thinking about personhood and the
status of the embryo 97
Assisted reproduction: questions and
resources 101
Antenatal screening and testing 103
Termination of pregnancy 104
Termination of pregnancy: ethical issues 106
Termination of pregnancy and the law 108
Choice and childbirth 111
Reproductive ethics and medical students 115
Core Concepts: Reproductive Ethics 116
Assessments: Reproductive Ethics in practice 116

Chapter 6 Minor Morality: Children and Adolescents 121

Introduction 122
The child without capacity 122
The older child or adolescent 124
The *Gillick* criteria 125
Consent and confidentiality 127
Paediatric ethics and medical students 128
Core Concepts: Paediatric Ethics and the Law 129
Assessments: Paediatric Ethics in practice 130

Chapter 7 A Meeting of Minds: Mental Health Ethics 137

Introduction 138
The mental health legislation 138
'Mental disorder' for the purposes of the
Mental Health Act 138
Assessment and treatment under the Mental
Health Act 139
Safeguards and the mental health legislation 141
Capacity, choice and treatment not covered
by the Mental Health Act 141
Whose disorder is it anyway? Feminist
ethics and eating disorders 144

Ethics and eating disorders in practice 146
Eating disorders and the law 148
Drug and alcohol dependency 149
Mental health ethics and medical students 151
Core Concepts: Mental Health Ethics and
the Law 154
Assessments: Mental Health Ethics in
practice 154

Chapter 8   I Blame My Parents: Genethics   159
Introduction 160
The nature of genetic information 160
Genetics before birth: saviour siblings 161
Genetic testing 163
Weighing the risks and benefits of genetic
testing 164
Genetic testing of those who lack capacity:
ethical perspectives 165
Sharing genetic information 167
Conclusion 169
Core Concepts: Genethics 170
Assessment: Genethics in practice 171

Chapter 9   Death, Distress and Decisions: End of Life   175
Introduction 176
Decision-making, autonomy and
responsibility at the end of life 177
Acts and omissions 179
The Doctrine of Double Effect 181
Suffering and futility 183
Who decides at the end of life? 186
End-of-life decisions and the law 187
Activities: End-of-Life in practice 190
Ethico-legal perspectives on palliative care 191
Referral to palliative care 191
The patient and clinician in palliative care 194
Palliative care and relatives or carers 196
Palliative care and teamwork 197
Dilemmas at the end of palliative care 199
Conclusion 201
Core Concepts: End of Life 202

End of life and medical students 203
Assessments: End-of-Life in practice 204

Chapter 10 Rights and Wrongs: Human Rights and Global Ethics 217

Introduction 218
Human rights and healthcare 219
The Articles of the Human Rights Act 1998 220
Global health and ethics 224
Cultural competence 224
Cultural relativism 226
Female genital mutilation: an example 227
Global health in practice: the medical
student elective 228
Core Concepts: Human Rights and Global
Ethics 233
Assessment: Human Rights and Global
Ethics 234

Chapter 11 Fallibility, Being Human and Making Mistakes 239

Introduction 240
Who is competent? 240
'Whistleblowing' 241
Complaints and Negligence 247
What is the clinical duty of care? 248
What is the standard of care in medicine? 249
What is causation in clinical negligence? 251
Clinical risk 252
Notes and records 252
Co-operation with other health professionals 254
Writing prescriptions 255
Conclusion 255
Looking after yourself as a medical student 256
Speaking out as a medical student 258
Giving voice to values: seven principles 262
Core Concepts: Competence, Whistleblowing,
Negligence and Clinical Risk 263
Assessments: Competence, Whistleblowing,
Negligence and Clinical Risk 264

Contents

**Chapter 12 Publish or Perish: Research and
             Publication Ethics**   **269**

Introduction   270
Research with human subjects   270
The validity and rigour of research   272
Balancing risks and benefits in research   274
Valid consent in research   277
Therapeutic and non-therapeutic research   280
Activities: research with human subjects   283
Guinea pigs as guinea pigs: the ethics of
using animals in biomedical research   283
The ethics of research involving animals   284
The regulatory framework for the use of
animals in research   287
Publication Ethics   289
Authors and Contributors   289
Research and 'salami slicing'   290
Conflicts of interest   290
Conclusion   290
Research and publication ethics and medical
students   291
Core Concepts: Research and Publication
Ethics   293
Assessment: Research and Publication Ethics   294

**Chapter 13 It's Another World: Healthcare Policy,
             Resource Allocation and Ethics**   **299**

Introduction   300
Resource allocation: the challenges   301
Ethical approaches to resource allocation   303
The law and resource allocation   306
Resource allocation and health policy   308
Resource allocation in clinical practice   310
Conclusion   312
Healthcare policy and medical students   312
Core Concepts: Healthcare Policy   313
Assessments: Healthcare Policy   314

Chapter 14 Putting It Together: Concluding Thoughts   **321**

**Appendix   A Literary Potpourri: Recommended
             Reading and Further Resources**   **325**

About the Publisher

BPP Learning Media is dedicated to supporting aspiring professionals with top quality learning material. BPP Learning Media's commitment to success is shown by our record of quality, innovation and market leadership in paper-based and e-learning materials. BPP Learning Media's study materials are written by professionally-qualified specialists who know from personal experience the importance of top quality materials for success.

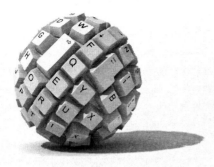

Free Companion Material

Readers can access more case studies and scenarios, with the author's commentary and links to relevant student guidance, for free online.

To access the above companion material please visit **www.bpp.com/freehealthresources**

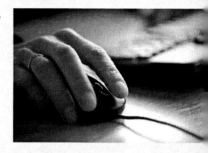

Abbreviations

A&E	Accident and Emergency
BMA	British Medical Association
BPAS	British Pregnancy Advisory Service
COPE	Committee on Publication Ethics
CPC	Choroid plexus cysts
CPR	Cardiopulmonary resuscitation
CQC	Care Quality Commission
DNAR	Do Not Attempt Resuscitation
DoH	Department of Health
DPA	Data Protection Act
DVLA	Driver and Vehicle Licensing Agency
ECHR	European Court of Human Rights
ECT	Electroconvulsive therapy
EMI	Extended matching items
FGM	Female genital mutilation
GAfREC	Government Arrangements for Research Ethics Committees
GMC	General Medical Council
GP	General practitioner
HFEA	Human Fertilisation and Embryology Authority
HRA	Human Rights Act
HMRC	Her Majesty's Revenue and Customs
ICU	Intensive care unit
INR	International normalised ratio
IVF	In vitro fertilisation
LPA	Lasting Power of Attorney
MCQ	Multiple choice question
NHS	National Health Service
NRES	National Research Ethics Service
OSCE	Objective structured clinical examination
PCT	Primary Care Trust

Abbreviations

QALYS	Quality-adjusted life year
RCP	Royal College of Physicians
REC	Research Ethics Committee
SAQ	Short answer question
SBA	Single best answer
SOAD	Second Opinion Appointed Doctor
TB	Tuberculosis
TOPs	Terminations of pregnancies
WHO	World Health Organisation

About the Author

Professor Deborah Bowman is Professor of Bioethics, Clinical Ethics and Medical Law at St George's, University of London. She has been involved in medical education at both an undergraduate and postgraduate level for over fifteen years. She has a longstanding interest in professional competence, and disputes in healthcare, with a particular emphasis on education. Deborah Bowman's interest in 'applied clinical ethics' enables her to work closely with policy organisations. She is also an accredited mediator working within the NHS. She has written widely, both in the academic and popular press, and is a regular commentator in the media, most recently as a programme consultant and panellist on the BBC Radio 4 series 'Inside the Ethics Committee'.

Dedications

This book is dedicated to all the students past and present, worried and otherwise.

Acknowledgements

This is a book that has been haunting my waking and sleeping hours for many years. Most days I have thought about what this book would be like and those thoughts have been shaped by innumerable conversations, encounters and observations. Many of the ideas that informed this book have their origins in the stimulating, encouraging and supportive environment of St George's, University of London, and St. George's NHS Trust, London. Students, staff and patients from across both institutions have contributed immeasurably, and often unknowingly, to this book and I am enormously grateful. There are colleagues and friends who have tolerated more of my thinking allowed than anyone should have to bear and special thanks are due to John Spicer, Leanda Kroll, Judith Ibison, Peter McCrorie, June Jones, Mary Gentile, Gwen Adshead, Lisa Schwartz and Suzanne Shale.

The science unit and broadcasters at the BBC taught me much about conveying complex ideas; particular gratitude is owed to Vivienne Parry, Beth Eastwood, Deborah Cohen, Pamela Rutherford, Michelle Martin and Joan Bakewell. The world of health policy has been a longstanding interest and Rosemary Field, Vicky Voller and Alastair Scotland were excellent guides to a mysterious world. My editor, Matt Green, has given new meaning to the word 'patient' as he responded with equanimity to unexpected crises and delays that meant this project took far longer than either of us anticipated. He is a gentleman in the world of publishing and his support, kindness and professionalism will never be forgotten. Finally, to my family whom I have ignored for far too many weekends: your love, tolerance and encouragement have made this book possible. Thank you.

Introduction

Medical students are often worried. It is unsurprising: medicine is a demanding training that expects much from those who embark upon the path of becoming a doctor. In over fifteen years of working with medical students of all ages and at all stages in their education, I have observed that ethics and law is one aspect of medical training that causes particular anxieties. What's more, it is not merely the matter of passing examinations in the subject that causes students to be concerned. As well as worrying about assessments in ethics and law, students are worried about how to apply what they have learned in practice. Given the diversity of learning environments, particularly clinical environments, students are likely to meet a wide range of role models, both positive and negative, and be called upon to draw their own moral boundaries.

Throughout my career, it has been my pleasure to work with, and learn from, many medical students, a lot of whom have sought advice and support when they have encountered, or been encouraged to participate in, what they perceived to be sub-optimal or ethically questionable practice. The challenge facing students in such situations is considerable and I have consistently been struck by how uncomfortable it can be as a medical student. As a result, I have long wanted to write a book for medical students that contained not only the essential information relating to the core curriculum and its assessment, but that also discussed the dilemmas that students can encounter in what is often described somewhat disparagingly to academics as 'the real world'. This is that book and it is dedicated to every student who has trusted me and shared their experiences of moral discomfort: I have learned much from each of you and the medical profession is all the better for you joining its ranks.

Chapter 1

Entering the Medical Moral Maze

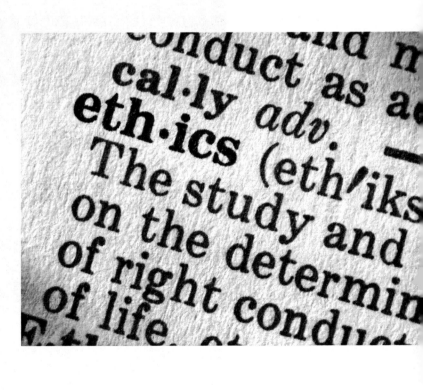

Entering the Medical Moral Maze

Introduction: what is the subject of medical ethics?

Whatever the content of a curriculum, ethics education incorporates knowledge; cognitive skills such as reasoning, critique and logical analysis; and clinical skills whereby abstract ethical learning is integrated with other clinical learning and applied appropriately in practice. Indeed, unless students and clinicians are able to draw on learning in ethics to enhance daily practice and better serve their patients, ethics education has ultimately failed.

How is ethics learned and taught?

Medical schools are given considerable flexibility in how they ensure that students meet the prescribed learning outcomes described by the General Medical Council in *Tomorrow's Doctors*.[1] Ethics is therefore, like other subjects, learned in diverse ways depending on the preferences of staff, the available resources, the educational philosophy of the course and practicalities. However, the most effective ethics learning is likely to occur when students experience a range of activities. Didactic, large group lectures are appropriate for sharing information efficiently, for example outlining the details of Mental Health legislation or the provisions for non-voluntary treatment in psychiatry. Small group tutorials or seminars enable students and tutors to discuss ideas in depth, to form and to challenge arguments and to explore intuitions. Clinical learning provides a window onto 'ethics in practice' as the neat, ordered and illusory clarity of textbooks yields to the uncertain, sometimes confusing and often memorable reality of daily practice. Individual mentoring allows students and their teachers the time to reflect on, discuss and explain the 'back story' to decisions, choices and practice. In short, if there is an opportunity to engage with the subject of medical ethics and law, seize it!

Ethical reasoning may sound terribly grand, but, in reality, it is nothing more than thinking through the available options (which, of course, depends on being sufficiently informed to know what

---

[1] *Tomorrow's Doctors*. London: General Medical Council, 2006.

options are available) and weighing the relative merits thereof in a logical and thorough manner. Whilst undergraduate education and training in ethics varies, one way of thinking about the process of learning in ethics is as shown below.[2]

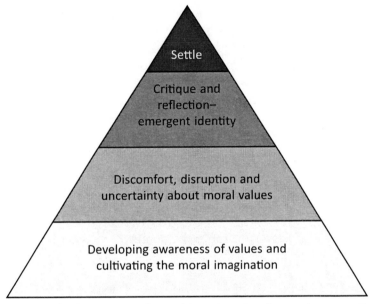

Figure 1.1 The four stages of an ethics education: learner's perspective

Why do students worry about ethics and law?

For most students, an ethical education will involve emotion, discomfort and perhaps irritation as personal responses are interrogated and constructively challenged with contrasting perspectives. All of us have our own values and opinions. A necessary part of learning in ethics and law is to become aware of the assumptions on which your personal values are based, to reflect on those values critically and to listen and respond to challenging or opposing beliefs. As Douglas Adams pointed out, assumptions are the things we don't know we're making. Over time, you will begin to realise that the 'intuitive' and apparently 'clear' response to an ethical dilemma is dependent on inherent assumptions and personal values that may never have made explicit before in education. As

---

[2] For detailed discussion of the origins and application of this model in ethics education, see Bowman, D. The Challenges of an Ethical Education in Europe. *Die Psychiatrie* 2005; 2(3): 158–164.

you progress, so you will become increasingly aware that there are varied ways of approaching disease. Likewise, the more you engage with the ethical dimensions of medicine, the more you will begin to see multiple perspectives on problems.

A frequently heard lament from medical students concerned about ethics is that there is *'no right answer'*. Whilst it is the case that ethics often incorporates diverse analyses leading sometimes to a number of different conclusions, there are ways of approaching an ethical issue which are dependent on an accurate understanding of the relevant law, professional guidance and clear elucidation of the relevant moral questions. In other words, there is information that you need to know and ways of expressing your views that provide structure and rigour. Your personal views are important, but you also need to acknowledge other perspectives, be supported by reasoning and located in an accurate understanding of the current law and relevant professional guidance. In other words, there are answers and often the way in which you express that answer will be as important as the content of your response. Like mathematics, ethics is a subject where you are required to show your working!

In contrast to learning the basic and clinical science of medicine, ethics can sometimes appear to challenge the core of a person's belief system and therefore identity. As such, sometimes even gentle debate, questioning and challenge can feel, if not personal, certainly uncomfortable. This is neither unexpected nor is it unique to medicine. Few people like to be challenged or relish having the weaknesses in their arguments revealed. It is exposing and, if not done carefully, can result in feeling alienated and inhibited. The key point is that uncertainty, complexity and plurality of approach are signs of ethical competence not incompetence. With practice, confidence grows.

Teachers and students should be aware of the significance of emotion and its effects on a learner's willingness to participate in, and apply, even the 'best' education. Rather than being an 'irrational' or undesirable response, emotion is helpful because it indicates an important issue or significant problem. Your anxiety is linked to your commitment to becoming and being 'a good clinician'. And that is an achievement to be celebrated.

The vignettes below are obviously caricatures, but you may recognise some of the traits demonstrated by these students. Don't worry: this is not a 'what type of medical student are you?' exercise. These vignettes are included to emphasise that these responses to ethics and law are normal, valuable and can be managed by both students and teachers alike to demystify the world of ethics and law.

Pragmatic Paul – 'What do I have to know to be safe?'

Paul is overwhelmed by the sheer volume of what there is to learn in medicine and takes a strategic approach to his learning. For Paul, the bottom line is all that matters and he knows that clinical negligence and complaints are risks. Paul can see that ethical discussion and the analysis of different perspectives might be interesting, but in a crammed timetable, he feels it is something of a luxury and really just wants to know *'what do I have to know so as not to be sued?'*

Paul is right to want to know the key messages about core topics and should not be criticised for seeking a bottom line. However, as Paul begins to learn more about the law and becomes skilled in critiquing relevant rules, guidelines, principles and approaches, he will see the how policy, regulation and ethics are inextricably linked. Paul will begin to see that being 'safe' usually involves reasoned and explicable decision-making. The shortcuts Paul seeks may be misleadingly appealing, even dangerous. Paul should use the relative space a medical student enjoys to develop reasoning and analytical skills so that he can bring a considered approach to his practice when he qualifies. Discussion with senior clinicians who have made difficult decisions, in which they make explicit their choices and the rationale for those choices, will also help Paul see that the notion of a single bottom line may be illusory but that does not mean decision-making is paralysed.

Sceptical Sima – 'What's the point of ethical reasoning if I'm going to get sued anyway?'

Poor Sima needs to know that it is not all doom and gloom! As with many other topical stories, tales of the litigation sword of Damacles hanging over the heads of all clinicians are much exaggerated and distorted. It remains relatively difficult to bring a successful clinical negligence action. In any event, defensive medicine is unhelpful and is likely to make Sima unhappy. Sima needs to know why people complain and sue their doctors. As she progresses through the course, Sima will begin to realise that she has a lot of power and responsibility to ensure her relationships are professional, thereby serving her patients and protecting herself. As well as thinking about the aetiology of clinical negligence, Sima should think about how she will practise in areas where there are many gaps in the law. For example, the law offers limited, broad headings only in respect of confidentiality, so Sima needs to find ways to work through how she will interpret these broad headings in practice. Legal precedent may guide her, but she needs recourse to ethical frameworks and structures to help her elucidate and analyse situations. Susan may enjoy tools such as David Seedhouse's ethical grid[3] which provide a structured approach to ethico-legal problems.

Moral Malak – 'Just because the law and the GMC say I have to do it, doesn't mean I should'

Malak is correct to acknowledge that there may be a difference between morality and legality. Sometimes the law explicitly codifies a moral position, sometimes it supplements it and sometimes it acknowledges that there is difference. For example, the Abortion Act 1967, as amended, regulates a practice that some consider to be immoral and acknowledges that although terminations may be lawful provided certain criteria are met, some clinicians believe terminations to be unethical and there is a right of conscientious objection.

However, conscientious objection for which the law makes explicit provision is different from accepting that personal ethics can or should override the law. Indeed, a doctor who acts outside the law that has been passed in a democratic society might be considered to be arrogant as well as professionally foolish. This is not to suggest that the perceived dissonance between law and morality that Malak cites is irrelevant or unworthy of discussion. On the contrary, much useful learning can come from exploring Malak's disagreements with specific legal provisions using structured reasoning and facilitated discussion with those who have a different perspective.

Confused Chris – 'Where does the BMA fit in?'

Chris is expressing a common difficulty for students who are encountering an entirely new vocabulary (in addition to the biomedical and scientific vocabulary with which they also have to become familiar). Chris needs exercises to explore boundaries between law, professional codes and guidelines and ethical principles and theory. As with all new skills, when explicit signposts, steps to work through and structures are helpful and as one becomes more confident, so the process becomes implicit and natural.

---

[3] Seedhouse, D. *Ethics: The Heart of Healthcare* (3rd ed.) Chichester: Wiley, 2009.

What does this book offer the worried student?

This book aims to be distinct from the many other titles competing for students' attention. Whilst the core curriculum in ethics and law is comprehensively covered, this title differs in that it reflects the preoccupations and concerns of the many students who have shared their experiences with me. Each chapter follows the same structure. First, the core concepts are discussed using illustrative activities and case studies to demonstrate reasoning and the application of key information to the clinical context. Secondly, there is a section dedicated to assessment of the topic in which sample Objective Structured Clinical Examination (OSCE) stations and written questions are provided. Finally, there is a discussion of how students might experience ethico-legal dilemmas prior to qualification. Whilst much of the information discussed in the pages of this book are based on conversations with students, care has been taken both to seek consent to use, and to anonymise, the material.

Ethical theories and frameworks

As the subject of ethics has evolved so too have theories and frameworks which are used to explain and structure moral analysis. Like any other part of your medical training, you are learning a subject where experts have theorised, debated and analysed problems. Theories and frameworks are simply approaches to ethical reasoning which can be useful and need not be feared. Crudely put, there are frameworks and tools that tend to focus on the application of ethical theory to clinical problems and they are mostly derived from ethical theories. The box below summarises the key ethical theories that a medical student may encounter.

Key ethical theories

Deontology	A rule- or duty-based approach to morality in which defined norms should be followed and obligations fulfilled without exception eg a deontologist would argue that one should always tell truth irrespective of the consequences. In Western ethics, deontology is generally said to derive from the work of Immanuel Kant.
Consequentialism	An approach that argues that morality is located in the outcomes or consequences. In bioethical terms, such

	an approach is evident in discussions of likely risks and benefits. In Western ethics, consequentialism is generally said to derive from utilitarianism and the work of Jeremy Bentham and John Stuart Mill.
Virtue Ethics	Offers an approach in which particular traits, characteristics or behaviours are identified as desirable and likely to lead to positive moral outcomes. It is sometimes described as a hybrid theory in that it combines the normative approach of deontology with reference to the positive consequences of virtuous characteristics or behaviours.
Rights Theory	Assesses morality with reference to the justified claims of others, most commonly individuals, against society or the provision of a service eg healthcare. Rights may be moral or 'natural' and arise from being human, or legal and therefore enforceable in court. Sometimes a distinction is drawn between positive rights that impose a duty on another to act, or negative rights which prohibit interference from others.
Narrative Ethics	An approach that counters the rationality claimed by deontologists and consequentialists depending on subjective and particular experiences. In narrative ethics, morality is embedded in the stories (note: these differ from medical histories) shared between patient and clinician. It is an approach that argues that moral choices should be informed by attention to multiple, even conflicting, perspectives on a situation.

How persuaded you are by a particular theory is an individual and personal response. You shouldn't be afraid to experiment with different approaches. Indeed, it is worthwhile understanding other ethical approaches, even in broad terms, as it will help you to see how others might approach the same ethical problem.

Methods for analysing an ethical problem or case

1. The four principles

Many students encounter 'the four principles' approach in medical ethics education. The framework was originally proposed by two

American bioethicists, Tom Beauchamp and James Childress[4], and it has become a dominant approach in Western medical ethics. Ranaan Gillon, one of the earliest advocates for ethics education in the United Kingdom, has published[5] a shorter and developed version of a principles-based approach to medical ethics which is preferred by some. The four principles being:

- Autonomy – literally 'self-rule' ie people are able to make their own choices and to decide what happens to them in healthcare
- Beneficence – to do good ie to act in a patient's best interests, as determined by the autonomous patient him or herself
- Non-maleficence – to avoid harm (derived from a well-known Latin instruction to doctors: 'first do no harm' or 'primum non nocere')
- Justice – to treat people equitably and fairly

The four principles represent 'mid-level' principles and are intended to enable structured analysis of diverse moral problems and specific situations. In any given situation, the four principles can be systematically considered to explore the ways in which individual choices and preferences can be informed, respected and protected; risks can be minimised and balanced against benefits (which are more than merely medical benefits); and fairness, equity and parity achieved.

Although the four principles approach is common, even dominant, in UK ethics teaching, it is not without its critics. The four principles approach has been criticised for its formulaic ubiquity in ethics education, leading one commentator to describe the approach as '*utterly fatuous*'.[6] There is undoubtedly a risk for those who come to rely too unquestioningly on the four principles as the default and sole method of analysing an ethical problem. There is neither any inherent moral magic in using the words 'beneficence' or 'non-maleficence', nor does the framework guarantee a comprehensive or intelligent analysis and resolution of an ethical issue. Often, particularly in written answers, students will write the principles

---

[4] Beauchamp, T. L, Childress, J. F. *Principles of Biomedical Ethics* (6th ed.) New York: Oxford University Press, 2008.

[5] Gillon, R. *Philosophical Medical Ethics*. Chichester: Wiley, 1985.

[6] Cowley, C. The Dangers of Medical Ethics. *JME* 2005; 31: 739–742.

down without explanation or even reference to the specific question. The four principles are a useful starting point but they are not the only way to approach an ethical problem. Indeed, most clinicians encounter bioethical problems in their daily work and rarely invoke the language of the four principles explicitly. Ideas and opinions about risk, benefits, fairness and personal choices inform discussions on the wards, but such discussions are not usually billed as 'applying the four principles'. This book aims to mirror clinical work and to demonstrate how judicious use of the four principles can be helpful whilst reassuring readers that the four principles is but one of many ways of approaching ethical dilemmas both in examinations and real life. As such, the language of the four principles is used in an applied way but only where it is directly relevant to the scenarios presented and discussed.

2. Structured case analysis

When approaching a problem, a scenario or a case study the following process might help order your thinking:

•   Summarise the case or problem
•   State the moral dilemma(s)
•   State the assumptions being made or to be made
•   Analyse the case with reference to:
−   Ethical principles/frameworks/theories
−   Consequences
−   Professional codes of practice or national guidelines
−   To the law
•   Acknowledge other approaches and state the preferred approach with explanation

3. The ethics 'work up' (Bowman 2010, after Jonsen, Siegler and Winsade 2006)

The American bioethicists Jonsen, Siegler and Winslade[7] identified four 'topics' that they argue are basic and intrinsic to every clinical encounter, namely:

---

[7] Jonsen, A. R., Siegler, M, Winslade, W. J. *Clinical Ethics: A Practical Approach to Ethical Decisions in Clinical Medicine* (6th ed.). New York: McGraw-Hill Medical, 2006.

- Medical indications – all clinical encounters include a review of diagnosis and treatment options;
- Patient preferences – all clinical encounters occur because a patient presents before the doctor with a complaint or problem. The patient's values are integral to the encounter;
- Quality of life – the objective of all clinical encounters is to improve, or at least address, quality of life for the patient; and
- Contextual features – all clinical encounters occur in a wider context beyond individual doctor and presenting patient, to include family, the law, hospital policy, national regulations, etc.

These four topics are present in, and pertinent to, every case or ethical problem. In the interest of consistency, the order in which each topic is considered should remain the same. However, no topic bears more weight than the others. Each should be evaluated as shown in the box below:

Medical Indications:	Patient Preferences:
Consider each medical condition and its proposed treatment: (i) Does it fulfil any of the goals of medicine? (ii) With what likelihood? How do I know? (iii) If not, is the proposed treatment futile?	What does the patient want? Does the patient have the capacity to decide? If not, can anyone advocate the patient? Do the patient's wishes reflect a process that is: • informed? • understood? • voluntary? • continuing?
Quality of Life: Describe the patient's quality of life in the patient's terms and from the care providers' perspectives.	**Contextual Features:** Circumstances that can either influence the decision or be influenced by the decision.

The four topics described above give you a map or visual overview of the case or problem ensuring that relevant perspectives are captured consciously and with structure. Having mapped the case or problem, a series of questions should be considered:

- What is at issue?
- Where is the conflict?
- What is this a case of? Does it sound like other cases you may have encountered?
- What do we know about other cases like this one? Is there clear legal or practice-based precedent? If so, it is a paradigm case ie one in which the facts are well-known and about which there is professional and/or public agreement concerning its resolution.
- How is the present case similar to the paradigm case? How is it different? Is it similar (or different) in ethically significant ways?

The law

There are three legal systems within the United Kingdom, namely the legal systems of i) England and Wales; ii) Scotland; and iii) Northern Ireland. Although in practice there is a great deal of similarity, it is important for students intending to move around the United Kingdom to remember that there are three distinct legal systems. This book focuses only English and Welsh law.

England and Wales operates a common law system which essentially means that law is made via judicial decisions in cases which establish precedents that are applied to future cases. Whether a judicial decision constitutes a precedent depends on which court made the decision with higher level courts having authority over the lower level courts. The diagram below is taken from Her Majesty's Court Service and shows the court hierarchy.[8]

Within the legal system, there are two broad categories, namely criminal and civil law. Whilst the majority of cases involving healthcare take place in the civil system, occasionally medical cases become criminal eg when a patient dies in circumstances

---

[8] www.justis.com/support/faq-courts.aspx

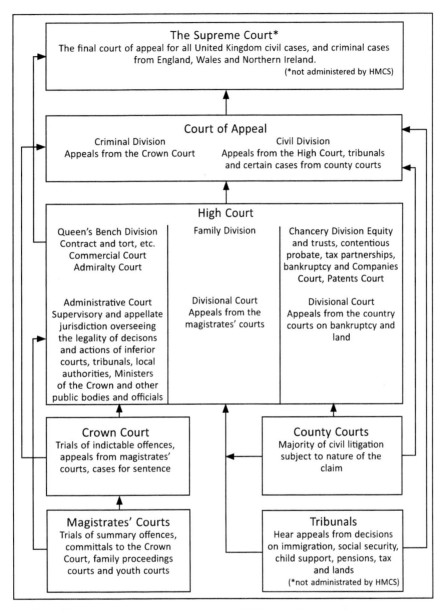

Figure 1.2 The court hierarchy system (© Crown Copyright, reproduced from the HMRC website under the Open Government Licence: www. nationalarchives.gov.uk/doc/open-government-licence)

that may constitute manslaughter. The burden of proof differs in criminal and civil cases. A criminal case must be proved beyond reasonable doubt in order for there to be a conviction, whereas in a civil case eg a claim of negligence, the claim must be proved on the balance of probabilities.

In addition to case law, you will also encounter Statutes or Acts of Parliament that set out law in particular areas of clinical practice such as the Abortion, Mental Health and Mental Capacity Acts. Statutes can be amended by parliament (eg the Abortion Act 1967 has been amended by the Human Fertilisation and Embryology Act 1990) consolidated into subsequent legislation or repealed by another Act of Parliament. A statute is described as primary legislation and will often be supplemented by implementation guidance in the form of Codes of Practice eg the Mental Health Act Code of Practice or delegated legislation such as statutory instruments.

When you encounter legal references, you are likely to be bemused. It can take law students many years to become familiar with the myriad referencing systems for cases. For most medical students, it is sufficient to know that court proceedings are transcribed and will appear in a 'law report'. Those law reports may be published in a newspaper, online in a legal database and in bound volumes. Law reports are referenced in abbreviated form immediately after the names of the parties and the date of the report. There are many different abbreviations depending both on the nature of the case and where it is published but you do not need to worry about those.

Reading about ethics and law

The amount of reading you do about ethics and law will depend on the nature of your course and your own interest in the subject. Students have often said that they find the subject fascinating in the teaching room but when they go off to do their own research they encounter papers that are impenetrable or, even worse, dull. Whilst there is limited advice to be offered about dull papers (apart from perhaps avoidance), it may be useful to have a structure in mind when reading a paper. Soon, these steps will become automatic, but at the beginning it can be useful to work through a checklist similar to that shown in the box below.

Reading an academic paper in ethics and law: a 12-step approach

1.	What is your first impression of the paper? Why?
2.	What are the key points made in the paper?
3.	What assumptions does the author make?
4.	What is the author's conclusion?
5.	How do the key points support his or her conclusion?
6.	What alternative perspectives does the author consider?
7.	Are there any inconsistencies in the argument(s)?
8.	How does the paper compare with other reading you have done on the topic?
9.	How would the author's approach be applied to a clinical case?
10.	Do you agree or disagree with the author? Why?
11.	What questions remain unaddressed or inadequately answered?
12.	If you had the chance to ask the author one question about the paper, what would it be?

Professional codes and guidance

As well as ethical theories and frameworks, and the law, you will also find standards and ethical guidance in codes of practice. Codes differ both in how much they are included in medical education and status. For example, the standards set out by the General Medical Council ('GMC') are the basis on which doctors are regulated. If a doctor falls below the expectations of the General Medical Council, he or she is vulnerable to disciplinary procedures irrespective of the harm caused or whether legal action ensues. Recently, the GMC has turned its attention to the standards expected of medical students. The publication *Medical Students: Professional Values and Fitness to Practise* is an important document and sets out how medical students are expected to behave and why.[9] In contrast, the Hippocratic Oath, although well-known, is outdated and something of an ethical curiosity meaning it is rarely, if ever, sworn. The symbolic value of taking an oath of some kind remains and significant numbers of medical schools expect students to make a declaration or commitment to maintaining ethical standards, often at graduation.

---

[9] The document, in common with all the ethical guidance from the GMC, is available at www.gmc-uk.org in the 'Education' section.

The student moral maze

A word that you are likely to hear often as a medical student is 'professional'. It is a term that can seem both dauntingly wide and frustratingly abstract. So what does it mean to be a 'professional' student? There are multiple definitions of professionalism. At the time of writing an internet search brought up a staggering 1,652,354 descriptions. You have been selected for your place at medical school in a highly competitive process for your potential. You already have the foundations of professionalism. Professional behaviour is not just something that is expected with patients. Your interactions with your peers too provide opportunities for you to reflect on, and demonstrate, professionalism. For example, clinical skills sessions provide not only an opportunity to learn practical skills but also an opportunity to learn how to maintain the dignity of the person with whom you are learning and obtain consent for conducting a clinical examination. Properly obtained consent, professional behaviour and respect for confidentiality in clinical skills sessions is likely to generate an atmosphere in which students feel sufficiently 'safe' to volunteer and participate fully.

The last decade has seen considerable increase in attention to professionalism at medical school. Papers abound on the most effective strategies for teaching professional behaviour, reliable assessments of professionalism and the relationship between professionalism at medical school and subsequent fitness to practise. Of the myriad publications, there are two notable projects. First, as mentioned earlier, the General Medical Council has issued guidance that is specifically applicable to medical students.[10] The GMC guidance has been followed by two initiatives: podcasts and an e-bulletin both aimed at communicating directly and regularly with medical students about professionalism and standards. Secondly, the King's Fund has been running a large medical student-led project called 'The 21st Century Doctor' via roadshows and Facebook. The project is ongoing at the time of writing[11] but its webpage makes interesting reading even in advance of the publication of conclusions. The subject of professionalism amongst medical students is considered in depth in Chapter 2: 'Morality Tales: Ethics and Medical Education'.

---

[10] The document, in common with all the ethical guidance from the GMC, is available at www.gmc-uk.org in the 'Education' section.

[11] http://www.kingsfund.org.uk/current_projects/the_21stcentury_doctor/

Assessments: the Ethical Examination

Written assessments

Written assessments of ethics and law come in many guises. Common approaches include short answer questions (SAQs), extended matching questions or items (EMQs and EMIs respectively) and single best answer questions (SBAs) often as part of an integrated examination covering the full range of subjects encountered by medical students. Less commonly, written assessments may consist of short or modified essays or multiple choice questions. In addition to written examinations that take place at the end of a module, term, semester or year, many medical students will encounter in-course assessments in ethics and law. Such in-course assessments may be essay-based, task-orientated or related to a portfolio. For example, in the author's own institution, students are, at different points in the course, required to write a reflective piece about the ethico-legal dimensions of their experiences in the clinical environment, work in groups to prepare and deliver a presentation on a topical ethico-legal problem or issue and write a letter to a journal. In addition to the core assessments, there are likely to be opportunities to student selected components or special study modules in ethics and law which offer the chance to explore a particular area in greater depth. Finally, a rising number of students choose to pursue intercalated degrees in ethics and law and in related disciplines such as philosophy and the medical humanities.

Whatever the specific format of the written assessment in ethics and law, there are some principles that are helpful to all types of questions. First, written assessments have three main aims, namely to:

1. Test your knowledge; and/or
2. Evaluate your understanding; and/or
3. Assess your reasoning ability

Keeping these three aims in mind when you are both preparing for, and completing, written assessments will help focus your revision, structure your answers and improve both your confidence and performance.

Questions in the MCQ, EMI, EMQ and SBA format obviously contain the answer, but a well-written question will also include convincing distracters. Those distracting items will be plausible options; indeed in the case of SBA questions where you are being asked to choose the single best option the distracters are often realistic, albeit sub-optimal, responses. To answer these types of questions, you need not only to know your stuff but also how to apply that stuff! You are being asked the ethico-legal equivalent of 'driving test' medicine ie to demonstrate best practice. As such, you need to be sure that you know the fundamentals and how those fundamentals relate to clinical practice. For example, in relation to young children, you need to understand the concepts of parental responsibility; the rationale for, and limits of, parental consent; and the role of the courts in medical conflicts involving children. The very act of identifying the fundamentals of a topic is an important stage in enhancing your understanding. To make the task easier, in this book, there is a box at the end of each chapter describing the core concepts relevant to the topic. In EMI, EMQ, SBA and MCQ questions, reasoning is implicit ie it is captured by the question but you are not being asked to explain your answer.

In contrast to SBAs, EMIs, EMQs and MCQs, short answer questions require you to answer in your own words. Pay attention to the number of available marks. I frequently mark papers where students have written three-quarters of a page in response to a question where there is only a single mark available. Conversely, it is not unusual to encounter two-word answers where there are ten marks available for that question. The number of marks is a clue as to the weight and time you should give to the question: it is intended to help! It is important to note the verbs used in questions. For example, if you are asked to 'list', it is likely that you are being asked to cite pieces of factual information, as in the question below:

Sample SAQ

Question List the four elements of consent. (4 marks)

Answer Consent should be:
    (i)   Made by a person with capacity;
    (ii)   Given voluntarily;
    (iii)   Sufficiently informed; and
    (iv)   Continuing.

If you are asked to 'explain' or 'discuss' a concept, this is an invitation to not merely say what you think or recite knowledge you have picked up about the topic, but indicates an expectation that you will give reasons for your response. The examiner needs to know why you are answering as you do. So, if there are relevant sources to support your answer such as the law, cases or professional guidance from the GMC and / or other influential organisations such as the Royal Colleges, you should cite those sources. Similarly if you are asserting a particular point of view, excellent answers will acknowledge alternative opinions and demonstrate reasoning. The question below demonstrates the skills required in a SAQ where you are asked to explain your answer:

Sample SAQ

Mr Dunston's wife, Mrs Susan Dunston, arrives at the renal unit, unaccompanied by her husband and asks to see the consultant. The consultant meets Mrs Dunston who explains that she is 'terribly concerned' about her husband. She tells the consultant that he *'won't tell me anything. I have no idea how ill he actually is, or what the future holds'*. She asks the consultant *'can you tell what's really going on? After all, I am his next of kin.'*

Question How should the consultant respond to Mrs Dunston's request. Please explain your answer. (4 marks)

Answer The consultant should explain that he is unable to discuss Mr Dunston's care with Mrs Dunston without explicit permission from Mr Dunston. The rationale for this is the duty of confidentiality which is embodied in both law and the GMC guidance on confidentiality and states that the duty to a patient is qualified only when:

- The patient has consented to sharing information;
- It is not possible to obtain the patient's consent to share the information but it is the patient's best interests so to do; and
- There is a serious risk of physical harm to an identifiable individual or individuals (*W v Egdell*).

In the scenario described, there are no grounds for the consultant to share confidential information without Mr Dunston's express consent which, regrettably, the consultant does not have.

In course assessments are typically longer pieces of work and may be reflective or academic in nature. The first rule therefore is to consider whether you are being asked to write something personal about your own experience of, and response, to ethico-legal issues in medicine or whether you are expected to produce a scholarly piece of work comprised of analysis and referenced argument.

Reflective writing requires you not merely 'to do', but 'to *learn* from doing'. To succeed in reflective work, you need to be alert to the human elements of your experiences eg what did you feel? How did the experience fit with or challenge your values? What has gone well for you and what challenges remain? What were your observations about the response of others? It is a hybrid task that requires you to write from both the personal and professional perspective. Many students are wary of, and anxious about, reflective writing. Such anxiety is not surprising: using the first person and talking about the subjective are alien to medical students who are trained to write in the dispassionate and objective tradition of the biosciences. I have never yet met a student who, without encouragement and reassurance that they *really are* being asked to write about themselves, and their feelings and thoughts, did not manage to write reflective pieces. What's more, the reflective writing that it has been my privilege to read has been among the most thoughtful, moving and thought-provoking work that students have shared with me. So, have a go, dive in and enjoy!

Academic writing for in course assessments may be in the form of essays, reports or even dissertations if you are doing an intercalated degree, although many courses, including my own, try to set imaginative tasks that are not essay-based. For example, over the years I have asked students to write a letter to a journal in response to a paper; to analyse a case; to critique guidelines on resuscitation decision-making; to write an editorial about a medical news item; to participate in a debate; to write a book review; and to make a conference poster. Whilst, the assessment options described above vary in format, each one requires that you demonstrate knowledge, understanding and reasoning ability. The box below describes the characteristics of strong and weaker answers in longer pieces of writing about ethics and law.

Stronger Answers	Weaker Answers
Accurately describe the relevant law, both statutory and case-based	Omit or misrepresent key pieces of legislation or case law
Appropriately and relevantly engage with ethical theories, models and frameworks, explaining why the approach has been chosen and its relevance to the subject	Does not demonstrate engagement with principal and relevant ethical theories, models or frameworks and/or does not explain choice of approach with reference to subject at hand
Constructs a reasoned argument that is convincingly argued and acknowledges alternate perspectives	Does not present a cogent argument, often preferring to invoke largely personal opinion and/or presents only a partisan analysis without acknowledging diversity of possible perspectives
Is fully and appropriately referenced demonstrating engagement with a range of materials, including seminal papers and professional guidance	Is poorly referenced and/or lacks evidence of attention to source materials, be it in ethics, law or professional guidance and codes of practice
Applies information to provide a specific response to the title, question or problem posed	Does not convincingly apply the ideas presented to the particular title, question or problem posed
Reaches a conclusion that is supported by the discussion in the piece	Does not offer a conclusion, or reaches a conclusion for which the discussion does not argue or sustain
Remains within the word limit and is without spelling and grammatical errors	Exceeds the word limit and/or is marred by poor grammar and spelling

Practical assessments

The most common form of practical assessment in ethics and law is the Objective Structured Clinical Examination (OSCE) station. In an OSCE, ethics and law are both integrated into stations and assessed as a discrete, stand-alone 'ethics and law' station; you will find that there are ethico-legal elements throughout an OSCE. For example, in any station requiring you to examine a patient or simulated patient, you are likely to be required to seek and obtain consent and to attend to the patient's dignity and comfort whilst also demonstrating your clinical examination skills. In addition, there are stations where the focus is predominantly or exclusively ethics and law which can cover any of the material presented in this book. Examples of how ethics and law can be examined in OSCE stations is included in each chapter of this title, but for now it is worth thinking about what you can do to enhance your OSCE performance both in relation to ethics and law, and more generally.

In nearly twenty years of assessing in OSCEs, I have observed that there are characteristics that are shared by those students who excel and those who struggle in OSCEs. The box below summarises what defines a stronger and a weaker performance in an OSCE.

Stronger OSCE Performance	Weaker OSCE Performance
A confident introduction and a clear opening that reflects what the student has been asked to do (rather than what she wishes she had been asked to do or what she has misread due to nerves)	Overwhelmed by nerves, resulting in panic, inappropriate giggling, 'rabbit in headlights' syndrome or tears
Focus on the task throughout	Failure to read the instructions properly or to perform the task as required by the instructions
Fluent and purposeful discussion of the task both with the patient and/or, if required, the examiner	Waffling, vague, poorly-directed and purposeless 'chats' with no obvious aim or organisational structure
Alert to the cues and concerns of the patient	Ignoring or otherwise disregarding the patient

Stronger OSCE Performance	Weaker OSCE Performance
Accurate knowledge and appropriate awareness of the limits of expertise, responsibility or experience	Poor or inaccurate knowledge and/or lack of insight into limits of expertise, experience or responsibility
Effective and sound communication skills	Poor or inappropriately-applied communication skills
Meaningful closure of station	No closure to station eg no management plan etc and/or running out of time

The OSCE: ten top tips

So how do you ensure that your OSCE performance is strong? The following top ten tips might help:

1   OSCE stations and instructions are carefully crafted, far more so than most students would believe. Nothing is incidental, nothing is superfluous. From the instructions, to the actor's script or patient briefing, everything is aimed at enabling you to show specific knowledge and skills. Trust the process and remember that the instructions are not there to catch you out and the patient or actor is trying to help you not to mislead you, so listen and respond to their cues.

2   Everyone has a bad time at some stage in an OSCE. It may not be visible to anyone else, but at some point, every candidate's mind will go blank, everyone will encounter a dreaded station or one for which they feel unprepared, each person will want to cry or shout with frustration and no one will escape believing it all went perfectly. The trick is not to let the emotions and anxieties that are felt by all students doing OSCEs overwhelm you. Although it is a tough trick to pull off, it can be done. By accepting that such emotions are normal and universal, you can begin to plan for how to manage in the exam. Some students visualise their most dreaded moments, others role play the 'blank' moment and some imagine the situation to be an unthreatening social event rather than anything formal or high stakes with examiners being replaced by supportive family members in their imagination. If you can be kind to yourself, think about how you manage stress in advance and remember it is a healthy response rather than a weakness: you *will* conquer those nerves.

3   Try not to 'carry' one OSCE station into another. Another tip that is easy to write and hard to implement but nonetheless essential. Sadly I have observed excellent students come into the station I am examining

in a tear-stained or despondent state which inevitably compromises their performance. Even sadder, often those students have not done nearly as badly as they fear on the preceding station. Remember, when you leave a cubicle, it is over and the only thing you can do is concentrate on the next station.

4   Read the instructions and then read them again. In times of stress, we can misread and it happens a lot in OSCEs. If the examiner redirects you to the instructions, he or she is trying to help you – reread the instructions!

5   The patient or simulated patient (SP) has a script and detailed instructions. Sometimes students worry that by allowing the patient or SP too much time to talk, they will run out of time. The patient or SP will not waffle, mislead or go off-script. On the contrary, what your patient or SP says contain cues and clues that are essential to performing well. So, invite the patient to talk, listen carefully, pick up on, and respond to, the patient's concerns and questions.

6   Remember that stations may feel unpleasant or uncomfortable but that doesn't mean you aren't doing it right. For example, an OSCE station where you are sharing unwelcome information with a patient may mean that you are greeted with anger, distress or hostility. It is not personal. You will encounter stations that are designed to assess how you work with angry or distressed patients.

7   Try not to be distracted by the examiner. Although it may be tempting to see if you can spot how many marks you have been awarded, it will distract you. Your focus must be on the task.

8   At some stage you will encounter examiners whom you know well. You may like them or not. You may respect them or not. They might have a fearsome reputation or be loved for their perceived generosity towards students. The important thing is to forget everything you ever felt or thought you knew about the examiner. This is *your* moment.

9   If your mind goes blank, you make an error, you remember something late in the station or you are feeling overwhelmed, take a moment. You will not lose marks for taking and deep breath and asking calmly if you can just think for a moment. It is normal for human beings to lose their train of thought and to forget things: the best people do it all the time and it will not compromise your OSCE performance.

10   Avoid OSCE post-mortems, always. Plan a post-OSCE treat, always.

Activities: Ethics in practice

1.   The doctor-patient relationship
Consider the questions below, giving examples where possible:
(a)   What duties does a doctor owe her patient?
(b)   Are these absolute or qualified duties?
(c)   Does a doctor owe the same duties equally to all her patients?
(d)   Could or should a doctor approach the following patients in the same way?
- A confused man of eighty-six years of age requiring treatment for diabetes;
- An informed woman in her thirties requesting a home birth; and
- A fourteen-year-old girl seeking oral contraception.

2.   On being an ethical medical student
(a)   Is being a medical student 'different'? If so, why?
(b)   What are the particular privileges and responsibilities that you have as a medical student?
(c)   What does it mean to be professional as a medical student?
(d)   What are the specific rules of professional behaviour that apply to medical students and doctors?
(e)   Are professional standards applicable only to encounters with patients or to educational sessions with fellow students as well?

3.   Personal values and professional behaviour
How realistic (or desirable) is it for doctors' relationships with their patients to remain professionally neutral? In certain cases it may be clear that a strongly-held personal belief will affect relationships with patients, eg a doctor who is opposed to abortion may legally conscientiously object to participation in terminations.
(a)   What examples can you cite of situations in which doctors' values might influence their relationship with a patient?
(b)   In what ways might doctors manage their values so as not to adversely affect relationships with their patients?

Conclusion

Education in ethics and law may sometimes be confusing, discomforting and unsettling. It is a very different type of subject from many of the others with which students are grappling. A response, even an uncomfortable response, indicates engagement; and from engagement, comes learning. And your teacher will be learning too: to teach ethics is to learn ethics – the process inevitably requires the 'teacher' to reflect on, develop and grow his or her own expertise, both in ethics and in clinical practice. If you can listen to others, accept that you will be asked to explain your views without it being a personal affront, and remain open to new ideas, you will reap the rewards of an ethical education: namely qualifying as a doctor who can accept uncertainty, make considered and well-reasoned decisions and by and large sleep at night.

Chapter 2

Morality Tales: Ethics and Medical Education

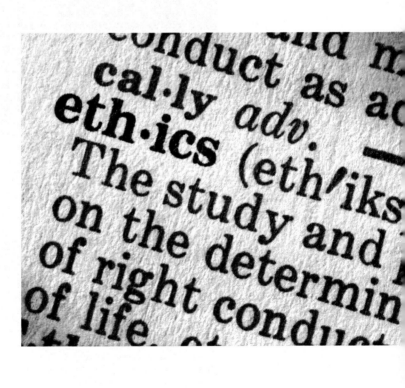

Morality Tales: Ethics and Medical Education

On being a medical student

As a student you will work in the clinical environment throughout your training and you will experience a range of practice. The majority of your experiences will be positive, perhaps even inspirational. However, sometimes you may observe, or be asked to participate in, something that concerns you or occasionally something that you know to be unethical. Such experiences can place students in a difficult position. In the busy clinical setting, students are at the bottom of the medical hierarchy and it is natural that you will want to fit in. Most people that medical students encounter will be positive role models. Unfortunately, medicine is not immune from negative role models and most students will meet someone in their training who serves more as a warning than an inspiration.

There are aspects of the clinical teacher-student relationship that can make it difficult for even the most robust student to respond appropriately to requests or even demands that ethical corners be cut.

- First, most students are acutely aware that there is an imbalance of power in their relationship with clinical teachers. Doctors who teach students are not only in charge in the clinical environment but they are the source of teaching and may even determine whether a student passes his or her attachment.
- Secondly, most students naturally want to achieve, see and do as much as possible on an attachment.
- Thirdly, it is much more pleasant to be accepted, liked and included on a clinical team; 'rocking the boat' is inevitably perceived as a threat to fitting in whilst working in the clinical setting.
- Fourthly, most people who act in a way that is ethically questionable are not 'bad' people. There is a range of explanations for why sub-optimal ethical practice occurs. In some cases, it is a pragmatic response to a busy, demanding and overwhelming job – it is simply quicker or easier to cut the consent process short or to explain a patient's symptoms

in the waiting room rather than in private. For others, the issue is a knowledge deficit. Ethics and law is a relatively recent addition to the undergraduate medical curriculum and remains taught in a widely variable level of detail, which means that there is a number of doctors practising who will not necessarily know the ethico-legal framework for their work as well as the students they are teaching. For those who have received teaching in the subject, things may have changed since they qualified.

- Finally, doctors who teach are keen that students see and experience as wide a range of practice as possible and, occasionally, that enthusiasm can compromise ethical practice. However, there is also an ethical obligation on qualified clinicians to support students when they are placed in a situation that conflicts directly with teaching they have received and professional standards. Although there are often understandable reasons for students being placed in a complex ethical position, it is nonetheless a discomforting and even painful experience for many. Students' educational experiences cause emotional responses that will shape their future learning and eventually their practice.

Ethical erosion and how to avoid it

Most students have high ideals and integrity when they start medical school. Yet, for many years, commentators have discussed the phenomenon of 'ethical erosion' which describes a decline in students' ethical standards and increasing cynicism as training progresses. Despite the emphasis on ethics in the curriculum, it seems that medical education and training actually makes some students less ethical than they were before they started medical school.

As well as learning the principles of sound ethico-legal practice, your medical education and training should provide the opportunity to discuss your own experiences of making ethical choices. At my own institution, the 'ethics roadshow' provides a safe environment for students to share their experiences of the clinical setting (the name of these events was not my choice but has stuck!). At these sessions, there are neither preset learning objectives nor lesson plans: it is nothing more complex than a small group of students and a trusted tutor discussing the dilemmas that clinical students experience daily but are rarely found in ethics textbooks. In nearly a decade of facilitating these 'ethics roadshows', particular themes recur: the question of if and how students are introduced to patients; the difference between learning from or on patients; the dissonance between 'classroom ethics' and observed behaviour in the clinical setting; and the effects of professional hierarchy, competition and insecurity on remaining true to ethical ideals have been discussed by every group, irrespective of location or specialty. In the armoury of strategies available to those seeking to avoid or correct the process of 'ethical erosion', the 'ethics road show' has proved to be an invaluable means of revisiting core values, sharing experiences, and empowering learners.

Many medical schools will encourage students to contact staff with questions or concerns about their clinical experiences. Understandably, many students worry about the 'safety' of disclosure or find it difficult to approach staff directly. One way in which I have tried to make the process of talking to members of staff easier is by developing the Educational Incident Form. The form is a mechanism by which students can log experiences of learning (anonymously, if they wish). It is confidential, and available online and in student handbooks. It is a confidential document that can be submitted without a name. Students who use the form describe it as less intimidating than making a formal complaint or seeking disciplinary measures. Importantly, the forms also inform staff development and discussion of standards in medical education, practice and training.

The educational incident form has been designed to be deliberately short, specific and simple. An educational incident is defined as an event in education or training that surprised or concerned the learner. When the student completed the form, it comes directly to one member of staff who acts according to the *student's* preferences and most students do not want to make their concerns 'formal'. The most common outcome is that the incident is logged and contributes to a collated, anonymised annual report describing the types and incidence of educational incidents in which no student is identifiable, but still communicates important information about the 'collective student experience' to staff responsible for education and training. In the decade that the educational incident forms have been used, some trends have emerged. First, older, female students are the most likely to complete an educational incident form. Secondly, the issues that most commonly recur concern inappropriate, humiliating and derogatory remarks or 'jokes' about patients, and introductions / consent for the student to be present or participate in patient care. Other issues that commonly crop up on educational incident forms involve perceptions of poor teaching and disregard for dignity. Occasionally (and certainly less often than I would like), the educational incident form is used to describe an experience that was inspirational, outstandingly positive or otherwise memorable for positive reasons.

How do students describe their experiences? The box below contains a verbatim example of one student's 'educational incident' which is reproduced with her generous permission:

A student experience – taken from an educational incident form

'I was in an ENT clinic with a consultant. He neither introduced me sought consent for me to be there. He told me firmly that I was "being stupid" asking patients if they minded me being there – it wasn't their choice. He said this whilst a patient was in the room. I decided to take the appointment cards out and call the patients myself so I could consent them beforehand. During clinic I became concerned with his hygiene. He used the same nasal spray nozzle twice – after which I changed it myself. He seemed to give a very small dose of anaesthetic (obviously this is an opinion but I've seen quite a few bronchoscopies and they gave five squirts where he was giving one, and he didn't tell patients to inhale or lean back etc to enhance the anaesthetic action). Each patient on whom he used a fibroscope was in obvious pain: discomfort is expected but I really thought they were in pain. Once, I suggested giving further anaesthesia but he gave up trying to do the scope; the patient was crying.

He twice dropped sterile equipment, then picked it up and used it on a patient. Once it was a nasal speculum, which only grazed the floor. The second time he completely dropped a forcep-like contraption which he then used to grasp a growth on a man's tonsils, ie right in the back of the throat. He didn't wash his hands once, nor did he wear gloves. I was shocked and intimidated and felt it was inappropriate to comment further.'

Conflicts of interest in education

Practical conflicts of interest regarding patient care and student learning reflect the tensions that can arise when seeking to meet the patient's interests, the clinician's goals and the learner's priorities. It is worth taking time to reflect on the impact of your desire and need to learn, the requirement that you seek consent properly, the expectation that you attend to the dignity and feelings of patients and that you remember the value of learning from patients, rather than on patients.

Emotional or interpersonal conflicts of interest, potential and actual, can occur in medical education. The feelings that arise between teacher and learner may not be explicitly acknowledged or considered, but nonetheless exist and can powerfully influence the effectiveness of the education. Most experienced teachers have students or juniors whom they remember fondly. Equally, but perhaps less commonly discussed in public, most experienced educators can readily recall the student or junior whom they found to be challenging or problematic – perhaps the 'arrogant' junior who lacked insight into his limitations or the student with apparent 'contempt' for the subject at hand. Likewise, students too will feel differently about, and respond variably, to teachers who may be teaching identical subject matter because of the feelings those teachers evoke in them as individual learners. Such emotional responses are inevitable. The trick is for teachers and students to remain alert to their own emotions and to consider how they may enhance or inhibit teaching and learning.

Role models and cautionary tales

Teachers in medical education, particularly clinical teachers, are role models for students and junior doctors. Ethnographic accounts have memorably captured the ways in which medical education and training is much more than a process whereby knowledge and skills are conveyed. Rather, medical education, and specifically the powerful effect of role models, communicates the values and norms shared by doctors, thereby indicating the so-called 'hidden curriculum'. When role models are sound, students have a valuable insight into ideal professional practice. Regrettably, when role models are questionable or simply negative, their influence will be equally enduring but considerably less desirable. As such, teachers have a significant responsibility to be good role models because it is one of the most powerful ways of teaching. Role modelling occurs constantly, whenever the student is able to observe his or her teacher. Teachers are role models to their students and juniors irrespective of whether they are interacting and whether the teacher realises he or she is being observed. One day you too will be a role model, probably before you even realise that you are. Take the time to think about the role models you meet and the role model you want to become – it says much about the sort of doctor you will be.

Chaperones and medical students

Chaperoning implicitly recognises the importance and integrity of the human body. The General Medical Council provides national guidance on chaperoning which is a useful starting point. However, the mere existence of guidelines does not act as an ethico-legal panacea, and challenges remain, particularly with regard to the place of judgement. For example, the use of chaperones during physical examinations is often only considered and discussed in medical training in relation to the obvious areas of practice eg female and male genito-urinary, breast and rectal examinations. It is worth finding out about the guidance on the use of chaperones both at your medical school and in any clinical setting in which you are working.

Medical students are often 'passing through' a clinical placement and may be unaware of the local practice regarding chaperones. Medical students also have unique status in that they are not employees and therefore may be considered potentially more vulnerable than clinicians who are employed and indemnified by the hospital or NHS Trust. The use of chaperones is not merely protective to, and therefore in the interests of, the patient, but has an important function in protecting doctors and students too. A chaperone should be considered (a) when practising clinical examination skills with a patient that could be described as intimate (which may extend beyond the standard definition to any situation where a patient has to undress) and (b) when the patient requests one, or you feel the situation demands one for your protection. An appropriate chaperone can be a peer or other member of clinical staff of the same sex as the patient, but not a friend or family member of patient. Chaperones should be offered irrespective of the sex of the student, thereby avoiding presumptions about sexual orientation. If you are asked to do something that makes you uncomfortable, or you find yourself in a situation that makes you feel uneasy, you should listen to your intuition.

Professional behaviour, the General Medical Council and medical students

It was a significant development in medical education when the GMC published guidance[12] for medical schools on what could and should be expected of medical students. Although the UK does not register medical students with the General Medical Council, all medical schools are effectively vouching for a student's suitability for provisional registration at graduation. Medical students commonly work with patients from the earliest days of their training and are privileged in the access they have to vulnerable people, confidential information and sensitive situations. As such, medical schools have particular responsibilities to ensure that students behave professionally and are fit to study, and eventually to practise, medicine.

The GMC publication explicitly demonstrates that medical students are different from other university students. That difference requires students to be aware of their professional obligations from the earliest days of their admission to a medical degree. The guidance is wide-ranging and discusses the standards of behaviour expected from medical students in the clinical setting, with their teachers, patients and fellow students, and in relation to health, integrity, trustworthiness and probity which may, in practice, extend to consideration of how students conduct themselves outside of the medical school environment. Ultimately, poor professional behaviour may result in a student being found unfit to study or practise and/or being refused provisional registration with the GMC (and therefore being unable to pursue a career as a doctor despite having graduated).

What sorts of behaviour would cause medical schools and/or the GMC to be concerned about a student's professionalism and suitability for medicine? The document 'Medical Students: Professional Values and Fitness to Practise': Areas of Concern indicates the areas that commonly prompt concern in relation to medical students (www.gmc-uk.org/education/undergraduate/professional_behaviour.asp).[13]

---

[12] Medical Students: Professional Values and Fitness to Practise. London: General Medical Council, 2005.
[13] At paragraph 76.

There is a wealth of literature on what constitutes professionalism (both in medicine and in general). One of the advantages of owning a book such as this is that you can rely on the author to engage with that voluminous literature so you don't have to! Most of those who write about professionalism spend a considerable amount of time defining it and this author is no different; the table below sets out my preferred 'six domains' approach to professionalism.[14]

The six domains of professionalism

1.	Competence
2.	Interpersonal Relationships and Emotional Function
3.	Awareness and Maintenance of Boundaries
4.	Consistency of Practice and Reliability
5.	Reflection and Learning
6.	Commitment to Service

None of us is perfect and, at some stage, we are all likely to behave in a way that is less than ideal. We all have bad days and make mistakes. Medical students are human and studying for a profession that is well-known for its stresses and pressures. In general, concerns about professionalism depend on a pattern of behaviour that is observed by a number of people. Guidance on professionalism is not a mechanism for excessive scrutiny or an unrealistic charter for perfectionism. On the contrary, both national and local guidance emphasise that medical schools should allow for growing maturity, adaptation to the particular environment of medicine, ill-health, personal problems and different approaches to learning. Admitting a mistake, taking responsibility and seeking help when you need it are markers of professionalism. No one who trains or works with you will be without their own fallibilities and foibles and everyone wants you to succeed. The vast majority of problems can be resolved and many students need a bit of additional support or advice at some stage in their medical education and training. Don't be proud – there will be members of staff, counselling services and pastoral provision that are available to you and are likely to have seen a lot of students who have gone on to have successful careers and happy lives. Seek them out – they want to help you.

---

[14] Bowman, D. *Professionalism: Dilemmas and Lapses*. London: National Clinical Assessment Service, 2009.

BPP LEARNING MEDIA

An ethical education in practice

Consider the two case scenarios that follow. In the first one, advise Hattie on how she should respond.

Scenario

Hattie is a fourth year medical student working on a respiratory firm. She is approached on her way into work by a young woman asking if she has a light. Hattie is sitting in on the cystic fibrosis clinic and is asked by her consultant to clerk Miss Kenyan, who has been a patient at the clinic since she was a baby. Miss Kenyan is 17 years old and the consultant, Dr Jaya explains that she is concerned that Miss Kenyan is not caring for herself properly. She has missed a couple of appointments at the clinic and the physiotherapist contacted the consultant to express concern about Miss Kenyan. Dr Jaya asks Hattie to find out whether Miss Kenyan is adhering to her treatment regime and report back before she sees her in clinic. When Miss Kenyan sees Hattie coming into the room, she groans *'oh no, just my luck. Now you know I'm smoking – please don't tell the other doctors'*. As the consultation progresses, Hattie learns that Miss Kenyan is smoking about 25 cigarettes a day, is no longer doing her physio regularly and has become erratic about taking her medication. Miss Kenyan pleads repeatedly with Hattie *'not to tell anyone, I'll be better about it all but please don't tell Dr Jaya. Anyway, isn't medical stuff supposed to be confidential?'* How should Hattie respond to Miss Kenyan?

You will find a detailed discussion of confidentiality in Chapter 4, but for now, it is sufficient to say that this is a situation in which complete confidentiality cannot and should not be offered. Miss Kenyan has shared information with Hattie that is medically significant (or may be: as a student you might not be able to make a judgement about the medical relevance or otherwise of information; even seemingly innocuous details can be of medical significance). Hattie should also consider the broader implications of incorrectly offering complete confidentiality to a vulnerable patient like Miss Kenyan. Hattie is a relatively inexperienced medical student and the potential implications of a well-meaning but misguided promise of confidentiality could be serious and considerable.

The ethico-legal rationale for sharing the information with Dr Jaya is that confidentiality is shared within a clinical team rather than being vested in a single individual. Hattie, as a medical student, is part of the clinical team and therefore has to share the information with those responsible for Miss Kenyan's care. Furthermore, where it is in the patient's best interests but you can't get consent, a doctor may breach confidentiality on a need-to-know basis. Miss Kenyan is non-adherent to treatment, possibly depressed and certainly vulnerable. Some readers might suggest that as Hattie had seen her smoking outside the hospital it was irrelevant to the interview, but Miss Kenyan has mentioned it again explicitly and repeatedly within the interview, and also admitted that she has neither been attending physiotherapy nor taking her medication.

The ideal response by Hattie would be to explain why Dr Jaya would consider the information that Miss Kenyan has disclosed important to her care, and encourage her to speak to Dr Jaya herself. However, if Miss Kenyan refused or challenged Hattie about her right to confidentiality, Hattie should explain about the shared nature of confidentiality (within the team) and tell her honestly but kindly that she will have to discuss her care with Dr Jaya, if Miss Kenyan will not do so herself.

In summary, for Hattie, a medical student who is passing through the clinical environment, offering to keep such essential information about this vulnerable young woman 'completely confidential' is not appropriate. The parameters of confidentiality should be explained and a rapport established with a view to persuading the patient to discuss her care with the consultant herself. If she continues to refuse to do so, Hattie should convey her concerns immediately to Dr Jaya (and tell Miss Kenyan that she will be doing that and why). It is risky in the extreme to start giving advice, however well-intentioned, for which a student is not qualified.

Finally, if you thought that Hattie should offer complete confidentiality, it might be worth thinking about what Hattie would have said when her consultant asked her to present the findings of her interview with Miss Kenyan. Would Hattie really have told the consultant *'It's a secret'*?! Presumably not, in which case Hattie would then be in the even more difficult position of having misled Miss Kenyan, albeit inadvertently, and having risked compromising her trust in her clinical care.

Scenario

Martin is a final year medical student. Whilst on the wards he observed a patient, Mr Hughes, experiencing an adverse drug reaction because the Foundation, Year 2 doctor, Dr Parveer, had made a mistake in the dosage. Dr Parveer admitted what had happened to Martin but said that the patient should be told that his discomfort was due to an allergic reaction. When Martin looked at the notes, there was no mention of the incident. At the next ward round, Martin listened to Dr Parveer presenting the patient to the consultant, Dr Linden, and noticed that once again the incident was not mentioned. What should Martin do?

The duty to apologise and explain when things go wrong has been embodied in medical codes of conduct since 1998. Mr Hughes has suffered some 'discomfort' and adverse effects. The GMC's guidance requires that the patient is advised of what has happened and offered a prompt apology and explanation. A further consideration for Martin is that the medical notes are a legal document and should be maintained scrupulously and honestly to provide a clear, contemporaneous, complete and accurate account of a patient's care. The omission or misrepresentation of events or information puts the patient at risk of future adverse events, and renders Dr Parveer's colleagues professionally vulnerable because they will not be in receipt of all the facts.

The ethical issues in this case are truth-telling and openness. However, if Dr Parveer is not willing to be honest in this situation, what are Martin's obligations as a medical student at the bottom of the professional hierarchy? Martin may feel considerable sympathy for Dr Parveer who is working within what has often been described as a culture of unattainable perfectionism. Medicine is demanding, complex and challenging, and camaraderie with, and sympathy for, one's colleagues who are trying to maintain the illusion of perfection and infallibility is natural. However, is it ethical?

Dr Parveer's conduct might be understandable but he has put a patient at risk and, if his dishonesty goes unchallenged, his own career may also be compromised by his willingness to lie and cover his tracks. If Dr Parveer does not learn to be honest and open about his mistakes and limitations, he is a dangerous colleague. He is likely to be reckless and cannot be trusted. These are important professional deficits and can only impede his clinical work. If

Martin recognises this, he may well minimise problems that could hinder Dr Parveer's career.

As a member of the team, Martin has a duty, in common with his colleagues, to ensure Mr Hughes' best interests are served. However loyal Martin may feel to Dr Parveer, his first and overriding duty is to Mr Hughes. The bottom line is that a career in medicine not only brings rewards, but also responsibilities that may not be easy to discharge: this is one of those responsibilities. However, as a student, Martin does not have to deal with this immensely difficult situation alone. Indeed, it may be inadvisable for Martin to approach Dr Parveer at all but to consider the sources of confidential support that might be available to him, including his clinical mentor, a personal tutor and senior medical school staff with a remit for student support. The important message is that Martin should not be managing this situation alone but it cannot be ignored.

Maintaining professional relationships

It is easy to assume that the ways in which we interpret core requirements such as courtesy, respect and effective communication are common. This exercise is designed to help you reflect on the assumptions and priorities you will be making when you work with others during your medical education and training. Grade each statement from 1–5 (where 1 = 'strongly disagree' and 5 = 'strongly agree'). It is a simple but powerful way to make the implicit and potentially destructive, explicit and constructive.

Statement	Grade 1–5
You should use a formal title until invited to do otherwise.	
You should check whether you are pronouncing unfamiliar names correctly.	
Nicknames at work are inappropriate.	
It isn't acceptable to raise your voice or shout at work.	
You shouldn't joke about anyone's appearance at work.	
You should introduce yourself to anyone you don't recognise in a clinic, theatre, ward or meeting.	
You should say 'please' and 'thank you' at work.	

Statement	Grade 1–5
Flirting at work is inappropriate.	
You shouldn't talk over, or interrupt, others.	
You shouldn't swear at work.	
To talk about others behind their back is gossip and unacceptable.	
If you have to give someone feedback, it should be done in private.	
If you are going to be late, you should phone ahead to apologise.	
If you have to criticise someone's work, you should find something positive to say as well.	
Emails should receive a response within 48 hours unless you are on leave or otherwise absent.	
You should return phone calls within 24 hours unless you are on leave or otherwise absent.	
Promises shouldn't be broken.	
If you are unwell, it is inconsiderate to come to work.	
It is unacceptable not to wear antiperspirant or deodorant.	
If you are unwell, it is inconsiderate to stay at home unless you really can't get out of bed.	
You should make an effort to ask after colleagues' families.	
It is impertinent to ask about colleagues' personal lives.	
You shouldn't talk to anyone with your arms crossed.	
You shouldn't look at your watch when talking to someone else.	
You should offer your hand when meeting someone for the first time.	
You should not touch a colleague at work.	
Items eg mugs, badges etc with a political slogan are unacceptable at work.	
You shouldn't sign an email to a colleague with a kiss.	
It is rude not to join colleagues for a drink if you are invited and available.	

Conclusion: the 'anti-Nike' approach to medical training: don't *'just do it'*

Ethics in the classroom may sometimes appear demanding, but it is in practice that it often becomes most challenging. One of the fundamental reasons we teach ethics is to improve clinical practice. Just as with clinical and communication skills, ethics has to be practised and understood as integral to what takes place on the wards and in clinics. Few medical students will encounter dilemmas involving genetic engineering or euthanasia, but almost everyone will, at some stage in their medical education and training, be invited to participate in an activity for which consent has not been sought, and observe behaviours that are unacceptable. The difficulty will not be in recognising these situations, but in responding appropriately and professionally.

Over the years, I have talked to many students who have spoken up when they were asked to act in a way that they felt to be inappropriate and, of course, to many more who were uncomfortable but remained silent. It is neither the case that those who speak out and remain true to their principles are inherently more 'ethical' or better-informed than their peers who did not challenge unethical behaviour, nor is it that those students who address inappropriate behaviour or requests are more outgoing, assertive or confident. Yet there are characteristics that the students who speak out share. First, many of them have had experience of standing up for their beliefs in other situations eg in a professional, campaigning or volunteer role prior to becoming a medical student. Secondly, many of these students have had experience either as a patient themselves or as a carer for someone who has been a patient. It seems therefore that practice at challenging behaviour and empathy for those who should be at the centre of healthcare – patients – are important when considering why some students speak out, and others remain silent, in the face of unethical or inappropriate behaviour.

In Chapter 11, I discuss in more detail the ways in which students can develop the confidence and skills required to enact and remain true to the ethical standards the vast majority have when they begin medical school. Just as your clinical skills will grow as you progress through your training, so too will your ethical skills. Learning about ethical theories and medically-related case law will be important, but there is much more to being an ethical medical student. Throughout your education and training, keep your ethical antennae finely tuned, reflect on what you see and do, seek support and advice when necessary and be kind to yourself and your patient. In short, throughout your training, try to adopt the 'anti-Nike' approach when asked to act in a way that is ethically problematic: don't 'just do it'.

Chapter 3

It's My Life: Capacity and Consent

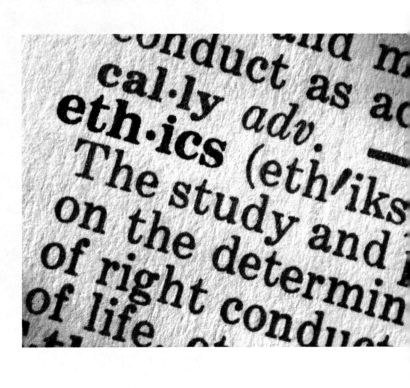

It's My Life: Capacity and Consent

Capacity: introduction

Capacity[15] is at the heart of ethical decision-making and it is the gateway to self-determination. People are able to make their own choices only if they have capacity. The assessment of capacity is a significant undertaking: a patient's freedom to choose depends on it. If a person lacks capacity, it is meaningless to seek consent. Although doctors carry out assessments of capacity, it is a legal rather than a medical concept ie its definition is drawn from the law. Therefore, you are required to understand the relevant law, particularly the Mental Capacity Act 2005. This chapter discusses the assessment of capacity in adults. Capacity and children is covered in Chapter 6.

The law

The Mental Capacity Act 2005 and its accompanying Code of Practice is the legal source of guidance on capacity for those over the age of sixteen. The legislation is based on the principles set out below:

Underlying principles of the Mental Capacity Act 2005

• Every adult has the right to make his/her own decisions and to be assumed to have capacity unless proved otherwise.
• Everyone should be encouraged and enabled to make his/her own decisions, or to participate as fully as possible in decision-making ie given help and support to make and express a choice.
• Everyone has the right to make apparently eccentric or unwise decisions.
• Proxy decisions should consider best interests, prioritising what patient would have wanted.
• Proxy decisions should be 'the least restrictive of basic rights and freedoms.'

---

[15] The word 'competence' is also used, albeit less frequently since the Mental Capacity Act 2005 was passed.

It is the Mental Capacity Act 2005 that sets out the criteria for assessing whether a patient has the capacity to make a decision. The criteria for capacity are shown below:

Criteria for adult capacity under the Mental Capacity Act 2005

The patient should be able to:

(i)   Understand the information relevant to the decision;
(ii)   Retain that information;
(iii)   Use or weigh that information as part of the process of making the decision, and
(iv)   Communicate his decision (by any means).

Assessment of capacity is not a single, one-off judgement. Capacity is often fluctuating and, in practice, patients may be somewhere along a continuum of capacity meaning that a patient might be capacitous to consent to one type of treatment but not another. It is important to be cautious about relying on previous assessments. Assessments of capacity should be regularly reviewed. The way in which a doctor communicates can enhance or diminish a patient's capacity as can pain, fatigue and environment. Practical considerations in assessing a patient's capacity are summarised below.

Practical issues in assessing capacity

- Starting point – adults are presumed to be capacitous. An assessment should only be carried out if there is doubt about a patient's capacity. The assessment must be made with reference to the patient's situation.
- Pre-existing diagnoses – the assessment of capacity is unrelated to any pre-existing diagnoses including diagnoses of mental illness or disorder. The assessment of capacity is concerned with function and not with diagnostic labels.
- Non-co-operation with assessment – if a patient refuses to co-operate with an assessment of capacity, it does not mean that he or she can be assumed to be incapacitous.
- Influencing factors – the way in which explanations are given, a doctor's manner and demeanour and the surrounding environment can enhance or diminish a patient's potential for capacity. Options that maximise a patient's understanding include treating underlying

conditions that may inhibit decision-making; writing down information; drawing diagrams; using educational models; videos and audiotapes; using translators; letting the patient choose a friend or relative to be present; and finding a private place for the consultation.

- Confidentiality –the perspectives of others may be useful when assessing the capacity. Such information should be sought if it is relevant, but with due regard to the principles of confidentiality.
- Documentation – assessments of capacity should be recorded in the medical notes.

If you conclude that a patient has capacity, he or she is able to make their own choices, even if their decisions appear to be irrational or may lead to harm or even death. However, that does not necessarily mean that you simply wave goodbye. Rather, the focus should be on explaining, without judgement or hyperbole, why you are concerned about the patient's decision and on encouraging the patient to return should he or she wish to do so. It is a frustrating and difficult situation, but you must remain calm and avoid frightening or interrogating the patient whom you believe to be acting unwisely.

Patients who lack capacity

Significantly, and for the first time in England and Wales, the Mental Capacity Act 2005 also provides statutory recognition of advance decisions, proxy decision-makers and advocacy services for those patients via the Independent Mental Capacity Advocacy Service. When a patient lacks capacity, decisions may be made on his or her behalf via:

- A Lasting Power of Attorney (LPA)
- An advance decision
- A determination of the patient's best interests

Lasting Power of Attorney

The legal recognition of proxies via the Lasting Power of Attorney provisions in the Mental Capacity Act 2005 is a significant change for clinical practice. Previously, third parties had been limited to taking over financial and legal affairs and had no remit in healthcare. Now, proxy judgement for people lacking capacity can be given by someone who has been granted a Lasting Power of

Attorney.[16] Once a person's lack of capacity has been registered with the Public Guardian[17] and the Lasting Power of Attorney granted, the person holding the LPA is charged with representing a patient's best interests. Therefore, it is important to establish whether there is a valid LPA in respect of an incapacitous patient and to adhere to the wishes of the person holding the Lasting Power of Attorney. The only circumstances in which clinicians need not follow the LPA is where the attorney appears not to be acting in the patient's best interests. In such situations, the case should be referred to the Court of Protection.[18]

There have been a number of publicity campaigns aimed at encouraging people to consider nominating a legal proxy for future healthcare decision-making. The ethical rationale being that 'prospective autonomy' is desirable and provides a preferable moral basis for care of the incapacitated patient than the clinical determination of 'best interests'. You might also consider whether it is part of the duty of care to raise the subject of future decisions when treating patients in whom capacity is likely to diminish. Understanding that advance decision-making and the nomination of proxies are legally possible potentially enables clinicians to work proactively to ensure that future healthcare is informed and chosen rather than well-intentioned but inferred.

Advance decisions

Advance decisions, sometimes colloquially called 'living wills', enable people to express wishes about future treatment or interventions. The decisions are made by capacitous patients in anticipation of a time when they cease to have capacity. Advance decisions are governed by the Mental Capacity Act 2005 and policies

---

[16] The role of the Lasting Power of Attorney replaces the Enduring Power of Attorney that was largely confined to acting for those lacking capacity in financial and property decisions.

[17] For guidance and further information on the role of Lasting Power of Attorney, see the Office of the Public Guardian website: www.direct. gov.uk/en/Governmentcitizensandrights/Mentalcapacityandthelaw/ Mentalcapacityandplanningahead/DG_186373

[18] The Court of Protection has the power to remove someone from the role of Lasting Power of Attorney if it is satisfied that the attorney is not acting in the best interests of the incapacitous person.

on advance decision-making are increasingly common in NHS Trusts since the Act came into force. There are criteria that must be met for a patient to make a legally valid advanced decision. Those criteria are shown in the box below.

Validity criteria for advance decisions

☑	Capacity: is the patient capable of making a decision?
☑	Voluntariness: is the patient doing this freely and of his or her own volition?
☑	Information: does the patient understand the implications of the choices and preferences he or she has expressed?
☑	Specificity: is the advance decision specific enough about possible future situations as to make clear what the patient wants in a given situation?
☑	Continuing nature: has the advance decision been superseded by the appointment of a LPA or is there any indication that the patient has changed his or her mind?

In practice, it is the requirement of specificity that is most difficult because of the inevitable uncertainty surrounding future illness and potential treatments or interventions.

An advance decision can be made to refuse treatment and to express preferences, but cannot be used to demand treatment. In general, no patient has the right to demand or request treatment that is not clinically indicated. Therefore it would be inconsistent to allow patients to include in their advance decisions request for specific treatments, procedures or interventions. The limits on requesting active treatment via advance decision-making were confirmed in the case of Leslie Burke[19] who has spino-cerebellar ataxia and wished to receive artificial hydration and nutrition even in circumstances that might be considered futile[20] by clinical staff. The Court of Appeal stated that the General Medical Council's guidance on life-sustaining treatment was lawful in vesting discretion in the clinical team to decide on the withdrawal or withholding of such treatment. Advance decisions may be made orally or in writing. However, for life-sustaining treatment, advance refusals must be in written form and witnessed. What's more, the decision should state explicitly

---

[19] R (Leslie Burke) v General Medical Council [2004] EWHC 1879.
[20] Futility is discussed in detail in Chapter 9.

that it is intended to apply even to life-saving situations. The more informal and non-specific the advance decision is, the more likely it is to be challenged or disregarded as being invalid.

An advance decision cannot be used to refuse basic care such as maintaining hygiene. Advance decisions should be periodically reviewed. Any amendments, revocations or additions can be made in the same way as a codicil is made to a will assuming, of course, that the person is still capacitous. Any changes must, of course, be communicated to all parties who have access to the advance decision eg the GP, any hospital departments, solicitors, relatives and carers, which highlights a further practical point in relation to advance decision-making, namely how to make the advance decision available to clinical teams who may be meeting a patient for the first time and / or in an emergency situation. The law requires only that clinicians make reasonable attempts to establish whether there is a valid advance decision in place and the presumption is to save life where there is ambiguity about either the existence or content of an advance decision.

The ethical rationale for the acceptance of advance decisions is usually said to be respect for patient autonomy. If capacitous patients are entitled to make a free and informed choice about healthcare, it is difficult to distinguish morally between the right to make free choices in the present and the extension of that right to future decision-making. Thus, advance decisions may be an effective way to extend someone's autonomy when capacity is lost. However, it could also be argued that none of us is capacitous to make decisions about our future care because the person we become when ill is qualitatively different from the person we are when we are healthy.

A further ethical challenge relates to the response of clinicians to patient choice. Doctors may be distressed or uncomfortable when faced with the patient who appears to favour death over life, but cannot allow personal discomfort or anxiety to compromise respect for the patient's autonomy. True respect for autonomy and the freedom to choose necessarily involves allowing people to make choices that others might consider misguided. It could be argued that patients who have had the opportunity to express their concerns, preferences and reservations about the management of their health are likely to trust their doctors and to enjoy a more honest and effective relationship with healthcare professionals.

At present, advance decisions remain relatively rare but are likely to become increasingly common. Indeed, there have been several high profile campaigns led by national organisations such as Help the Aged and The Alzheimer's Society to encourage people to plan ahead and consider future healthcare, making it an area of increasing ethico-legal importance.

Determination of best interests

Where a patient has neither made an advance decision nor nominated a proxy via a Lasting Power of Attorney, the ethical task is to weigh what is in the patient's best interests. In practice, the determination of best interests (which are more than merely best medical interests) is likely to involve a number of people eg members of the healthcare team, professionals with whom the patient may have had a longer term relationship and relatives and carers. However, third parties in such a situation are not making determinative judgements, rather they are being asked to give an informed sense of the patient and his or her likely preferences.

The Independent Mental Capacity Advocacy service[21] exists to provide Independent Mental Capacity Advocates in situations where a person lacks capacity but does not have family or friends to represent their interests in relation to decisions about health or social care. The Independent Mental Capacity Advocacy service must be involved where significant medical decisions are being considered or in relation to accommodation decisions where a patient has been in hospital for more than 28 days. The Advocates are not proxy decision-makers but act as independent facilitators to inform the determination of a patient's best interests.

---

[21] For a clear and accessible summary of the IMCA service and its work, see *Making Decisions: The Independent Mental Capacity Advocate (IMCA) Service*. London: Department of Health, 2009.

Capacity and medical students

Questions of capacity arise for medical students from the earliest days of training. The first stage in seeking consent to talk to, take a history from or examine a patient is to assess whether he or she has got capacity. The vast majority of patients will be able to choose whether they wish to participate in medical education. However, there are patients where there is doubt about their capacity and, of course, those who lack capacity, for example, because they are unconscious. Students also encounter inconsistency in how capacity is regarded in clinical practice: students report encountering patients in the clinical environment who have been deemed insufficiently capacitous to consent to treatment, but are simultaneously considered to be sufficiently capacitous to agree to medical students being involved in their care. How then should a medical student react where there are either doubts about a patient's capacity or a patient clearly lacks the capacity to make choices about involving students in his or her care?

Where a patient's capacity is in doubt, the first question a student might ask is '*do I need to take this history/do this procedure/perform this examination on this patient now?*' Is this really the only opportunity to practise a skill? If it is possible to seek consent from another, less vulnerable, patient whose capacity is not in doubt, then you should do so. If, however, there is a case for wanting to involve a patient without capacity in your learning, how should you proceed? Carefully and considerately is the answer. As you will recall from earlier in this chapter, where a patient lacks capacity, there are several bases on which decisions can be made, namely advance decisions, the LPA and the determination of best interests. The LPA is the easiest way for medical students to ensure consent is properly sought for involving a patient without capacity in their education because it allows consent to be explicitly sought from the legally appointed proxy. However, LPAs remain relatively uncommon and it is unlikely that an advance directive would include detail about a patient's wishes regarding medical students. As such, most students need to consider whether it is in the patient's best interests to be involved in medical education.

On what basis might it be in a person's best interests to be involved in medical education? One way to assess an incapacitated person's views about including medical students in their care is to ask those who are close to and know the patient well, just as the team should do when making treatment decisions. The question of whether it is in a patient's interests to have a student present also depends on what the student is present *for* ie is what is being done to the patient necessary and an integral part of care? For example, it may be in an unconscious patient's interests for a student to contribute, under close supervision, to suctioning a tracheotomy tube but not for six students to perform a rectal examination.

The question of the extent to which students should be included in the healthcare of patients who lack capacity remains vexed and uncertain.[22] All students should have regard to the vulnerability of all patients (irrespective of capacity). Where a student encounters a patient about whom there are questions, be those questions of capacity or other factors such as tiredness or comfort, the student should consider whether it is appropriate to approach that person at that time. There will be circumstances when a student can only learn key skills from an incapacitated patient. In such situations, if possible, consent should be sought at a time when the patient has capacity eg prior to a patient being anaesthetised before surgery. If however, the patient will never have capacity, the extent to which it is acceptable to be involved in care is a judgement. That judgement should be informed by those who know the patient, the necessity of the intervention, the student's competence and the degree of supervision available. Taking the time to think through the options and make a considered decision about your involvement will ensure you develop two crucial elements of clinical competence, namely ethical awareness and professional integrity.

---

[22] The question was the subject of an Institute of Medical Ethics Conference on 24 June 2010 at which a Professor of Medical Law argued that an intensive care consultant had acted unlawfully in teaching medical students involving unconscious patients without obtaining consent.

Core Concepts: Capacity

Capacity is presumed in adults and a capacitous decision cannot be overridden.
Capacity is at the ethical heart of clinical practice because from it flows autonomy ie the freedom to choose or refuse care.
Capacity is a legal concept.
The relevant law relating to capacity in adults is found in the Mental Capacity Act 2005.
Incapacity can only be assumed where a patient is unconscious.
Capacity is a dynamic and decision-specific concept that can fluctuate.
The Mental Capacity Act 2005 sets out the criteria to be met for a patient to have capacity ie the ability to i) understand information; ii) retain information; iii) weigh up information; and iv) communicate a decision.
Capacity is a fluid concept and doctors can do much to enhance, or impair, capacity.
Assumptions about capacity based on diagnoses should not be made
Advance decisions can be made under the Mental Capacity Act 2005 for consideration at a time when a patient no longer has capacity
An ethical rationale for recognising advance decisions is autonomy ie that they foster 'future' autonomous decisions.
People may nominate a proxy under the Mental Capacity Act 2005 via a Lasting Power of Attorney.
Where patients lack capacity and have no advance decision or legal proxy, they are treated in their best interests, which are broader than merely best medical interests, and should be as minimally restrictive of rights and freedoms as possible.
The Code of Practice that supplements the Mental Capacity Act 2005 sets out in greater detail the ways in which clinicians can evaluate a patient's best interests.
The Independent Mental Capacity Advocacy Service exists to serve the interests of those patients who lack both capacity and a third party to represent their interests.

Assessments: Capacity in practice

1. Assessing capacity to consent to an injection

> You are working as a medical student in a rheumatology outpatient clinic. Michael Wyndham has come for a steroid injection to increase mobility and decrease pain in his knee. He is 72 years old, living in warden-managed accommodation and somewhat forgetful. The consultant has asked you to assess his capacity to consent to the injection.

Guidance notes

- The task in this scenario is to assess Mr Wyndham's capacity by using appropriate communication skills to explore whether he meets the criteria of legal capacity, namely can he:
    - Understand information he is given about the injection;
    - Remember the information for a sufficiently long time to make a decision;
    - Weigh up the information so as to reach a considered decision; and
    - Communicate his decision to you and the clinical team?
- You should begin with an appropriate introduction, telling Mr Wyndham your full name and role and checking his identity and preferred form of address before asking Mr Wyndham to explain why he is attending. By allowing Mr Wyndham time to share his expectations and understanding, you will be able both to gauge what he already knows and to offer appropriately relevant information at the right level of detail.
- Depending on his understanding, further information can be offered explaining that the injection is intended to alleviate Mr Wyndham's pain and increase his mobility. As well as discussing the purpose of the procedure, you should explain that there are some possible disadvantages of the injection eg sometimes the

pain may worsen before it improves and joint injections are not always successful in managing pain/mobility problems.

- There are several ways in which you can demonstrate that you are checking Mr Wyndham's comprehension and retention of the information you have given him. For example, you might use phrases such as *'I realise I've given you a lot of information, what are your thoughts so far?'* and *'is there anything you would like explained further?'*

- The next task is to explore whether Mr Wyndham can weigh information in the balance so as to reach a considered decision. All that the rather arcane legal language means is that you should have some sense of Mr Wyndham using information to make a decision. A simple way to explore this aspect of capacity assessment is to ask *'how do you feel about the injection now that we've discussed it a bit?'* or *'now you've heard more about the injection, what are your thoughts?'*

- The final requirement is that Mr Wyndham communicates his decision: a step that is often overlooked in capacity assessments. Having explored whether Mr Wyndham is capacitous to make a decision, don't forget to give him the opportunity to communicate whether he has actually reached a decision! It is also good practice to summarise the consultation, invite further questions and explain that you will share your discussion with your consultant.

- As with all encounters with patients, throughout you should take time to verify Mr Wyndham's understanding, be alert to both verbal and nonverbal cues and invite questions.

2. Advance decisions under the Mental Capacity Act 2005

Ms Prima Japhur is a 52-year-old woman who has motor neurone disease. She is under the care of the neurology team which you have recently joined as a clinical student. Ms Japhur has come to the clinic because she *'wants to discuss her future care with people'*. Establish specifically why she has come to the clinic and offer Ms Japhur appropriate advice.

Guidance notes

- The principal aim of this scenario is to assess your ability to provide accurate information about making an advance decision in an empathic and professional manner. Although to do so you will have to discuss Ms Japhur's motor neurone disease, this is *not* the primary aim of this assessment. Don't worry: the actor playing Ms Japhur will have been briefed on the extent to which she should steer the station. As always, don't forget the basics: begin with an appropriate introduction telling Ms Japhur your full name and role and checking her identity and preferred form of address.

- Talking about the degeneration of a serious neurological condition is a sensitive issue: Ms Japhur is facing the possibility, even the probability of deterioration and eventually death. It seems that she has come to seek advice on the issue of advance decisions but you should explore sensitively what Ms Japhur wants to discuss. The starting point for the consultation is to discover what Ms Japhur both knows and wants to know.

- Once the issue of advance decisions arises, you should explain that it is possible to make an advance decision. The Mental Capacity Act 2005 sets out the legal framework in which advance decisions are made and applied. In particular, you need to explain that there are criteria (as described earlier in this chapter) for making a valid advance decision. Take time to explain each of the criteria and to explore Ms Japhur's wishes. First, an advanced decision must be made by a capacitous person. Ms Japhur appears to have capacity and, as adults are presumed to have capacity, you need not spend time assessing capacity. However, it is sensible to explain that for an advance decision to be implemented there has to be certainty that it was made by a capacitous person and voluntarily. You might therefore discuss ways in which Ms Japhur can demonstrate that her decision was made voluntarily and when she had capacity. For example, by suggesting that an advance decision is written and witnessed by someone who can attest to her capacity. You might ask whether Ms Japhur has, or will, discuss the issue of making an advance decision with her family. Listen carefully to the patient's response and explore the options for sharing information without judging or passing comment on what a partner should or shouldn't be told, when and by whom – that is not your role.

- You need to spend time exploring Ms Japhur's specific concerns eg feeding, resuscitation, and treatment of infections and her preferences. It is neither necessary nor possible to cover every eventuality. So long as you demonstrate awareness a valid advance decision must be informed and specific to situations likely to occur in Ms Japhur's future that will suffice. You should also assure Ms Japhur that she can take her time in drafting the decision and that she can change her mind at any point. You might also point out that some people choose to nominate a third party via the LPA process to act on their behalf when they lose capacity. If Ms Japhur prefers the LPA option, that should be incorporated into any advance decision and she should be aware that a valid LPA will supersede an advance decision.

- This consultation is likely to be complex and has potent emotional resonance for Ms Japhur. It is essential therefore to pace the discussion. Information should be offered in discrete chunks, checking for understanding and leaving time for Ms Japhur to take in what is being said and ask questions. No matter how accurate or valuable the information provided, Ms Japhur may feel overwhelmed and emotional. Remain alert to verbal and nonverbal cues, allow her space for questions and demonstrate empathy where appropriate.

- It is unlikely that most people would be able to decide whether and how to make an advance decision during a single meeting in an outpatient clinic. You should acknowledge the difficulty and significance of the choices Ms Japhur may make and offer appropriate follow-up as she makes her decision eg subsequent appointments, involvement of GP, discussion with family, patient-led organisations and written literature. Summarising, offering time to think and reminding Ms Japhur that she is welcome to discuss matters further at future appointments is a good way to close the consultation.

3. Proxy decisions under the Mental Capacity Act 2005 – Lasting Power of Attorney

> Mr Rafi is 83 years old. He has not been in good health for the last decade. He has diabetes mellitus, mild dementia, early signs of heart failure and was recently diagnosed with colorectal cancer. Mr Rafi has been living in a nursing home for 11 months. On receiving the diagnosis of colorectal cancer, Mr Rafi asked his solicitor to advise him on how his daughter, Mrs Geeta Patel, could take over the *'difficult decisions'*. A Lasting Power of Attorney was duly granted. Mr Rafi was admitted to the intensive care unit (ICU) three days ago with pneumonia. He is intubated and unconscious. Mr Rafi is not responding to treatment. The clinical team needs to decide how to proceed and want to talk to Mrs Patel.

Guidance notes

- This is exactly the sort of situation where the LPA that Mr Rafi arranged for his daughter to hold applies. Mrs Patel is, by virtue of the LPA that has been granted under the Mental Capacity Act 2005, empowered to act as Mr Rafi's proxy. As such, her representation of her father's best interests has legal force equivalent to any capacitous patient.
- Ideally, Mrs Patel and her father discussed the possibilities of deterioration in his health when establishing the LPA. Nonetheless this is likely to be a difficult conversation. Mrs Patel may feel the burden of doing the right thing for her father and is being asked to make significant decisions when she is probably distressed and tired. As with any capacitous patient, the task is to explain clearly and compassionately what is happening to Mr Rafi outlining the treatment he has received and the available options. Remember that what medical students and clinicians take for granted may not be known or understood by Mrs Patel. It is increasingly rare for people to see the dying process and, understandably, many are afraid of what is unknown. Gentle explanation of how Mr Rafi is likely to respond if treatment is withdrawn and what constitutes 'a good death' may be useful for Mrs Patel.

• Remember that merely because the legal issue is 'solved' by Mrs Patel being the nominated proxy, ethical practice requires patience, honesty about both what is known and unknown, empathy and skilful communication. Mrs Patel may want time to reflect before making a decision. She may wish to ask questions either immediately or later. She may want to involve other family members. The point is that the meeting with Mrs Patel should be paced according to her wishes and needs. Establishing and maintaining an effective relationship is as essential as the Mental Capacity Act in enabling Mrs Patel to fulfil her role as her father's proxy and represent his best interests.

4. Capacity and communication

Sample SAQ

Mr French is a 27-year-old man with learning difficulties. He has been brought to hospital by his mother following a fall at home. The team wonders if he has capacity to make choices about his healthcare.

(a) What criteria would you use to determine whether Mr French has capacity? (4 marks)
(b) If Mr French lacks capacity, on what legal basis should decisions be made about his care? (4 marks)
(c) Under what circumstances, if any, could Mr French's mother give consent or refuse treatment on behalf of her son? (2 marks)

Guidance notes

Part (a)   The criteria for capacity require that time be taken to assess Mr French's ability to:

• Understand information sufficiently;
• Remember information (not indefinitely but long enough to make a decision);
• Weigh up information to make a considered decision; and
• Communicate his decision by words, sign language, drawing or other means.

Capacity is specific to the decision that has to be taken, so it may be that Mr French is able to make some decisions about his care but not others. Similarly capacity can fluctuate and doctors can do a lot to enhance someone's capacity by, for example, paying attention to the environment and their demeanour when talking to patients.

Part (b) Where a patient lacks capacity, the Mental Health Act 2005 provides guidance on how to proceed. It may be that someone has made an advance decision indicating wishes for future care and/or appointed a proxy with a LPA. However, both an advance decision and/or a LPA require that they were made by a person with capacity. If Mr French has never had capacity, he will not have a valid advance decision and/or LPA. In that case, decisions should be made in Martin French's best interests (which are not merely his best medical interests). Mr French's mother and others who know him well may inform the determination of Mr French's best interests but they are not acting as a proxy; rather they are providing an insight into Mr French's needs, preferences and interests.

Part (c) Mr French's mother would only be able to act as a proxy ie to make treatment choices about her son's care if she had been granted a LPA at a point when Mr French had capacity (it should not be assumed that because he has a learning disability, he lacks capacity).

5. Capacity and choice

Sample EMI

Mrs Oates is 74 years old. She has Parkinson's disease and has contracted pneumonia.

She has told the clinical team that she does not want any further attempts at cardiopulmonary resuscitation (CPR). Mrs Oates develops respiratory failure and deteriorates. When she lapses into unconsciousness, her two sons both insist that treatment should continue and that they want *'everything possible'* done for their mother. The consultant, Dr Makin, commences CPR.

EMI: Questions

From the following list, please select the single best answer to the questions below:

A   Dr Makin has acted correctly

B   The Mental Health Act 2007

C   Mrs Oates' sons are entitled to insist that their mother should be ventilated

D   The Homicide Act 1957

E   Mrs Oates is entitled to ask the team not to resuscitate her again

F   Dr Makin has acted paternalistically

G   The Mental Capacity Act 2005

H   Dr Makin should disregard Mrs Oates' request because it was not made in writing

I   The Mental Health Act 1983

J   Dr Makin has acted beneficently

K   People over the age of 65, such as Mrs Oates, are not entitled to make decisions about their resuscitation status; it is a decision for the healthcare team

L   The Suicide Act 1961

M   Unless there is a valid Lasting Power of Attorney, no third party can consent to, or refuse, treatment on behalf of another but family members can advocate a patient's interests

N   People can demand to be resuscitated and clinicians must follow their wishes irrespective of the clinical situation.

1.   Which statement from the list above describes the role a capacitous patient has in resuscitation decision-making?

2.   Which statement from the list above reflects the ethical model Dr Makin is adopting by attempting to resuscitate Mrs Oates?

3.   Which statement from the list above describes the position of Mrs Oates' sons in respect of decision-making about her care?

4.   Which statute in the list above provides the legal framework for determining whether Mrs Oates can make decisions about her care?

EMI: Answers	
1.	C
2.	D
3.	M
4.	G

Consent: introduction

Consent is integral to ethical and legal practice. Obtaining informed consent is the legal basis on which patients make free choices and gives meaning to autonomy. Autonomous decisions are made by people who have capacity, are adequately informed and are acting voluntarily. If a patient makes an autonomous, but seemingly bizarre, decision that satisfies the capacity, that decision must be respected even if harm or death occurs. To act without, or in opposition to, a patient's valid consent is to commit an assault or the tort of battery.

Whilst there are established processes for seeking consent in clinical practice, merely signing a consent form does not necessarily equate to meaningful agreement and understanding. To achieve meaningful consent depends on the ways in which doctors work with patients to ensure that informed choices can be, and are being, made. One way of structuring your thinking about consent is to break it into its constituent parts as shown in the box below.

Criteria for meaningful consent

For consent to be valid it should be:

☑ Given by a patient who has capacity to make a choice about his or her care
☑ Voluntary ie free from undue pressure, coercion or persuasion
☑ Sufficiently informed
☑ Continuing ie patients should know that they can change their mind at any time

Seeking consent

Whilst it is common and good practice for written information to be provided to patients, it does not abrogate responsibility to talk to the patient. All patients should be able to ask questions, explain their own preferences and priorities and discuss the risks and benefits of an intervention as part of seeking consent.

Consent forms can often seem obsessed with risks. Disclosure of risk is, of course, an integral part of obtaining consent. Risk disclosure is assessed in accordance with the standard of care test (discussed in depth in Chapter 11) that applies to any aspect of clinical practice ie did the doctor disclose risks in a way that accords with the practice of a reasonable body of his peers? And does the degree of risk disclosure withstand logical analysis? Essentially, the information given to a patient should be that which a 'reasonable person' would require whilst being alert to the particular priorities and concerns of individuals. The content of the information shared should cover: risks and benefits; possible consequences of treatment and non-treatment; options and alternatives; and delineation of both what is known and not known about the patient's care. Disclosure of uncertainty should be as much part of the discussion as sharing what is well-understood. And it is a discussion: patients should be given the opportunity to ask questions and express their concerns, priorities and preferences rather than being subjected to an uninterrupted clinical monologue.

Legal actions involving consent often claim that disclosure was either inadequate or misleading. However, as well as demonstrating that the provision of information fell below the standard of care expected, a claimant also has to show causation ie that the inadequate consent process directly contributed to foreseeable damage or loss. Even if risk is not disclosed or it is insufficiently well-disclosed, the patient has to demonstrate that had risk been disclosed, his or her decision to proceed would have been different. Following the case of *Chester v Afshar*,[23] a further layer has been added. In that case, the House of Lords held that a patient did not need to demonstrate that he or she would never have had treatment, but only that the he or she would have delayed having treatment to another time and sought care from another clinician.

---

[23] *Chester v Afshar* [2004] 4 All ER 587, HL.

Consent in medical education and training

Much of medical education and training takes place in the clinical environment. Future doctors have to learn new skills and apply their knowledge to real patients. However, patients have a choice whether they wish to participate in educational activities even if they are in a 'teaching' hospital. It is easy to overlook the precepts of ethical practice when you are keen to learn and your teachers are enthusiastic about sharing their expertise. However, demonstrating ethical practice is as integral to professional training as observing procedures and eliciting signs.

For medical students, the most common situation in which consent is sought is when seeking patients' agreement to participate in learning. The principles of seeking consent for educational activities are identical to those applied to clinical situations. Look at the following scenarios and consider whether valid consent has been obtained. It may help you to consider (i) what information has been exchanged and by whom; and (ii) the extent of any agreement.

Scenario

Mrs Gould walks into Dr Anselm's surgery to find Felicity, a second year medical student, in the room. Dr Anselm greets Mrs Gould saying *'Hello, you don't mind if Felicity sits in, do you?'*

Scenario

Ms Kapoor has been a patient on the antenatal ward for seven weeks. She has pre-eclampsia. Dr Wilkes takes two third year students, Henry and Kate, to see Ms Kapoor. Dr Wilkes talks to Henry and Kate about pre-eclampsia and Ms Kapoor's case. He then suggests that they should each have a go at taking Ms Kapoor's blood pressure and turns to Henry saying *'you go first'*.

Core Concepts: Consent

Valid consent is the legal translation of the importance of the ethical principle of autonomy.
There are four components of valid consent: (i) capacity; (ii) voluntariness; iii) sufficiency of information; and iv) continuing nature of consent.
Seeking consent may, in itself, have therapeutic value and is an opportunity to build a relationship with the patient.
Consent need not be written but documentation may provide evidence of the consent process.
If a patient lacks capacity, it is a legal nonsense to seek consent.
A capacitous patient is entitled to refuse treatment and express a preference between options, but cannot demand treatment.
To proceed in the face of a capacitous patient's refusal or without valid consent is to commit an assault or the tort of battery.
It is important to be honest both about what is known and what is uncertain when providing patients with information to seek consent. Furthermore, information should cover both the risks/benefits of treatment and non-treatment.
Seeking consent from patients to participate in teaching or training is an essential part of clinical education and subject to the same principles as seeking consent for treatment.
Refusal of treatment ie refusal to give consent may appear unwise or even bizarre, but if the criteria for seeking valid consent are met, such refusal cannot be overridden.

Assessments: Consent in practice

1. Seeking consent for an investigation

> Mr Bellow is 53 years old. He has been referred for an endoscopy with a history of dyspepsia which has not responded to treatment with antacids and H2 antagonists. Helicobacter pylori has been excluded. Mr Bellow attends the endoscopy unit and you are asked to accompany the Foundation, Year 2 doctor to obtain Mr Bellow's consent for the endoscopy.

Guidance notes

- Capacity can be assumed. Mr Bellow is an adult and there is nothing in the scenario to indicate that he may lack capacity to make his own decisions. The first task is to establish what Mr Bellow understands about the referral and planned endoscopy. It is easy to assume that Mr Bellow's GP has explained why he is being referred for an endoscopy but it is essential to find out from the patient himself how he perceives his situation: a simple, open question asking Mr Bellow to share what has been happening will be invaluable.
- Having asked for Mr Bellow's account, the aim is to be responsive and to develop a proper dialogue.
- Patients' worries can be surprising and may be unanticipated by those for whom an endoscopy is a 'routine' investigation. Risks should be contextualised and discussed with reference to benefit. When advising Mr Bellow about the principal risks of endoscopy eg bleeding, perforation etc., it is important also to discuss the likely benefits and its value in managing his poorly-controlled dyspepsia.
- Mr Bellow should understand that he has a choice. A referral, even within the monolithic NHS, does not preclude patients from choosing care at each stage. If the task of seeking consent has been well done so far, Mr Bellow will have received a lot of information. Inviting questions and reminding Mr Bellow that he can change his mind are simple but necessary ways

to capture the essential concepts of voluntariness and ongoing consent.

- Only when the consultation has reached the point at which Mr Bellow has no further questions, should the consent form be introduced. It is good practice to talk Mr Bellow through the form and to be prepared to answer any further questions he may have. A signed copy should be placed in the notes before the procedure begins.

2. Capacity, consent and the medical student

> Javick is a third-year medical student on a medical firm. Dr Master, the consultant, asks Javick to examine Mrs Alhami, aged 86, who has been admitted with abdominal pain. Specifically, Dr Masters tells Javick that he should *'have a go'* at performing a rectal examination. Javick has never performed a rectal examination before, although he has practised on models in the clinical skills cubicles. Mrs Alessi seems confused and appears distressed when Javick approaches her. How should Javick proceed?

Guidance notes

- The first issue to consider is whether Mrs Alhami has capacity to give or refuse consent for Javick to perform an examination. The fact that Mrs Alhami is confused may raise some doubt about her capacity. If Mrs Alhami does not have capacity, then any examinations, interventions or treatment must be in her 'best interests'. The request for an examination, including a rectal examination, is problematic in the context of 'best interests'. Whilst the rectal examination is likely to be a routine part of Mrs Alhami's care, it is unlikely that Javick's findings alone would be relied upon. What is being proposed is for educational rather than therapeutic purposes. If Mrs Alhami is unable to consent because she is lacks capacity, it is difficult to make the case for Javick carrying out the rectal examination for the first time. Some might argue that because the ability to perform a rectal exam is a necessary skill for a medical student to acquire, educational examinations can be carried out on incapacitated patients. However, there should be a strong case for conducting the procedure on a vulnerable patient rather than on someone who is able to choose whether to participate in student education. For instance, it might be that one can only learn to take a history from a psychotic patient without consent, but a rectal examination can be performed on capacitous patients.

3. Refusal of treatment: a Jehovah's Witness patient

> Miss Townsend, aged 26, is brought to A&E following a road accident. She has heavy blood loss as a result of her injuries. Miss Townsend is conscious and tells you that she is a Jehovah's Witness and *'must not receive blood products under any circumstances'*. Miss Townsend adds that you will find a card in her purse which she carries at all times to ensure, even if she were to be found unconscious, that no one would give her blood products.

Guidance notes

- Although Jehovah's Witnesses are often discussed separately in the ethico-legal literature, the correct analysis of this scenario draws on the fundamental concepts of capacity and consent that are discussed in this chapter. Remember, irrespective of the reasons for refusal, if a patient has capacity he or she is entitled to refuse treatment. Miss Townsend is an adult who is refusing medically-indicated treatment. Therefore the first question is whether she is capacitous. As an adult Miss Townsend should be presumed to have capacity, although depending on her injuries and their effects, there may be a case for assessing her capacity formally. If her capacity is assessed, the question will be whether Miss Townsend can understand, retain and weigh up information about her circumstances and then communicate her decision. If so, she has capacity to choose and refuse treatment like any other adult.
- Patients, like Miss Townsend, who have beliefs that may affect medical treatment, may carry documentation to confirm their wishes. Such documentation should be considered as an advance decision and therefore assessed in accordance with the criteria for validity set out in

the Mental Capacity Act 2005. Whether the card Miss Townsend is carrying is valid pivots on whether it was made at a time when she had capacity, with adequate information and is specific to the current situation. If those criteria are met, it is a valid, written advance decision and must be respected. The only caveat is that as Miss Townsend is refusing potentially life-saving treatment, her advance decision should be witnessed and signed. However, given that she is conscious and assuming she has capacity enabling her to confirm her wishes verbally and in real time, the advance decision is neither required nor determinative.

- Cultural and religious sensitivity is required and it is essential not to make assumptions. For example, there is a range of views, as occurs in other religious groups, amongst Jehovah's Witnesses regarding the acceptability of blood products. It may be acceptable to some Jehovah's Witnesses to receive minor processed blood fractions or certain components.[24] In some areas, a hospital liaison committee will exist to facilitate greater understanding between the Jehovah's Witness community and clinicians. Such committees may be a valuable resource in difficult cases, time and circumstance permitting. Miss Townsend needs the same amount of information that would be given to any patient. The need and probable urgency for blood transfusion following extensive blood loss should be accurately explained without exaggeration.

- Ultimately, it is Miss Townsend's decision whether or not she receives blood products. She has expressed her wishes both verbally and in writing. Such a decision may be incomprehensible or distressing, but it is Miss Townsend's decision to make. The clinical team will have done its job by ensuring she makes a capacitous and informed choice. It is best practice to ensure, wherever possible, that consultants are involved in cases such as Miss Townsend's and that the decision process is accurately documented.

---

[24] *Management of Anaesthesia for Jehovah's Witnesses.* (2nd ed.) London: Association of Anaesthetists of Great Britain and Ireland, 2005.

4. Refusal of treatment and self-discharge

> Mr Prior, aged 55, attends A&E with his wife who, he says, *'made him come because she is making something out of nothing'*. Mr Prior had what he describes as *'indigestion'* following a heavy meal the previous evening but his wife insists it was *'not just indigestion'*. Mr Prior took some antacids but reports that he is still a bit *'uncomfortable'*. When it is explained that an ECG and further investigations are indicated to exclude a myocardial infarction, Mr Prior says that he *'has had enough of all this nonsense. It was just a nasty bout of indigestion'*. On discussion, it becomes clear that Mr Prior is keen to leave the hospital to go to work where he is due to be tendering for a new contract with a potential client.

Guidance notes

- There is no reason to doubt Mr Prior's capacity. Remember that a capacitous patient, like Mr Prior, has the freedom to accept or reject medical treatment even where that choice is unwise or frustratingly ill-advised. Ultimately, patients who have capacity can self-discharge against medical advice. Although Mr Prior may appear to be making a decision that seems foolish, there is a balance to be struck between explaining why it would be advisable to remain in hospital and acknowledging that the choice is ultimately Mr Prior's to make.
- There are important points to remember when a patient wishes to self-discharge against advice, namely:
  - Building a rapport with Mr Prior is essential. He has apparently come to the hospital reluctantly and his concerned wife remains present. Remember though that you know nothing of the couple's relationship and should therefore ask neutrally whether Mr Prior would prefer to talk alone or with his wife present.
  - What is Mr Prior's actual understanding of risks and the potential consequences of refusing an ECG and other investigations? Merely because something has been said, understanding cannot be assumed to follow. Explore what Mr Prior understands about his experience so far. Is he aware that there are some significant unanswered

questions regarding his heart? What does he understand about a myocardial infarction, if anything? In order to make a meaningful autonomous decision, Mr Prior needs to know the risks and potential consequences of his choice. Explaining why you are concerned and why the investigations are indicated is essential to ensuring that Mr Prior is sufficiently informed. The possibility of his chest pain being cardiac has to be explained to Mr Prior, but he should not be confronted in a bullying or alarmist way. Empathic acknowledgement of the inconvenience of his symptoms at such an important time in his working life, exploring whether there are other solutions and demonstrating a willingness to listen are crucial.

- Although Mr Prior has identified an important work commitment as the reason he wishes to discharge himself, it may be that he is afraid, in denial or simply unaware that he is potentially at risk. Being alert to the verbal and nonverbal cues from Mr Prior is likely to lead to a better understanding of his wish to leave the hospital.

- Compromise may be possible, but if not, be sure to explore the options for the patient should the symptoms worsen and ensure that you have 'safety-netted' eg advising Mr Prior of changes in symptoms that warrant urgent attention, suggesting alternative sources of care and communicating with his GP.

- Patients should feel that they can return should they change their mind or the situation worsens. If Mr Prior doesn't feel judged or reprimanded, he is more likely to return to the hospital should he reconsider his decision or if the pain worsens. You should encourage Mr Prior to return should he deteriorate or simply change his mind and remind him that there are a number of ways of accessing care quickly eg NHS Direct, GP and A&E etc.

- Inform Mr Prior in a non-judgemental way that if he chooses to leave without receiving the recommended care, the hospital will ask him to sign a form to confirm that he understands that he is choosing to leave, even though the clinical team would like him to stay.
- As a medical student, you should seek senior advice, ideally from the consultant in charge before the patient leaves. Document all discussion in the notes comprehensively and clearly, and cross-refer to the self-discharge form.

Chapter 4

Trust Me, I'm a Medical Student: Confidentiality

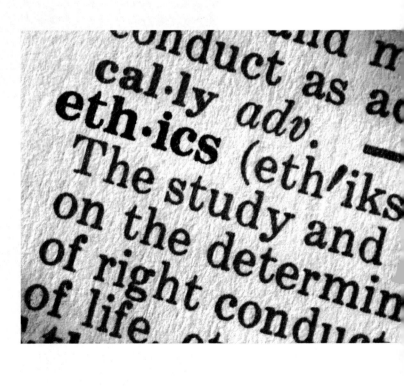

Trust Me, I'm a Medical Student: Confidentiality

Introduction

Confidentiality is considered a somewhat strange area medico-legally. It is clearly a highly valued area of medical practice, much emphasised by the professional codes of conduct and governing bodies. Doctors working for the NHS do not have a contract with their patients; a duty to keep confidences is inferred at common law ie via case law. Therefore, doctors and medical students working in the clinical environment have a legal obligation not to divulge information that they obtain during the course of their medical relationship. The case law on confidentiality is relatively limited; there are few remedies for breach of confidence and it tends to be a matter for professional discipline rather than legal redress.

Most doctors would agree that whatever the legal basis for their duty of confidence, there are strong moral reasons that confidences are respected. Trust depends on confidentiality. Patients are able to discuss embarrassing subjects and cross physical taboos because the environment is sufficiently safe to allow them to be vulnerable. Yet, there are many inadvertent breaches of confidentiality on a daily basis. Clinical conversations, often with identifying details, take place in lifts, corridors, coffee shops and cafes. Even within appropriate settings, confidentiality is systemically compromised by the proximity of beds, the number of staff on a ward round and the curtains that we pretend are soundproof as we draw them to protect patient privacy.

The duty of confidence: extent and qualification

Whilst acceptance of a duty of confidentiality is almost universal amongst doctors, the extent to which this duty is absolute or may be compromised is not necessarily a matter of agreement. There are several widely-accepted common law justifications for breaking confidentiality. There are three broad categories which encapsulate the qualifications that exist in respect of the duty of confidentiality as shown in the box below.

Categories for the qualifications to the duty of confidentiality

- Consent
- In the patient's best interests but it is impracticable or unreasonable to seek consent
- In the public interest

The three categories above are useful as a way to think about the extent of the duty of confidentiality but there is considerable ethical discretion in practice. In addition, there are several statutory provisions that require disclosure of confidential information in certain circumstances.

Consent to share confidential information

At first sight this appears to be the most straightforward circumstance in which confidences may be divulged. Indeed, the GMC recognise that a certain amount of consent must be implicit in the sharing of information between health professionals[25] who are assuming clinical responsibility for the patient.

It is easy to assume that relatives and a patient's next of kin will be involved in care, but it is essential to remember that you must not share confidential information with anyone, even a spouse, partner or close relative, unless you have the patient's permission. Clinicians may become used to seeing family members on a ward or in clinic. Such familiarity does not alter the fundamental principles of confidentiality that apply to every patient. The decision whether to share information with relatives is the patient's alone (assuming he or she has capacity). It may seem surprising for a patient to wish to keep information private, but it is his or her choice to make and should not be judged or compromised by well-meaning but misguided clinicians. Even when consent to share information with a relative has been given by a patient, the scope of that consent can be problematic and worthy of comment. Consider the scenario below.

---

[25] Who are all, irrespective of profession, bound by confidentiality.

Scenario

You are attending your placement at a local general practice and sitting in on Dr Mahoney's morning surgery. Maddie Ayling, aged 15, is the second patient of the morning. She is accompanied by her mother. Dr Mahoney asks Miss Ayling if she is happy to have her mother present and Miss Ayling confirms that she *'has no problem'* with her mother's presence. You notice that Dr Mahoney discreetly moves the computer screen away from Mrs Ayling's sightline. Dr Mahoney diagnoses a bacterial throat infection and wants to prescribe Amoxycillin. However, Dr Mahoney realises that she will need to warn Miss Ayling about the possibility of an interaction that will reduce the effectiveness of the oral contraceptive that she prescribed three months ago.

While Miss Ayling has consented to her mother being present in the consultation, Dr Mahoney cannot assume that she has consented to her mother discovering that she is taking the contraceptive pill. Hence, Dr Mahoney discreetly moving the computer screen showing Miss Ayling's current medication and pausing when she wishes to prescribe Amoxycillin. It is essential to consider the extent of the consent that someone has given to sharing confidential information and to proceed with caution.

A patient may consent to information being shared amongst medical professionals, but this does not mean that he or she is consenting to all potential uses of the information. Consider the scenario below.

Scenario

Ms Baine attended a large teaching hospital for a termination of pregnancy. Whilst at the hospital, she had signed a form agreeing that her cases notes could be used as part of a research project into the complications of termination of pregnancy. Six months later, Ms Baine returned home with her boyfriend and switched on the answerphone to hear the following message:

'Good afternoon, this is Dr Sami at St Jude's hospital. I am a specialist in obstetrics and gynaecology and I am doing research on termination of pregnancy. Your notes seem incomplete and I'd be grateful if you could call me back on 0120 0304050 and answer a couple of simple questions. Thank you and I look forward to hearing from you.'

Ms Baine's boyfriend had no idea that she had been pregnant with their child and he ended their relationship. Ms Baine complained to the hospital and threatened legal action.

When calling patients, careful regard should be had to confidentiality. If, as is common, a doctor has to call a patient on the phone without knowing whether the number is one on which the patient will be available and able talk privately, it is sensible to be cautious. Even though a patient has given a telephone number, there can be pitfalls for the unwary. It is good practice when asking for a telephone number to check with the patient if it is a personal line, whether there is a good time to talk privately and if it is acceptable to leave a message if the patient is not available. In all situations, doctors should be circumspect in giving information over the phone. Ask the name of the person to whom you are speaking before identifying yourself. If you have not reached the patient, politely saying that you will call back is the best option. Should you reach an answerphone or voicemail service, it is preferable not to leave a message. Occasionally, it may be important to make contact with the patient as soon as possible, in which case, a neutral message asking for the person to call you and leaving a telephone number is probably the most pragmatic solution, as the potential breach of confidentiality has to be weighed against the need to contact the patient. In the scenario above, it was not sufficiently urgent to justify leaving a message for the patient on an insecure answering machine.

Confidential information and the patient's best interests

A further circumstance in which a doctor may divulge a confidence is where she considers it to be in the patient's best interests so to do, and when it is undesirable on medical grounds to seek consent. This clearly raises the issue of medical paternalism and the extent to which that is acceptable has changed considerably in the last 15–20 years. However, there are still circumstances where information is shared about a patient who cannot give consent such as the patient who lacks capacity due to severe dementia. In such circumstances the rationale for sharing the information is that it is not possible to obtain the patient's consent but it is in his or her best interests that family and/or carers are informed of what is happening.

Disclosure of confidential information in the public interest

This is the final category that may be justify a breach of confidence. The case of *W v Egdell*[26] is the source of the law and professional guidance on what constitutes the 'public interest'. W was a patient in a secure hospital. The hospital intended to transfer W to a regional secure unit and sought an independent opinion from a psychiatrist, Dr Egdell, regarding W's suitability for such a transfer. Dr Egdell wrote a report that was unfavourable to W and, as a result, the transfer was abandoned. A routine review of W's detention was also due and Dr Egdell became concerned that his report would not be included in W's notes, meaning that a decision might be taken with inadequate medical information about the risk to the public. Dr Egdell sent copies of his report to the medical director of the hospital and the Home Office. W brought an action in contract and in equity alleging breach of confidence on the part of Dr Egdell.

The Court of Appeal held that only the 'most compelling circumstances'[27] could justify a doctor acting contrary to the patient's interests in the absence of consent. However, Dr Egdell had a legitimate fear of a real risk to public safety that entitled him to take reasonable steps to inform the appropriate authorities of his concerns. The case initially caused disquiet amongst those who perceived the decision as condoning a serious breach of confidentiality and giving doctors discretion to determine the 'public interest'. However, such concern seems to have been somewhat overstated, as clear principles were enunciated to guide professionals in how to use their discretion. Those principles are shown in the box below.

Confidentiality and defining the public interest

- The risk must be real and serious rather than fanciful;
- The risk must be of physical harm rather than any other sort of harm;
- An identifiable individual or individuals must be at risk; and
- Disclosure must only be to those who are in vital need of the information

---

[26] [1990] Ch 359; [1990] 1 All ER 835.
[27] Per Lord Bingham at p. 378.

Consent should be sought wherever possible and disclosure on the basis of the 'public interest' should be a last resort. Each case must be weighed on its own merits and a clinician who chooses to disclose confidential information on the ground of 'public interest' must be prepared to explain how he or she has balanced serious risk with the professional obligation of confidence. Even where disclosure is justified, confidential information must be shared only with those who need to know ie appropriate sources.

Is there a duty to warn?

If there is perceived public interest risk, does a doctor (or medical student) have a duty to warn? The legal answer is that in England and Wales there is no professional duty to warn others of potential risk. The judgment in *W v Egdell* provides a justification for breaches of confidence in the public interest but it does not impose an obligation on clinicians to warn third parties about potential risks posed by their patients. The closest the English courts have come to considering whether there is a duty to warn arose in a case involving a sex offender who abducted, assaulted and murdered a young girl, Rosie Palmer.[28] The perpetrator was a psychiatric outpatient who had disclosed to healthcare professionals that he was thinking about harming a child. Rosie Palmer's parents brought an action claiming negligence. The action failed and the Court of Appeal held that there was insufficient proximity between Rosie Palmer and the Health Authority because Rosie Palmer had not been specifically identified as the focus for the perpetrator's intentions.

Students and clinicians often worry about risk to others in the context of patients with sexually transmitted diseases, in particular HIV. Counselling and advice in sexual health clinics will routinely address such risks. However, it may be the case that a patient refuses to tell his or her sexual partners about his or her HIV status. In such situations, what is the healthcare professional's obligation? The position regarding confidentiality and disclosure of a patient's HIV status has not been definitively resolved. At present, if a patient who is HIV positive refuses to inform his or her sexual partner, a doctor may use the *W v Egdell* criteria and the GMC's professional

---

[28] Palmer v Tees Health Authority [1998] All ER 1980.

guidance on confidentiality to inform his reasoning but it is still a judgement on the part of an individual clinician.

The GMC guidance on confidentiality[29] and disclosure of communicable diseases[30] reflect the judgment in *W v Egdell* and the priority afforded to confidentiality. The GMC states that doctors are entitled to disclose information about a patient's HIV status (or information relating to other serious communicable diseases) to his or her sexual partner(s) if they believe the patient has not, or will not, disclose and there is a real risk of serious harm. You should attempt to persuade the patient to inform his or her partner(s) before disclosure and advise the patient of your intentions to contact his or her partner(s) if it is safe and practicable to do so. Finally, you should anonymise disclosure, wherever possible, to third parties and not identify the patient.

The GMC guidelines accord with the common law and state that whilst there may be cases where a doctor is justified in breaching confidentiality, there is no duty to do so. Judgement is required and the decision whether to disclose information is left to the individual doctor albeit with the reminder that he or she should be prepared to justify his or her decision. As a medical student you should understand the principles of confidentiality and when breaches are justifiable. You must also ensure that you always seek the advice of a senior member of staff when faced with complex questions of confidentiality.

Specific statutory provisions on disclosure of information

The common law exceptions to the general duty of confidentiality sit alongside several statutory provisions that cover specific areas in which disclosure of medical information may be mandatory. The statutory requirements include the notification of births (including stillbirths) and deaths, termination of pregnancy, poisonings and serious work accidents. In addition, regulatory bodies and public inquiries may require access to healthcare records in order to

---

[29] *Confidentiality*. General Medical Council, October 2009.
[30] *Confidentiality: Disclosing Information about Serious Communicable Diseases*. General Medical Council, September 2009.

make a judgement about a practitioner's competence or fitness to practise. The statutory provisions of which you should be most aware as a medical student are those relating to notifiable diseases. Notification should be made in the correct form to the consultant in communicable disease control when you encounter a patient with a notifiable disease such as tuberculosis (TB). For a doctor to fail to advise the consultant in communicable disease control promptly of a patient with a notifiable disease is a criminal offence. National guidance is available to provide clinicians with ready access to best practice in the management of TB.[31] Locally, most NHS Trusts will have guidance on how to involve the infectious disease team when a patient is suspected to have, or diagnosed as having, a notifiable and/or communicable disease.

Confidentiality and police requests

There is no statutory obligation for a doctor to supply confidential information to the police. In law, the police have no more general right to confidential medical information than anyone else.[32] However, there are certain statutory exceptions to this general rule, eg information following traffic accidents and relating to terrorism.[33] Clearly, the lack of a general obligation to furnish the police with confidential information does not permit a doctor to act as an obstruction to a police investigation. The default position is that, in the absence of a court order requiring disclosure, the consent of the patient should be sought before any personal or clinical details are disclosed to the police. Where requests are received from the police for clinical information or access to medical records, most NHS Trusts have protocols for how such requests should be made and by whom they should be handled.

The British Medical Association (BMA) has issued guidance which covers co-operation with the police.[34] This advice suggests that disclosure of confidential information should only be considered in the case of *serious* crimes whilst recognising that the term of severity is open to interpretation. The guidance suggests that

---

[31] *Tuberculosis: Clinical Diagnosis and Management of Tuberculosis and Measures for its Prevention and Control.* London: RCP, 2006.

[32] *Sykes v DPP* [1962] AC 528, per Lord Denning at 564.

[33] Prevention of Terrorism (Temporary Provisions) Act 1984, s 18.

[34] *Confidentiality and Disclosure of Health Information Toolkit.* BMA, July 2008.

confidentiality may be breached where crimes such as murder, manslaughter, rape, treason, kidnapping and abuse of children or other vulnerable people have been committed. Furthermore, the guidance proposes that serious harm to the security of the state or to public order and serious fraud also fall into the category of crimes where information may be shared with the police. In contrast, the BMA notes, in cases of theft, minor fraud or damage to property where loss or damage is less substantial, a breach of confidence would not generally be justifiable.

Sometimes the police will seek, and be granted, a court order under the Police and Criminal Evidence Act 1984 permitting access to healthcare records as part of the investigation of a crime. It is good practice to ask the police if they have obtained a court order enabling them to access medical information. If a court order has not been sought, it is wise to wait until a decision about such an order has been made before granting access to medical information; judges do not always grant court orders. However, if a court requires it, confidential clinical information must be disclosed.

Particular problems of confidentiality

Certain categories of patient present recurring and particular problems of confidentiality. Consider the following groups:

The impaired driver

Driving carries particular risks when patients have diagnoses or symptoms that potentially compromise their control of the vehicle. The Driver Vehicle and Licensing Agency (DVLA) has a specialist unit, the Drivers' Medical Group, which is responsible for establishing fitness to drive.[35] The DVLA uses a system of expert panels to set standards and to advise on the implications of driving with specific symptoms or conditions. The categories covered by the DVLA panels are shown in the box below.

---

[35] See also the DVLA publication *At a Glance Guide to the Current Medical Standards of Fitness to Drive*.

Medical advisory panel categories

- Alcohol Drugs and Substance Misuse and Driving
- Cardiovascular System and Driving
- Diabetes Mellitus and Driving
- Disorders of the Nervous System and Driving
- Psychiatric Disorders and Driving
- Visual Disorders and Driving

It is a criminal offence for a person not to disclose a relevant medical condition to the DVLA and the onus is on the patient to contact the DVLA. However, doctors cannot rely solely on patients to make the appropriate disclosure. Doctors have a specific professional obligation to ensure that the DVLA is aware of anyone who may be medically unfit and unsafe to drive. If a patient refuses either to contact the DVLA or to allow a doctor to do so on his or her behalf, a clinician should advise the patient that he or she will contact the medical advisor at the DVLA.

The patient with gunshot or knife wounds

Gunshot and knife wounds have special status and form a distinct category in professional guidance on confidentiality. The advice from the General Medical Council[36] is that doctors should notify the police where a patient has a gunshot wound or wounds. Disclosure involves a two-stage process. The first step requires clinicians to inform the police when a patient arrives with a gunshot or knife wound but without identifying the patient. Accidental and self-harm injuries with knives are usually excluded from the notification process. The second stage asks doctors to consider whether patients who arrive with a wound from a gun pose a serious risk of harm to others ie is it a situation that falls within the scope of the 'public interest' qualification to the duty of confidentiality? As with other cases where confidential information can justifiably be shared with a third party, the details disclosed should be limited to that which is essential to avert risk and only given to those who need to know.[37]

---

[36] *Reporting Gunshot and Knife Wounds.* London: General Medical Council, September 2009.

[37] Frampton, A. Reporting of Gun Shot Wounds by Doctors in Emergency Departments: A Duty or A Right? Some Legal and Ethical Issues Surrounding Breaking Patient Confidentiality. *Emerg Med J* 2005; 22(2): 84–86.

The drug dependent patient

Prescribers of controlled drugs are required to return prescribing data to the drug misuse database. Otherwise, the duty of confidentiality to a drug abusing patient is the same as for any other patient ie it can be qualified by (i) the patient's consent; (ii) the patient's best interests where it is impracticable or impossible to seek consent; and (c) where there is a serious risk of physical harm to an identifiable person or persons.

The abused patient

When an adult patient is experiencing domestic violence, it can seem difficult not to intervene. However, provided that he or she has capacity and no one else is at risk you cannot disclose information about his or her situation to a third party. Neither does that mean you should not try to build rapport and trust, nor does it prevent you from encouraging him or her to seek support. The situation differs when faced with potential abuse of a child. Child safeguarding and protection are discussed further in Chapter 6.

The sexually active minor

Although there may be other conditions that a minor (most often a teenager) would seek to conceal from his or her parents, it is usually sexual activity that proves the most sensitive. The right to confidentiality is inextricably linked with the capacity to consent to the way in which such confidential information is used. A case brought by Susan Axon[38] confirmed the position regarding confidentiality and capacitous minors. Mrs Axon challenged the Department of Health guidance on confidentiality and argued that parents should be informed if teenagers under the age of consent had an abortion even if they had capacity. The court held that there was no right for parents to know that capacitous adolescents had sought a termination of pregnancy and that the same obligation of confidentiality applied.

Patient access to medical information

Patients who have capacity can ask for a copy of the data that is held about them in medical records, reports, letters and any other

---

[38] *R (on the application of Axon) v Secretary of State for Health* [2006] EWHC.

format without giving a reason. Requests can be made informally. There is no provision in law that prohibits doctors from showing patients their records but many NHS Trusts prefer that a formal request is made in writing and a fee may be charged. There are circumstances under which a request to see healthcare records can be refused; for example, if the records identify a third person and if disclosure is likely to adversely affect the patient's mental and/or physical health.

Confidentiality and death

The final area of concern in matters of confidentiality is death. From an ethical perspective, a doctor's duty of confidence remains the same after death. However, once again, practicalities ensure that this is not, in fact, the case, eg a death certificate is a public document and copies can be easily obtained. Interestingly, the law takes a different view from the GMC and the legal duty ends with the death of the patient.

Confidentiality and medical students

Confidentiality is essential from the moment that a medical student begins his or her course. Even when you have been impeccably professional about explaining to patients that you are a student, many people will not distinguish between students and qualified healthcare staff meaning that patients expect students to treat information as confidential.

There are number of distinct situations that you might encounter as a medical student that warrant attention. First, patients may confide more readily in students either because they seem more approachable or spend more time with patients. What should you do if a patient tells you something and ask you to withhold the information from the team? For example, if a young woman with diabetes confided that she had not been taking her insulin regularly or a man with bipolar disorder told you that he was not regularly taking his lithium. The answer is that you do need to share the information and it cannot remain between you and the patient. As a medical student who is 'passing through' the clinical setting, you cannot keep significant pieces of information to yourself. Students are not responsible for care and to keep information from those who are is dangerous. You may not know the significance of what a patient tells you and it is for a qualified practitioner to make a judgement about its relevance or otherwise. The expectation is that you will share information and refer appropriately within the team. The correct response to a request to keep information 'secret' is to explore why the patient is reluctant for you to share what they have said; for example, patients may be worried about 'getting into trouble'. You should reassure the patient and encourage him or her to speak to the team perhaps asking if there is someone with whom they have a particularly good relationship. If the patient refuses to tell any of the clinical team, you should explain that as a student you are not able to keep the information to yourself and you will have to talk to the clinical team to ensure that the patient gets the right care.

The second factor that is particular to medical students is confidentiality and academic work. What is the position when you use patient information in your coursework eg as part of projects, case studies or portfolios? Ideally, you seek consent when you use patient information as part of education, even if it is anonymised. It does not need to be onerous or complicated: a simple explanation that you would, if the patient agrees, like to use the patient's experiences in your work which will be shared with your tutors. If you produce work that is of publishable standard, it will be important to declare at submission stage that you had permission to use the patient data or to justify why permission was not sought; a fact that unfortunately catches many students (and their supervisors) out.

Finally, it is worth mentioning a few of the ways in which students have been caught out regarding patient confidentiality. Sometimes you will encounter people you know in the clinical setting and therefore have access to personal information. If it is possible, you should ask the individual concerned whether he or she objects to you being involved in his care. Obviously you should be seeking consent anyway, but by acknowledging your social relationship with the patient you demonstrate empathy and enable him or her to make a proper choice. It goes without saying that you must never access the medical information of friends, family or your peers. Similarly, any medical information about fellow students or staff that comes to light when you are in clinical skills or other educational settings should be confidential. The line between the professional and the personal can be blurred on social networking sites. Status updates about the '*nightmare patient*' you clerked or the *'exciting postpartum haemorrhage'* you saw are risky and potentially compromise professionalism and trust. Think carefully about what you share, even if you are confident that your security settings are such that only your friends are seeing your words – they can come back to haunt you.

 # Core Concepts: Confidentiality

Confidentiality is integral to the development and maintenance of trust.
Confidentiality is not an unfettered duty and there are three broad common law justifications for sharing confidential information, namely: • consent; • in the patient's best interests but unable to obtain consent; and • in the public interest.
The public interest was legally defined in a case called *W v Egdell* as the risk of serious physical harm to an identifiable individual or individuals.
The public interest qualification amounts to a justification for breaching confidentiality, but does not equate to a duty or obligation to do so.
Even where there is a public interest justification for breaching confidentiality, it is preferable to seek and, if possible obtain, patient consent prior to sharing information.
Relatives, partners and next of kin have no greater right to confidential information than any other third party.
There are several statutory requirements to share confidential information eg notifiable diseases, gunshot injuries and knife wounds.
It is easy to breach confidentiality inadvertently and the phone can present particular risks.
Access to healthcare records and medical notes is governed by the Data Protection Act 1998, and it is good practice to write notes as if each patient were to seek access to their records.
Requests for information from the police are common. In general, such requests are legally governed by the common law qualifications to confidentiality and the requirements of the Police and Criminal Evidence Act 1984. However, there are also specific statutory exceptions requiring information to be provided eg terrorism and certain road traffic offences.
Notifiable diseases must be reported in accordance with the Public Health legislation and failure to do so is a criminal offence.

Assessments: Confidentiality in practice

1. The impaired driver

> You are a on a placement in the neurology outpatient clinic. Mr Kellaway, aged 33, has grand mal epilepsy. Despite several changes in treatment, Mr Kellaway's epilepsy remains poorly controlled and he continues to have fits. The notes show that Mr Kellaway has been advised to stop driving and to inform the DVLA of his diagnosis. You recognise Mr Kellaway immediately as the man who parked his car next to yours that morning. You are certain that Mr Kellaway was alone and driving. Mr Kellaway has come in for a clinic appointment.

Guidance notes

- This is a scenario that inevitably involves conveying information that will not be welcome. Talking about driving reminds Mr Kellaway of the impact of his disease which is likely to be difficult. You should expect that the patient will become emotional, perhaps angry. Effective communication will convey the essential message about the unacceptability of Mr Kellaway continuing to drive whilst acknowledging the impact on his life. The first task is to acknowledge that you have seen Mr Kellaway driving. This should be addressed factually and neutrally once the initial introductions have been made: avoid being or appearing judgmental, or worse, confrontational.

- You should explore what Mr Kellaway has been told about driving whilst his epilepsy is poorly-controlled. Although the notes record that the issue has been discussed with him, you should not assume how the information has been received. You will need to listen carefully to Mr Kellaway because what he says will reflect what he knows and believes to be the risks of continuing to drive. Information about risk should be explained calmly and factually. Alarmist, patronising or chiding approaches should be avoided.

- If Mr Kellaway refuses to inform the DVLA, you should explain that where a patient presents a serious risk of physical harm to others, confidentiality can be breached. However, you should explain that breaching confidentiality is a last resort for clinical team and continue to encourage Mr Kellaway to approach the DVLA himself. The discussion with Mr Kellaway should be documented accurately and the consultant informed as soon as possible. Try to remain non-judgemental, avoid 'scolding', acknowledge the impact of not being able to drive and remain calm.

2. Confidentiality and relatives

> You are on a placement at the oncology outpatient clinic. Miriam Jensen has come alone. Her husband was diagnosed with acute myeloid leukaemia last week. Mrs Jensen is visibly upset. She says that she is *'very concerned'* about her husband. He is pale and tired but he has *'barely said a thing'* about what is going on. She knows that Mr Jensen came to the hospital for some *'sort of blood tests'* but nothing more. Mrs Jensen found the clinic's appointment card in her husband's jacket and has come in today because she is *'out of her mind with worry'*.

Guidance notes

- This scenario assesses not only whether you know that confidentiality cannot be breached without the patient's permission, but also how well you can handle a difficult situation with an anxious and upset relative. In addition to explaining to Mrs Jensen why the team is unable to share information about her husband's care with her without his permission, the consultation has to be conducted in a way that acknowledges Mrs Jensen's distress, explores options for facilitating a discussion with her husband and ameliorates rather than exacerbates her emotional state. It is a challenging situation and your communication skills may either inflame or diffuse the situation depending on the extent to which Mrs Jensen feels heard, understood and supported. Mrs Jensen is sufficiently anxious to have tracked down the details of the clinic, travelled to the hospital and waited without an appointment. It is essential that her anxiety, fear and concerns are heard and acknowledged. It is possible to empathise and support Mrs Jensen whilst not breaching her husband's confidentiality.

- First, the relationship of Mrs Jensen to the patient ie her husband should be confirmed. You should verify whether she is alone and if her husband is aware of her visit. There is a fine line between exploring why Mrs Jensen's husband is apparently refusing to talk to her and making uninformed judgements or inadvertent but damaging comment on her relationship. Phrases such as *'is everything alright in your marriage?I It seems odd to me he won't talk to you'* or *'this is a situation which makes me think you ought to consider marriage guidance counselling'* should be avoided! Alternative ways of discussing her husband's reluctance to talk to her might include phrases such as *'You are obviously and understandably very worried. Does your husband know how concerned you are?'* or *'it sounds as though it is a particularly difficult situation for you because your husband won't talk to you. Do you have any thoughts about why that might be?'*

- You will have to tell Mrs Jensen something that she does not want to hear ie that confidentiality cannot be broken even though she is the patient's wife and in obvious distress. Mrs Jensen may respond with frustration and become more upset, possibly even angry. Allowing Mrs Jensen to express her feelings whilst remaining calm is crucial.

- The scenario is simple in terms of ethico-legal content if not in terms of the communication challenges. Without Mr Jensen's permission, no information can be shared with his wife. Consent has not been given by Mr Jensen and the task is to explain the position to Mrs Jensen.

- Throughout this consultation, you may feel frustrated and even upset – no one likes to be in a situation where they are unable to help and feel ineffective. It is important that these feelings are not conveyed to Mrs Jensen. The unwelcome information may need to be repeated clearly and calmly. Time permitting, you might explore whether discussion between Mr Jensen and his wife could be facilitated. Suggestions might include:

- Mrs Jensen returning with her husband for a joint consultation;
- Exploring with Mr Jensen, at his next appointment, the impact of his diagnosis on his family life. Perhaps 'reality testing' and gently checking the sustainability of not involving his wife;
- Involving the family's GP and reminding Mrs Jensen that the GP is available to support her through this difficult time; and
- Asking sensitively whether there are friends or family who may be sources of support.

- At the end of the consultation, you might reiterate regret that you have been unable to help Mrs Jensen as she asked. An appropriate closure would be to summarise the possibilities for encouraging a discussion with her husband, reminding her of ways the clinical team may be able to support them.

Short answer questions

The following are examples of two short answer questions on confidentiality.

Sample SAQ

The duty of confidentiality owed by a doctor to a patient is not unqualified. Under what circumstances can confidential information be disclosed?   (6 marks)

Guidance notes

The circumstances under which a doctor can breach confidentiality are derived from common law, professional guidance and statute. The common law provides three broad categories when a doctor can breach confidentiality, namely (i) with the patient's consent (being careful as to the extent of the consent); (ii) where it is in the patient's best interests to share the information but you can't obtain consent eg where a patient has impaired capacity and his carers need to know how to look after him; and (iii) in the public interest which is specifically defined as where there is a serious risk of physical harm to an identifiable person or persons. In addition, there a several statutes that require disclosure, for example, the public health legislation covering notifiable diseases such as TB. Finally, the GMC has guidelines that require a doctor to share information in particular circumstances eg gunshot wounds and knife injuries (apart from those caused by self-harm or accidentally) should be reported to the police, albeit without identifying the patient unless there is a legitimate public interest reason to do so.

Sample SAQ

Dr Milner is working as a community psychiatrist. One of his patients, Ms Hollins, has become fixated on a member of staff at her college: Mr Kavanagh. Ms Hollins confides in Dr Milner that if she *can't have him, no one will*. Dr Milner is concerned about Ms Hollins' obsession with Mr Kavanagh but maintains patient confidentiality and does not discuss Ms Hollins with anyone. Three days later Ms Hollins attacks Mr Kavanagh's wife with a knife and she is seriously injured. Discuss Dr Milner's role in the above scenario with specific reference to confidentiality and risk to others.   (10 marks)

Guidance notes

Dr Milner owes Ms Hollins a duty of confidentiality. Trust between patient and doctor is essential in all specialties but perhaps is particularly resonant in psychiatry where patients may be marginalised and experience feelings of suspicion towards 'the system' and its agents. Where a patient presents a potential risk to a third party, a clinician faces a particular ethico-legal dilemma: how to balance the rights and interests of an individual (in this scenario, Ms Hollins) with those of a third party with whom Dr Milner does not have a therapeutic relationship and perhaps the wider interests of society at large (although it must be remembered that society has an interest both in responding to risk and to ensuring the doctor-patient relationship is based on trust and confidentiality).

There are circumstances in which Dr Milner could disclose what Ms Hollins has shared with him but both the law and professional guidance are open to interpretation about the extent to which Dr Milner can be expected or required to breach confidentiality. The two legal cases that are of particular relevance are *W v Egdell* and *Palmer v Tees Health Authority*. *W v Egdell* sets out guidance about how the 'public interest' should be defined, although the case emphasised that consent should be sought wherever possible and that situations should be assessed on their own merits. The guidance from *W v Egdell* states that a breach of confidentiality in the 'public interest' should be considered where there is a real and serious, rather than 'fanciful', risk of physical harm to an identifiable individual or individuals. The first question therefore is whether Dr Milner felt that Ms Hollins presented a real and serious risk not only to Mr Kavanagh but also to his family. Without further information it is difficult to know whether her remark was a significant threat. Some psychiatrists might say that their work is characterised by apparent threats and that patients are encouraged to be open about their darker feelings for therapeutic reasons.

Even if Dr Milner believed that Ms Hollins presented a real and serious risk to Mr Kavanagh and his family within the principles provided by the judgment in *W v Egdell*, does that equate to a duty to warn? The case of *Palmer v Tees Health Authority* confirmed that doctors do not have a duty to warn where a patient apparently threatens a group rather than a specific individual (in the Palmer case, young girls were threatened but not Rosie Palmer). The rationale was that there was not sufficient proximity between Rosie Palmer and the Health Authority and the court recognised the policy difficulties of requiring psychiatrists to warn of risk.

In addition to the *Egdell* and *Palmer* cases, the GMC guidance on confidentiality states that a doctor is entitled to disclose information if there is a real risk of serious harm, although doctors should seek consent and/or advise the patient if it is safe and practicable. Finally, disclosure to third parties should, wherever possible, be anonymised and not identify the patient. The GMC guidelines reflect the common law in stating that there is a justification for disclosing information, but not a duty or obligation. The law and the professional guidance require Dr Milner to exercise judgement and the decision whether to inform any one about Ms Hollins is ultimately left to him, albeit with the caveat that he should be prepared to justify his decision. Dr Milner has to weigh the risk of harm to others against the principles of confidentiality. If he concludes that a breach of confidence was justifiable, he might seek advice from the Trust legal team and/or his own defence union to ensure that he doesn't act impulsively and has an opportunity to explore his reasoning in this complex area of practice.

Chapter 5

New Beginnings: Reproductive Ethics

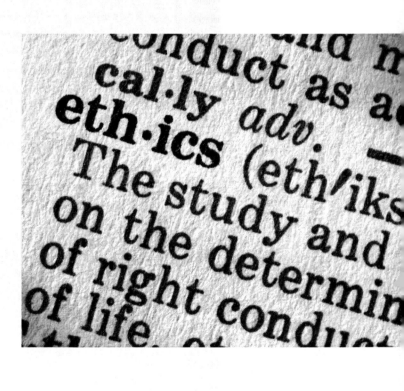

New Beginnings: Reproductive Ethics

Introduction

The area of assisted reproduction is probably the one that has most changed since I began my career. First, there has been a proliferation of techniques as technology, and its potential application, evolves. Secondly, the regulation and review of assisted reproduction has developed and altered considerably since the Human Fertilisation and Embryology Authority (HFEA) was established in 1990. Recently, the Conservative-Liberal Democrat coalition government in the UK announced its intention to abolish the HFEA as part of its review of non-governmental organisations. The decision to abolish the HFEA has been met with opposition by commentators concerned about the effect on effective discussion, debate and regulation of assisted reproduction.[39] Whilst the future regulation of assisted reproduction remains in question, there remain concepts and questions that are constant in any discussion of reproductive medicine. For a student therefore, the task is to understand what makes this area of practice unique and how ethical commentators have thought about the questions that are posed with each new scientific development and biotechnological advancement. The moral questions that were asked in the earliest days of creating 'test tube babies' in the 1970s continue to shape contemporary debates about cloning and stem cell research.

Personhood and slippery slopes

The ways which you understand and interpret the concept of personhood, and the status of the embryo, are essential to ethical analysis of assisted reproduction techniques (and, by extension, might inform your perspective on the status of the embryo and antenatal interventions such as screening and termination of pregnancy). Essentially, if you believe that human life is characterised in such a way as to afford the embryo human status or personhood, it will be difficult, if not impossible, to conclude that many reproductive medicine techniques are morally acceptable.

---

[39] Baroness Ruth Deech, speaking on the *Today* programme, BBC Radio 4, 24 September 2010; Parsons, J., Savaas, M. Why We Shouldn't Abolish the HFEA. *Bionews* 578, 4 October 2010.

Personhood refers to the ways in which we define what it is about human beings that makes them distinct, and is often the starting point for ethical arguments about what we should or shouldn't do in respect of those who have personhood. Personhood is the subject of a vast philosophical literature, but for the purposes of most medical students, especially the worried ones, it is sufficient to understand why personhood is an ethically significant concept and to be able to describe some of the ways in which personhood has been defined or explained. The box below sets out some of the commonest approaches to understanding personhood that are discussed in the field of ethics.

Ways of thinking about personhood and the status of the embryo

- Persons are characterised by their rationality or capacity for relationships as opposed to mere sentience.[40]
- Personhood depends only on existence: human beings have intrinsic value that creates moral status and warrants protection.
- The defining characteristics of personhood are relationships, emotions (either expressed and/or inspired in others) and interpersonal interactions.
- Personhood is linked to viability: once a foetus is capable of living outside the womb it has moral status and should be protected.
- Embryos have the potential to become a person and should therefore be afforded the status of persons from the moment of fertilisation.[41]
- Personhood is a matter of faith-based or religious teachings (which vary considerably in the conclusions that are drawn about when a person, with concomitant moral status, is created).
- Personhood is a gradual process of development and accordingly the status afforded to the embryo, foetus and eventually child will increase incrementally from conception through pregnancy until birth.[42]

In contrast to the contested ethical perspective on personhood, the law adopts arbitrary and different definitions of a person

---

[40] Harris, J. *The Value of Life*. London: Routledge, 1985; Singer, P. *Practical Ethics*. (2nd ed.) Cambridge: Cambridge University Press, 1993. Singer offers some interesting comparative perspectives on the status of humans and animals.

[41] Locke, J. *Second Treatise on Government*. Oxford: Blackwell, 1966.

[42] Dworkin, R. *Life's Dominion*. New York: Vintage Books, 1994.

depending on the particular legal context.[43] For example, for the purposes of research on embryos, day 14 is the limit beyond which research cannot be permitted,[44] the rationale being that is the embryological stage by which the neural crests have developed. It is a legal convenience and provides a pragmatic limitation on embryo research but it has been criticised as 'neuralist'.[45] A further example of the way that the law affords different levels of protection to the foetus can be found in the abortion legislation which is discussed later in this chapter.

It is, of course, only possible to determine which arguments you find to be the most cogent and convincing after a period of consideration and your conclusions are likely to shape how you respond to ethical questions arising from assisted reproduction. For example, if you conclude that the status of the embryo is morally equivalent to that of a person, it may be difficult for you to be persuaded that it is ethical to discard surplus embryos created as part of the IVF process. To destroy that which you believe to have personhood, even for positive ends, may be to ignore the Kantian precept that all persons should be ends in themselves, and never means to ends, no matter how compelling that end may be.

Even if you reject the notion that embryos have a status that is morally equivalent to a person, it does not render the practical tasks inherent in reproductive medicine comfortable or easy. If, having reflected upon and considered the arguments pertinent to the status of the embryo, you conclude that the embryo does not have status that is morally equivalent to a person, analysis may turn to the morality of the goals or consequences of assisted reproduction. What is a morally sufficient justification for permitting the creation, selection or disposal of embryos? Many people, both clinicians and lay people, could list a number of conditions that they believe would warrant selection using a technique such as pre-implantation

---

[43] Cf: Abortion Act 1967, ss 1–5, *AG's Reference (No 3 of 1994)* [1997] 3 All ER 936, *St George's Healthcare NHS Trust v S, R v Collins, ex parte S* (1998) 44 BMLR 160, CA.

[44] Human Fertilisation and Embryology Act, s 3(4).

[45] Saunders, P. (1997). Personal Submission from the General Secretary of the Christian Medical Fellowship to the Human Fertilisation and Embryology Authority and the Advisory Committee on Genetic Testing: Pre-implantation Genetic Diagnosis (www.cmf.org.uk/publicpolicy/submissions/?id=31).

genetic diagnosis. Such 'shopping lists' of justifications for selection techniques commonly include disabling or life-shortening conditions such as muscular dystrophy, Huntingdon's chorea and Diamond-Blackfan anaemia. However, there is unlikely to be consensus regarding the conditions that justify selection, leaving many 'grey' areas. For example, is the fact that a disease is late-onset rather than congenitally symptomatic a morally persuasive rationale for selecting embryos and discarding the unselected?

By exploring the intentions or aims of reproductive medicine, we are moving towards another key concept in the ethical debate, namely that of the 'slippery slope'. Slippery slope arguments are common in ethics[46] and evident in discussions about choosing characteristics, including the sex of any future baby, as part of pre-implantation technologies. Many commentators support sex selection for to prevent sex chromosome-linked diseases. The ethical debate becomes more difficult when sex selection is being discussed for so-called 'social' or non-medical reasons. For many, the selection of particular characteristics such as sex or eye colour raises the spectre of 'designer' babies. In contrast, for a smaller number of writers, sex selection is simply another version of family planning and it is disingenuous to object to sex selection given the highly organised way in which most couples in the Western world determine the timing and size of their families. In the UK, the HFEA has taken a conservative and cautious approach to sex selection for non-medical reasons as evidenced by the response to a couple who were denied IVF to create a female foetus. The couple's only daughter died aged three in a Bonfire Night accident and the family has four boys. The HFEA concluded that sex selection in such circumstances was unacceptable.

When considering the ethical aspects of employing assisted reproductive techniques in the context of disease, is there a distinction to be drawn between screening out a specific disease and screening in for a tissue match to donate to an existing child or, less commonly, a specific impairment? When screening out disease during assisted reproduction, the embryo, foetus and

---

[46] For example, the debate about euthanasia and assisted dying is often informed by slippery slope arguments ie the view that to formalise some forms of voluntary euthanasia would inevitably lead to undesirable and unintended extension of the practice into involuntary euthanasia; see Chapter 9.

future person are one and the same ie the technique is being used to prevent suffering in the embryo, foetus and future child. In the case of screening for a tissue match, it is specifically undertaken to improve or even end the suffering of another child. Furthermore, the creation of embryos and so-called 'saviour siblings' may even present physical and emotional risks to the child that is eventually born eg gathering stem cells may be considered to be largely harmless but marrow transplants do carry risks and we know little of the emotional legacy of children created specifically to help siblings. Returning to the most basic of ethical principles and to use the language of Kant, creating embryos and selecting particular characteristics challenges the notion that human beings should not be means to another's end. Although, it is important to point out that Kant was concerned with the use of others *solely* as ends and could not have imagined the world of assisted reproduction in nineteenth century Germany! It is worth thinking carefully about society's approach to parenthood when making moral judgements about assisted reproduction. For example, could all children be said to be means to their parents' ends to some extent? What is the moral difference between choice via reproductive techniques and chance ie natural conception resulting in a match?

Any assessment of whether a particular genetic condition is a sufficient justification for selection or disposal of embryos is a value judgement to a greater or lesser extent, reflecting personal assumptions about the condition in particular and the meaning of 'disability' in general. In which case, why should the value judgement of a clinician or expert in reproductive techniques be considered any more persuasive than those of the putative parents? The HFEA recommends that information about clinical conditions and the reality of living with a disability should be available to those seeking pre-implantation techniques. The acknowledgement that the medical approach to disability is limited and cannot substitute for personal experience is admirable, and acknowledges the difference between the biomedical understanding of a particular disease and the social reality of how a disease affects an individual. However, there are multiple realities that cannot ever be comprehensively represented. For some, the experience of having a child with a particular impairment may be represented as a lengthy and lonely struggle but for others it may be a rewarding and enriching experience. These multiple realities have somehow to be discussed with potential parents and that is perhaps one of the greatest ethical challenges facing those working in reproductive medicine.

Once embryos have been created, there are specific rules setting out what can and should happen. Concerns about the increased risks of multiple births led the HFEA to reduce the number of embryos that can be implanted from three to two and there have been calls recently for the number to be further reduced to one. Embryos that are preserved must be allowed to perish at the end of a five-year period unless there is a reason for keeping the embryos for treatment purposes in cases of medical need, so long as this period does not extend beyond the woman's fifty-fifth birthday. Embryos that have been stored by clinics have been discussed in a few high profile legal actions. It has been suggested that consent for the future use of embryos should be vested in the female partner, as she is the person for whom the embryos were intended. However, the law requires that both parties consent to the use of embryos and neither woman nor man is able to override the other party's wishes.

Assisted reproduction: questions and resources

Policies on access to fertility treatment used to vary widely around the country, prompting the National Institute for Clinical Excellence (NICE) to issue national guidance to health authorities in an attempt to end what was popularly described as a 'postcode lottery'.[47] The aim was to standardise the provision of assisted reproduction nationally. The guidance is lengthy and for those who are interested, you can read the full document at the NICE website.[48] Its key recommendations were that women between the ages of 23–39 years in whom there is a history of more than three years of sub-fertility should be given three cycles of publicly-funded IVF. The policy change is underpinned by a fundamental ethical question: is there a right to reproduce? And, if you believe that there is a right to reproduce, does that right create a duty on the part of the State to provide assisted reproductive services? Fertility

---

[47] The variable provision led to a number of legal challenges about the limitations put on the availability of IVF, eg the use of upper age limits that were held to be justifiable in a resource-limited NHS in the case of *R v Sheffield AHA ex p Seale* (1995) 25 BMLR 1.

[48] www.nice.org.uk

services have often been treated as 'special' but constructing assisted reproduction as distinct has moral consequences. For some, it leads to special pleading for fertility services. In contrast, treating fertility services as different can lead to discrimination.

Those seeking assisted reproductive techniques are subject to more scrutiny that those who conceive without medical assistance.[49] Historically, doctors have been required to take social factors into account when evaluating suitability for assisted reproduction and to consider the welfare of any child that might be created. Whilst it is understandable that it is considered morally desirable to reflect on the welfare of a child that might be born as a result of assisted reproduction, there are a couple of points to note. First, it requires doctors to consider the wellbeing and best interests of a future person rather than just the patient presenting for treatment. Secondly, it is not a judgement that doctors are neither trained nor qualified to make. Consideration of the welfare of a future child has led to significant debate about what it means to be a family. Initially, when the Human Fertilisation and Embryology Act was debated in parliament, there was pressure from some political quarters to limit IVF to married couples. A compromise was eventually reached: section 13(5) of the statute required those referring couples for, and providing, assisted reproductive techniques to consider the welfare of the child including *'the need of that child for a father'*. In the years that followed, there was much discussion about the appropriateness of the provision. Eventually, there was a review of the requirements relating to the welfare of the child resulting in new guidance from the HFEA. A welfare risk assessment must be conducted before treatment is provided. The presumption is that treatment will be offered save for situations in which there is deemed to be a risk of serious harm to any child born as a result of reproductive technologies. The guidance states that where a child born as a result of assisted reproductive treatment will be raised solely by a woman, consideration should be given to the woman's *'ability to meet the child's needs and the ability of other persons within the family or social circle willing to share responsibility for those needs'*.[50]

---

[49] Although comparisons are often made with adoption; a process which also involves prospective parents being closely scrutinised.

[50] *Welfare of the Child and the Assessment of those Seeking Treatment.* London: Human Fertilisation and Embryology Authority 2009.

Reproductive medicine is rapidly changing and occasionally, the ethico-legal analysis has sometimes appeared to lag behind, failing to anticipate, elucidate or respond in a timely way to moral questions. However, it isn't necessary to reinvent the ethico-legal wheel each time there is an innovation. Many of the ethico-legal questions that arise as a result of assisted reproductive techniques are fundamental and recurrent. The themes of personhood, resource allocation and discrimination recur and the basics of good ethical practice, such as regard for properly sought consent, protecting confidentiality, and treating patients in context, apply as much in relation to assisted reproductive medicine as elsewhere in clinical practice. Thinking about your views on the questions posed in this section and practising expressing your perspective in the face of differing opinions and challenging arguments will enable you to adapt and respond to whatever technological developments may occur in the coming years.

Antenatal screening and testing

Antenatal screening and testing are routinely offered to women in the UK. Indeed, so routine is the availability of antenatal screening that it is easy to overlook basic ethical questions. For some, the first and most fundamental ethical question is whether the aim of antenatal screening is in itself morally defensible? If so, what does it mean for antenatal screening and testing to be 'successful'? On a more practical level, if consent is to be meaningful, discussion between clinicians and patients must consist of more than simply quoting statistics on risk and should enable the patient to make an informed choice about screening and diagnostic testing. There is a range of screening options available: some are indicative and provide a risk profile whilst others are diagnostic. For example, a nuchal translucency scan will give a woman an estimated risk of having a child with Down Syndrome based on the measurement of the fluid under the nuchal fold and a woman's age. In contrast, chorionic villus sampling or an amniocentesis will, by karyotyping, reveal definitively whether the foetus has Down Syndrome (or other chromosomal abnormality).

As ultrasonography has developed and hospitals, both in the private and public sector, offer patients the opportunity to buy images and videos of their ultrasound scans, some commentators have questioned whether women presenting for the 'routine'

scan understand that their pregnancies are being screened for abnormality. It has been suggested by a minority that the use of ultrasound in pregnancy is so routine that consent should be considered 'implied'. However, such a position does not accord with the GMC guidance or the law on consent. Furthermore a move towards implied consent would not recognise the chain of events that may be put into place by a 'routine' ultrasound. The question of choice in pregnancy screening is fraught. Once a woman agrees to undergo 'routine' screening she is, perhaps unwittingly, taking the first step in a potential chain of further investigations and procedures, some of which carry risk. If a woman is recommended to undergo an invasive test as a result of a screening, is her choice to undergo the invasive test free? Antenatal screening usually leads to conversations about probabilities not certainties. The way in which these probabilities are communicated is crucial. It sounds quite different to tell a woman that there is a 10% chance that her child will have a disability rather than a 90% chance that her child will be healthy. Screening cannot provide absolute answers and this fact should form part of the conversation with patients when seeking consent. There will be both false positives and false negatives. It is also easy to overlook the fact that, despite the increasing sophistication of antenatal screening, there are significant conditions that cannot be screened for or diagnosed during pregnancy.

Just as women are not obliged to undergo any screening or testing in pregnancy, there is no right or entitlement to prenatal testing any more than there is a right to any other form of medical investigation or treatment. However, if a doctor refuses to perform a test he or she must consider whether it would unreasonable or illogical in the eyes of others so to refuse the patient the test requested. If so, the doctor could be vulnerable to a claim for negligence.

Termination of pregnancy

You may already have strong feelings about termination of pregnancy – in my experience, it is more likely than not that you know where you stand on the issue. When I teach on the subject, I ask at the beginning how many people have opinions about abortion. The vast majority reply that they have a personal view of termination and it is only a handful of people who are unsure. It can be useful to think about where your views, whatever they might be, originate and how you approach the subject of termination. The following self-assessment questionnaire is designed to help you to explore your own views on termination of pregnancy and to begin to engage with the ethical arguments that are commonly raised when discussing abortion.

Termination: self-assessment questionnaire

1. Do you have definite views about whether abortion is morally acceptable? If not, please go straight to question 5.

2. If, you do have definite views on whether or not abortion is morally acceptable, please identify which ethical concept(s) inform your views:
   (a) A woman's 'right to choose'
   (b) The 'sanctity' of human life
   (c) Pregnancy as a 'morally neutral' state
   (d) A balance of risks and benefits
   (e) Teachings of religion or faith
   (f) Other (please state)

3. Using your answer to question 2, please consider the questions below which corresponds to the ethical concept(s) on which you justify your views (indicated by letter) eg if your answer to question 2 was that you believe women have a right to choose, please answer question (a) below:
   (a) Does a woman have an unlimited right to choose to terminate pregnancies to the extent that she can terminate pregnancies infinitely as a form of contraception?
   (b) When does 'human life' begin? How do you know? Do you object to other contragestive forms of contraception eg post-coital hormone treatment or IUDs?
   (c) How can there be moral equivalence between a choice to end a pregnancy and the potential for human life that exists therein, and other choices about health eg the removal of an appendix or gall bladder?
   (d) Why is it appropriate for anyone other than the woman involved to weigh risks and benefits? If the outcome is poor, does this make a moral act immoral? Conversely, if the outcome is good, does this make an immoral act moral?
   (e) Is it morally acceptable to subject others to the beliefs of your religion or faith? If it is, why? If it is not, how do you reconcile your belief in the immorality of abortion with accepting that, for society, abortion is acceptable?

---

4. What is/are the moral argument(s) on which you base your views on abortion? How would you explain choosing this moral position over those described in questions (a)–(e) above?

5. If you do not have definite views on abortion, please consider the following moral concepts that are commonly invoked in the abortion debate and state which you find most convincing and why:

   (a) All women have the 'right to choose' a termination because of the principles of self-determination and autonomy.

   (b) An embryo and foetus are living entities and therefore should be afforded protection because of the fundamental 'sanctity' of human life.

   (c) Pregnancy is a morally neutral state and the choice to end a pregnancy is not morally different from the choice to have an appendix or gall bladder removed.

   (d) Abortion is morally justifiable because the risk of mental or physical harm to a woman who does not wish to proceed with a pregnancy overrides the harms to an unborn and undeveloped foetus. The needs of an adult are not equivalent to those of a foetus.

   (e) Religion or faith teachings are clear that all living beings (of which a foetus is clearly one) must be protected and not harmed – abortion is morally unjustified.

   (f) Are there any other common arguments you have heard in the abortion debate? If so, what were they? Were they convincing (please explain)?

6. Can the difference drawn in the Abortion Act 1967 between terminations of pregnancies (TOPs) performed prior to 24 weeks and those performed after 24 weeks' gestation be morally justified? If so, on what grounds?

7. Will you, as a future clinician, elect to exercise your right of conscientious objection and not participate in terminations as provided for under s 4(1) of the Abortion Act 1967? If so, why? If not, why not?

Termination of pregnancy: ethical issues

As the self-assessment questionnaire above illustrates there are myriad ways in which to approach the morality of abortion. The box below summarises the principal arguments that recur in the abortion debate.

Ethical arguments about termination of pregnancy

•   Moral status of the foetus and personhood
•   Feminist and liberal perspectives on choice
•   Rights-based arguments that often put maternal-foetal interests in opposition
•   Virtue-based approaches to clinicians and others working in the field
•   Scope of the moral regard given to the foetus and availability/conduct of terminations at law

Personhood and the status of the embryo and/or foetus have been discussed earlier in this chapter. You might want to return to that section and see how your views on personhood inform your perspective on termination of pregnancy. You might also consider the question of scope. Even if you believe that at some stage between conception and delivery the foetus acquires the moral status of a person, questions might still remain as to the extent to which you conclude terminations can be justified. For example, do your views on the moral status of the embryo mean that you believe that an abortion can never be justified, even in emergencies? Conversely, if you support termination, does circumstance or gestational age have any relevance when considering the provision of abortion?

Liberal approaches to termination focus on the freedom of a woman to determine what happens to her body. Feminist perspectives look at the provision of healthcare through the lens of paternalism, sexual inequalities, gender roles and oppression. Ethical arguments that adopt a liberal and/or feminist perspective commonly argue that access to safe abortion supports women's choices enabling them to retain control of whether and when to have children. Such accounts of the ethical aspects of abortion tend to focus on freedom, individual self-determination and choice and are in keeping with the value placed upon autonomy in contemporary Western medical ethics.

Rights-based analyses of abortion illustrate the tension between a woman and the foetus. Such arguments usually conclude that a foetus's rights, if they exist at all, cannot 'trump' the rights of the woman. It is an approach that appears to be endorsed in the law in the UK which provides that a termination of pregnancy should take place if the situation is an emergency and the woman's life is in danger. Such situations, at least in the UK, are relatively rare and may not be the only way to think about the relationship between maternal-foetal rights. For example, some have concluded that a foetus should not be put at risk of avoidable harm. In parts of the US, such a view has led to the passing of controversial laws that set out how pregnant women should behave and penalise those who choose to take part in risky behaviour eg drinking alcohol and taking drugs.

A less common way of looking at abortion is to draw on the virtue ethics literature. Remember virtue ethics is the branch of moral reasoning that explains what is right, to be preferred or desirable according to the characteristics of those involved. It is worth considering how the virtuous doctor (or medical student) would behave in relation to termination. Irrespective of your personal views, are there particular behaviours that are desirable and unacceptable when working with patients who seek abortions? A virtue ethicist might suggest that whatever the private views of the clinician, as a minimum, he or she should treat patients who request terminations with fairness, kindness, honesty and respect. Indeed, the virtuous approach does seem to be embedded within professional guidance on abortion for doctors. Even if a doctor conscientiously objects to abortion and exercises his or her right not to refer or participate in terminations of pregnancy, he or she is still required to be non-judgemental, open and responsive to women seeking a termination. Referrals to other doctors must be timely and made without criticism irrespective of an individual's own beliefs about abortion.

Termination of pregnancy and the law

The law relating to abortion is to be found in the Abortion Act 1967, as amended by the Human Fertilisation and Embryology Act 1990. The key aspects of the law to note are shown in the box below.

Key aspects of the law on termination of pregnancy

- Abortions can be carried out only on approved premises;
- Terminations must be approved by two doctors (in practice this usually means the referring doctor and the clinician who carries out the abortion) except in an immediate emergency where a single doctor will suffice;
- Prior to 24 weeks, an abortion may be lawfully conducted if there is a risk to woman's mental or physical health and/or to existing children;
- After 24 weeks, a termination may only be conducted in cases of *'serious handicap'* or where there is a risk of death or *'grave permanent injury'* to a woman's physical or mental health;
- The law has been clarified to allow for the selective reduction of embryos in a multiple pregnancy, provided the standard criteria for a termination are satisfied; and
- Clinicians have a right of conscientious objection and do not have to participate in terminations save for emergencies; see the Abortion Act 1967, s 4. The right of conscientious objection has been confirmed by the Department of Health to extend to medical students.

There is also a body of case law relating to termination of pregnancy that further clarifies the legal position. For example, legal precedent has established that whilst nurses enjoy the same right of conscientious objection as doctors,[51] that right does not extend to administrative staff responsible for writing referral letters.[52] Case law has also confirmed that male partners do not have any rights in relation to abortion.[53] A well-publicised case brought by a curate, the Reverend Joanna Jepson, is of particular note. Reverend Jepson became aware of a termination that had been carried out at 28 weeks gestation where the foetus had a cleft lip and palate. She brought an action for judicial review of the decision not to prosecute the clinical team that had conducted the abortion arguing that it was an unlawful termination because a cleft palate does not constitute a 'serious handicap' such as to justify an abortion at 28 weeks. However, in 2005 the court held that the doctors involved had acted in good faith and the Crown

---

[51] *Royal College of Nursing v DHSS* [1981] 1 All ER 545.

[52] *Janaway v Salford AHA* [1989] 1 AC 537, HL.

[53] *Paton v BPAS* [1979] QB 276; *C v S* [1987] 2 FLR 505.

Prosecution Service confirmed that they would not be prosecuting those involved in the termination.

Most recently, there has been a legal attempt to change the law regarding early medical abortions.[54] At present, the Abortion Act requires that women having a medical abortion take two doses of medication under clinical supervision. The British Pregnancy Advisory Service (BPAS) brought an action to challenge the requirement for supervision arguing that the UK was out of step with other jurisdictions and that, in practice, the majority of women leave immediately after taking the second dose of medication and are not therefore 'supervised' in any meaningful sense. The BPAS action failed and the requirement for supervision of early medical abortions remains.

There have been efforts by those on different sides of the abortion debate to change the law, most recently in 2007 to mark the 40th anniversary of the legislation. Examples that illustrate the range of proposed changes include changing the requirement that two doctors authorise a termination so that the approval of only one doctor is required; introducing a 'cooling off' period for women requesting a termination; acknowledging the increasing use of medical rather than surgical techniques; and reducing the gestational age before which non-emergency and serious handicap terminations can be provided.

Finally, it is worth summarising the empirical data on abortion. According to the most recent Department of Health statistics,[55] in 2009, there were 189,100 terminations (a 3.2% decrease on previous year). Of terminations carried out in 2009, 91% occurred before 13 weeks and 75% took place before 10 weeks. In the same year, 40% of terminations were medical rather than surgical. Whilst 94% of abortions were funded by the NHS, only 60% took place in the independent sector under NHS contractual arrangements.

---

[54] *British Pregnancy Advisory Service v Secretary of State for Health* [2011] EWHC 235.
[55] *Abortion Statistics, England and Wales: 2009*. London: Department of Health, 25 May 2010.

Choice and childbirth

Pregnancy and childbirth present particular ethico-legal questions. In law and until the baby has been delivered, there is only one legal person to consider, namely the woman. However, as already discussed in this chapter, for many people, the foetus warrants moral consideration. In practice of course, most decisions in obstetrics aim to serve the interests of both woman and foetus. As a woman's pregnancy progresses and delivery is imminent, ethical practice is increasingly informed by the wish to achieve a positive outcome. Yet, what constitutes a positive outcome can be differently interpreted by all those involved, specifically:

- Models of midwifery and medicine may describe contrasting, and sometimes conflicting, perspectives on ethical practice in childbirth eg in relation to the ways in which a woman's labour progresses.
- Policy reforms increasingly emphasise maternal autonomy with concomitant implications for choice in childbirth eg the 'named midwife' policy and the emphasis on choice of location for childbirth are both illustrations of policies that were difficult, if not impossible, for many NHS organisations to implement.
- There is a body of case law that turns on the capacity of a woman to make choices in labour which has significant implications for what it means to practise ethically. These cases and the implications are discussed later in the chapter.
- Clinical negligence has had a significant influence in obstetrics which is considered to be a high-risk specialty. As a result, there may be a defensive approach to clinical practice which can lead to decision-making being informed by the professional's interests. Britain has one of the highest caesarean section rates in the developed world[56] and many believe that there is an association between the perceived risk of litigation and the numbers of caesarean sections performed.

Whilst it is important not to generalise and stereotype professional difference, it is the case that midwifery emphasises the normal, whereas obstetrics is concerned with the pathological and

---

[56] The rate was reported as 24.8% of births in 2009-2010; see *Hospital Episode Statistics: NHS Maternity Statistics 2009–2010* (www.hesonline.nhs.uk).

management of abnormal.[57] All deliveries have the potential to become pathological, often in a way that is unpredictable and serious. It is therefore difficult to draw the boundary between the unwarranted medicalisation of childbirth and acting responsibly to avert an obstetric emergency. Irrespective of professional difference, both doctors and midwives have a duty of care to the woman which means putting her interests above professional disagreement about clinical territory. From a virtue ethics perspective, the requirement is to be humble, respectful and honest. Such an approach is likely to ensure that both midwives and doctors are able to work together rather than in opposition to provide an environment for childbirth that is safe, welcoming and effective.

Health policy has consistently emphasised continuous care and maternal choice in childbirth. In this respect it is no different from any other aspect of healthcare where Western ethics has stressed the entitlement of individuals to self-determination. It is worth pausing for a moment to consider how you, as a future doctor, can and will facilitate maternal choice. Are there circumstances under which you would disregard maternal choice? One of the commonest ways in which women are encouraged to express their preferences is via a 'birth plan'. Some have suggested that the birth plan is a form of advance decision. However, that is a curious interpretation because women are presumed to have capacity in labour (something that has been confirmed by a significant body of important case law which is discussed later). As such, most women are able to express their wishes during childbirth and do not need to rely on an advance decision. In rare cases where a woman loses capacity in labour, a birth plan has the potential to be an advance decision provided it meets the criteria of the Mental Capacity Act 2005. In practice, just as with other advance decisions, the birth plan's validity may be compromised by the specificity criterion and, in any event, it can be used only to express preferences and refuse treatment but not to demand a particular approach to childbirth. For example, a woman might use a birth plan to express a preference to remain mobile and use Entonox but she could not demand that she has access to a birthing pool or insist on an epidural.

---

[57] For a fascinating study of obstetric training and practice, see Scully, D. *Men Who Control Women's Health: The Miseducation of Obstetrician-Gynaecologists*. New York: Columbia University Press, 1994.

An important case that illustrated the unchanging nature of capacity in women who are pregnant and about to give birth was the case of *St George's Healthcare NHS Trust v S, R v Collins and others, ex parte S*.[58] Ms S, who was 36 weeks pregnant, attended a GP surgery for a registration appointment where she was found to have pre-eclampsia. Ms S explained that she had a strongly-held aversion to all medical intervention and that she understood that if she didn't receive treatment for her pre-eclampsia she or the baby may die. Ms S was admitted for assessment under the Mental Health Act and she subsequently had a caesarean section following a court order. The Court of Appeal made three clear and significant points.

First, a foetus is not a legal person (confirming the law on the status of the foetus). Secondly, capacity in pregnancy should be presumed just as it should be for any other adult. Where there is legitimate doubt (and it is not acceptable to doubt a patient's capacity merely because he or she is disagreeing with clinical advice) about an individual's capacity, the criteria for assessing the capacity of a pregnant woman are the same as for any other adult. Prior to the Court of Appeal's judgment, more than one judge had questioned whether women in labour had capacity on the basis that such women were, in the opinion of these judges, emotional, stressed and in pain. The case of Ms S clearly stated that pregnant women were to be treated like any other adult. Ms S's case preceded the coming into force of the Mental Capacity Act 2005, but for medical students and doctors in 2011, the principles and criteria set out in that Statute should be followed when assessing anyone's capacity. The final point made by the Court of Appeal was that compulsory treatment under the mental health legislation is for the alleviation of a mental disorder (which Ms S was found not to have) and does not encompass physical interventions: in this case, a caesarean section. The point about what compulsory treatment could be given under the Mental Health Act was particularly significant because pregnant women had previously been given physical treatment on the basis of a mental disorder. For example, a pregnant woman who had schizophrenia was obliged to have a caesarean section because a stillbirth would be debilitating for her and once she had delivered, she could resume taking her

---

[58] *St George's Healthcare NHS Trust v S; R v Collins and others, ex parte S* [1998] 3 All ER 673.

medication for her schizophrenia which would improve her mental health.[59] The hospital argued inducing labour and performing a caesarean section was legitimate treatment for her mental disorder under section 63 of the Mental Health Act 1983 and, as such, the woman's consent was not therefore required. The court accepted that argument. However, following the Court of Appeal's decision in the case of Ms S, the passing of the Mental Capacity Act 2005 and the amendment of the mental health legislation, it is highly improbable that a caesarean section could ever again be considered treatment for a mental disorder.

Moving away from cases where women have refused caesarean sections, the issue of choice in obstetric care also arises in situations where women request caesarean sections. As has already been noted, the caesarean section rate in the United Kingdom is high: approximately 1 in 4 births are by caesarean section.[60] In response to concerns about the numbers of caesarean sections, the National Institute for Clinical Excellence has examined elective caesarean section rates.[61] The NICE guidelines conclude that caesarean sections should not be available on request, but that there should be clinical reasons for performing a caesarean section. The next question is inevitably: what constitutes a clinical reason sufficient to justify a caesarean section? Some readers may feel that is a question that is entirely a clinical matter, but it has an inescapably moral dimension. Embedded in judgements about whether a caesarean section is justified are professional values, personal biases and individual preferences. The ways in which different obstetricians respond to requests for caesarean sections are likely to reflect, often at an unspoken or even subconscious level, the ways in which the doctor-patient relationship is understood, the effects of the power imbalance between a woman and her doctor; an individual's tolerance for risk; professional beliefs about patient autonomy; and personal views about the extent to which 'clinical' decisions encompass the broader social, psychological and emotional aspects of care. A good clinical decision acknowledges and attends to the ethical dimensions of that decision.

---

[59] *Tameside and Glossop Acute Services Trust v CH* (1996) 1 FLR 762.

[60] For the most recent data, see *Hospital Episode Statistics: NHS Maternity Statistics 2009–2010* (www.hesonline.nhs.uk).

[61] National Institute of Clinical Excellence. *Clinical Guideline 13: Caesarean Section, April 2004* (http://guidance.nice.org.uk/CG13/Guidance).

Reproductive ethics and medical students

As a medical student, you are unlikely to have much exposure to specialist assisted reproduction services. However you will meet people making decisions about fertility, pregnancy and delivery. This chapter has thus far focused on the general ethico-legal issues that arise for clinicians working in reproductive medicine or practising in obstetrics, but this section will discuss some of the specific experiences that a medical student may have in relation to situations involving fertility, pregnancy and childbirth.

First, you may find, particularly if you a male student, that experience can be harder to come by than you would like. Understandably, reproductive issues are amongst the most personal and private. Along with sexual health services, there might be a higher rate of people refusing to allow you as a medical student to observe or participate in their care. Whilst this can be immensely frustrating, it is not the time to cut ethical corners. Being involved in people's lives is a privilege and you should only be involved if they are willing. I am unaware of a single student who has graduated without seeing a range of obstetric practice and, if you are courteous, honest and respectful, you *will* have the experience you seek but it may take a little longer in this specialty than in others.

The second issue for medical students to consider is abortion; specifically whether you wish to express your right of conscientious objection. As stated earlier, the conscientious objection provision extends to medical students and you are entitled to refuse to participate in terminations if you wish. If that is to be your position, you will want to think about how you are going to explain your choice to your team in anticipation of placements. Many students, including those who conscientiously object, will encounter women requesting referral for a termination in general practices. You must, of course, be non-judgemental and respectful in such consultations irrespective of your personal views.

Finally, medical students who are willing to work at night and spend time with midwives (and midwifery students) are likely to have a much richer experience than those who limit themselves to daylight hours and the obstetric team. Most deliveries are lengthy and things happen on labour wards at night! By working with the midwives, you will not only learn an enormous amount about that tricky boundary between the normal and the pathological in obstetrics, but you will also forge effective professional relationships that will endure long after qualification.

Core Concepts: Reproductive Ethics

Assisted reproduction technologies and medicine have been regulated by the Human Fertilisation and Embryology Authority since 1990. However, in the recent government review, the HFEA is scheduled to be abolished. It is unclear how the need for regulation will be met.
The notion of personhood is a significant ethical concept in reproductive ethics and can be understood to be inherent, linked to form, function, relationships and/or emotion.
Antenatal screening should take place with consent that encompasses the uncertainty and implications of the information that screening may reveal.
The relevant law relating to termination of pregnancy is found in the Abortion Act 1967, as amended by the Human Fertilisation and Embryology Act 1990.
Before 24 weeks, two doctors can authorise an abortion on the basis of risk to the mental and/or physical health of a woman and/or existing children.
After 24 weeks, a termination may take place on the grounds of emergency (grave and permanent injury or loss of life) or serious handicap.
Women should be assumed to have capacity in pregnancy and labour.

Assessments: Reproductive Ethics in practice

Case Analysis

Harriet and Philip Jackson have been trying to conceive for two years. Investigations have revealed nothing abnormal in either Harriet or Philip and their apparent infertility is 'unexplained'. Harriet is 35 years old and Philip is 47 years old. Consider each stage of their experience and identify the key ethico-legal issues.

Stage 1

Harriet and Philip attend the surgery of their GP, Dr Ryan, and ask to be referred for IVF on the NHS.

Are they entitled to publicly-funded IVF?

Stage 2

Harriet and Philip meet Liza Kay, the infertility counsellor at the clinic. Liza Kay has a number of concerns about the relationship between Harriet and Philip. The relationship has not been happy for over two years. Harriet and Philip separately described regular and bitter arguments. Each partner has had a brief affair.

How should Liza Kay respond?

Stage 3

Harriet and Philip agree to attend counselling, their relationship improves significantly. The clinic is happy to proceed with IVF treatment. At this point, Harriet discloses that her only brother has severe autism. Harriet explains that she knows that autism is more common in males and *'having seen how devastating severe autism is for families, I would far prefer to have a girl.'*

Is Harriet's desire to have a female child social or medical? Is sex selection acceptable in any circumstances? If so, what distinguishes the examples you considered?

Stage 4

Harriet and Philip's second cycle of IVF results in four embryos. The clinic explains that it can only transfer two of the embryos and that it would prefer to implant a single embryo. Harriet and Philip ask the clinic to replace two embryos. Should there be limits on the number of embryos that can be transferred or should patients be allowed to make autonomous decisions?

What should happen to the embryos that are not transferred?

Stage 5

A successful pregnancy results for Harriet. At her 20-week scan, the radiographer notices three bilateral choroid plexus cysts (CPCs). CPCs are soft markers which are not themselves thought to be of major importance for the health and development of the foetus but which can indicate a problem, especially a chromosomal abnormality. The obstetrician, Dr Okuno, invites Harriet and Philip to discuss the findings. As soon as Harriet comes in to the room she bursts into tears and says *'there's something awfully wrong with our baby, isn't there?'*

How would you respond to Harriet's immediate question? What information do Harriet and Philip now need to help them to decide whether or not to have further diagnostic tests?

Stage 6

Harriet and Philip refuse further testing and the pregnancy progresses well. At 37 weeks Harriet tells her clinical team that she would like to give birth at home. Her consultant, Dr Okuno, is unhappy about her choosing a home birth because he does not believe that such a delivery is suitable given that she expecting twins and it is her first pregnancy.

How should Dr Okuno respond to Harriet's request for a home birth?

1. Termination of pregnancy

Sample SAQ

Sally Birch is 21 years old and presents at her GP, Dr Baslow's surgery, after doing a home pregnancy test that was positive. Dr Baslow confirms that Sally is approximately seven weeks pregnant. Sally explains that the pregnancy is unplanned and she is unsure whether she wishes to proceed.

(a) On what legal basis could Dr Baslow refer Sally for a termination of pregnancy? (4 marks)

(b) If Dr Baslow has a conscientious objection to terminations of pregnancy, how should he proceed if Sally requests a termination? (1 mark)

(c) The legal criteria for terminations change as pregnancy progresses. At what gestational age do the legal criteria for termination change and how do the criteria change? (3 marks)

(d) If Sally's partner were to approach Dr Baslow to try and persuade him not to refer Sally for a termination, how should Dr Baslow respond? (2 marks)

Guidance notes

Part (a)   Under the Abortion Act 1967, s 1(1)(a) Dr Baslow can refer Sally to a doctor registered to perform terminations of pregnancy on the grounds that she is less than 24 weeks pregnant and there is a risk to her mental or physical health (or that of any existing children) that is greater than the risk of the termination itself. At seven weeks' gestation that is the most likely provision of the Abortion Act 1967 under which a referral could be made. This provision is the most common for terminations in the UK. His referral should be supported by a second doctor who will verify that these terms apply to Sally. At seven weeks, Sally may be able to have a medical rather than a surgical termination of pregnancy but the same principles apply, including the requirement for medical referral and supervision of the process.

Part (b)   Doctors are permitted a right of conscientious objection under the Abortion Act 1967, s 4(1). Dr Baslow should refer Sally Birch to another doctor in a timely and non-judgemental way.

Part (c)   Under the Abortion Act 1967, terminations can occur in emergencies or for reasons of grave permanent injury, risk to life and 'serious handicap' beyond the 24-week gestational limit. Terminations in these circumstances are rare (approximately 1% of TOPs occurred post-20 weeks according to Department of Health statistics) and it is the interpretation of 'serious handicap' that has caused most controversy. There is no statutory guidance on what constitutes a serious disability such as to warrant a termination, and the provision was the subject of a legal challenge by the Reverend Joanna Jepson who discovered that a pregnancy had been terminated after 24 weeks apparently because the foetus had a cleft lip and palate. Her action failed and the Crown Prosecution Service did not prosecute anyone involved in that case.

Part (d) Male partners do not have any right to intervene to prevent a termination. Although it may be difficult, Dr Baslow cannot discuss Sally's care with her partner for reasons of confidentiality unless he has Sally's express consent to do so.

2. Fertility services

Sample SAQ

The National Institute of Clinical Excellence recommended in its guidance on access to fertility treatment that all women should receive three publicly funded cycles of IVF treatment.

Suggest four ethical arguments for and against universal access to fertility treatment in the NHS (10 marks)

Guidance notes

Fertility treatment can be constructed as a need or want. It would be helpful to acknowledge this point in your response.

Points in favour of universal access to fertility treatment include	Points against universal fertility treatment include
It is discriminatory to treat fertility treatment as different from other healthcare needs	Fertility treatment is a non-essential intervention
Universal access is equitable and ensures there isn't a postcode lottery	It is disproportionately expensive and has limited success
It removes discretion and therefore the potential for inappropriate social judgements from doctors and local healthcare providers	It removes the freedom from doctors to consider their particular patient's needs whilst imposing uniformity inappropriately eg the wide age band
It ensures transparency in the service	It has not been voted for, or chosen, by democratic processes but rather implemented by a government body
Human reproduction is a right and embodied in the Human Rights Act 1998	

Chapter 6

Minor Morality: Children and Adolescents

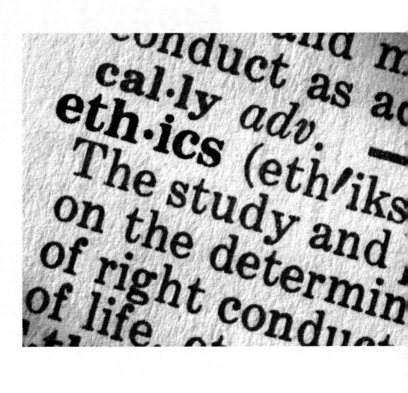

Minor Morality: Children and Adolescents

Introduction

Paediatrics has been the specialty in which some of the most high profile ethico-legal cases have arisen. It is unsurprising that the care of children prompts strong emotion and sometimes disagreement. This chapter will discuss the questions that occur in paediatrics focusing both on children who are too young to make their own decisions and older children who may be able to make their own choices about healthcare.

The child without capacity

Young children are unlikely to have sufficient understanding to make a choice or decision for themselves. Where a child does not have the capacity to make decisions about his or her care, treatment will usually depend upon obtaining proxy consent from someone with 'parental responsibility' as defined by the Children Act 1989.[62] Parental responsibility is now automatically acquired and shared between parents although until 2003, it was linked to marriage and unmarried fathers had to apply for parental responsibility.

Those who have parental responsibility do not have an unfettered right to make decisions on behalf of a child. It is expected that those who have parental responsibility will act in the child's best interests. Where there is doubt about whether someone is acting in a child's best interests, parental consent or refusal can be challenged.

What is the position if parents disagree about healthcare? Unless a court order has been made limiting the right of a parent to give consent, unilateral consent will suffice assuming that each party is acting in the child's best interests, although a doctor does not have a duty to proceed with treatment where there is parental disagreement, and the courts have acknowledged that it presents an ethical dilemma.

In emergencies, treatment can be given without consent on the basis of 'best interests'. The extent to which the power to act without

---

[62] s 2(1).

parental consent can be exercised depends on the welfare[63] or best interests of the child; this is inevitably a facts-based determination. The courts are prepared to override genuine and strongly-held religious or conscientious beliefs on the part of a parent vis-à-vis necessary medical treatment on the basis of the child's best interests. It is important to stress that such cases are treated on an individual basis and the concept of best interests does not mean merely best *medical* interests. For example, in the case of *Re T*, the parents of a child suffering from biliary atresia were held, by the Court of Appeal, to be entitled to refuse a liver transplant which would have lengthened the child's life. The court was clear that a child's best *medical* interests are not necessarily the same as a child's best *overall* interests which should take account of *quality and* quantity of life.

The cases of David Glass and Charlotte Wyatt further illustrate how difficult paediatric cases can be. David Glass was born with significant mental and physical impairment and required 24-hour care. Disagreement had arisen between David's family and the clinical team with regard to the treatment that was in David's best interests. In particular, David's family was concerned by the prescription of diamorphine and that a Do Not Attempt Resuscitation (DNAR) order had been made without their knowledge.[64] The European Court of Human Rights (ECHR) which held that David Glass's right to respect for a private life had been compromised and awarded damages. The court stated that where there is abject and consistent disagreement between families and clinicians, advice from the courts must be sought. The judgment was also critical of the largely medical approach taken to determining David's best interests.

In contrast, giving judgment in the case of Charlotte Wyatt, Mr Justice Hedley supported the clinical perspective of 'best

---

[63] The concept of 'welfare' is not defined in the Children Act 1989, but there is a checklist to be considered. Practitioners must consider (i) the ascertainable wishes and feelings of the child (s 1(3)(a)); (ii) the child's physical emotional and educational needs; (iii) the likely effect of a change in circumstances; (iv) harm suffered or likely to be suffered; (v) the age, gender and background of the child; and (vi) the child's background.

[64] Resuscitation decisions, including DNAR orders, are discussed in detail in Chapter 9.

interests'. Charlotte Wyatt was born at 26 weeks and had organ damage, respiratory, hearing and sight problems. Charlotte had been resuscitated several times. However, the clinical team caring for Charlotte was reluctant to ventilate her should she require resuscitation again believing it not to be in her best interests. The Wyatt family disagreed. Mr Justice Headley supported the clinical team's decision in a judgement that some commentators have argued disregarded the broader aspects of best interests. Subsequently, the declarations from the original hearing permitting doctors not to resuscitate Charlotte were lifted, although the judge stressed that clinicians need not *act against their conscience* and expressed the wish that Charlotte's family and her clinical team would work together to form an effective therapeutic relationship that would be in Charlotte's best interests. In so doing, the judge reflected that responsibility for children who lack capacity is shared and that recognition of this shared responsibility is important in reducing conflict and promoting ethical decision-making.

Even where a child does not have the capacity to make his or her own decision, clinicians should respect his or her dignity by discussing the proposed treatment with the child. Whilst the presenting patient is the child, doctors are dealing with a family unit. Sharing decisions and considering the needs of the child as a member of an established family are essential.

The older child or adolescent

As children grow up, the question of whether a child has capacity to make his or her own decisions turns on principles derived from a case called *Gillick v West Norfolk and Wisbech Area Health Authority.* In brief, Mrs Victoria Gillick challenged the implementation of a Department of Health circular concerning the prescription of contraception to girls under the age of sixteen. The case was eventually heard in the House of Lords.[65] The House of Lords, by the narrowest of majorities, found in favour of the Health Authority.[66] The principles that emerged from the judgment gave rise to the term '*Gillick* competent' and established that a child can

---

[65] At that time, the House of Lords was the highest court in the land; now it is the Supreme Court; see Chapter 1.

[66] *Gillick v West Norfolk and Wisbech Area Health Authority* [1986] 1 AC 112, HL.

make a choice about his or her health if a clinician considers that the criteria shown in the box below are satisfied.

The *Gillick* criteria

☑	The patient, although under 16, can understand medical information sufficiently;
☑	The doctor cannot persuade the patient to inform, or give permission for the doctor to inform, his or her parents;
☑	In cases where a minor is seeking contraception, the patient is very likely to have sexual intercourse with or without adequate contraception;
☑	The patient's mental or physical health (or both) are likely to suffer if treatment is not provided; and
☑	It is in the patient's best interests for the doctor to treat without parental consent.

There has been some debate about the use of the term '*Gillick* competence'; the phrase '*Fraser* competence'[67] is also sometimes used. Aside from the fact that 'capacity' is now preferred to 'competence', the interchangeable use of the terms '*Gillick*' and '*Fraser*' competence is incorrect. The term '*Gillick* competence' describes how young people's capacity is assessed in healthcare, including but not limited to sexual health advice and treatment. The 'Fraser guidelines' describe the practical application of '*Gillick* competence' when an adolescent seeks contraception.

The *Gillick* decision recognised that children differ in their abilities to make decisions and established that function (ie ability to understand), rather than chronological age, is the prime consideration when considering whether an older child can give consent. Situations should be approached on a case-by-case basis taking into account the individual child's level of understanding of a particular treatment. It is possible (and perhaps likely) that a child may have capacity to consent to one treatment but not another. The law is broad and discretion has been left to the clinician. It has been suggested[68] that whilst *Gillick* was frequently described as marking the demise of paternalism, the decision represented demise in *parental* rather than medical paternalism. The level of discretion created by *Gillick* ensures that medical paternalism remains.

---

[67] Lord Fraser was one of the judges in the House of Lords hearing the case.
[68] Teff, H. *Reasonable Care* at pp 146–152 Oxford: Oxford University Press, 2004.

The more serious and urgent the circumstances of a situation, the greater the likelihood of children's choices being challenged: for example, two teenagers who were practising Jehovah's Witnesses[69] and refused treatment with blood products for terminal conditions were deemed not to understand the consequences of their refusal and therefore could not be considered *Gillick* competent. Significantly in one of these cases[70], the boy continued his opposition to the treatment, and when he was an adult (and therefore able to exercise the right to refuse treatment previously denied to him as a minor), he died.[71] There have been subsequent cases, however, where teenage Jehovah Witnesses refused treatment and their wishes were respected. Either way, these are difficult and divisive situations.

Those cases may be contrasted with a decision involving a fifteen-year-old girl who refused to be admitted for assessment as an inpatient.[72] The evidence of the psychiatrist was that she might not be capable of making a wise decision. However, Douglas Brown J held that this did not render the girl incompetent, applying the *Gillick* test. It should, he said, be remembered that an evaluation using the *Gillick* criteria is not intended to determine whether a minor will make a wise choice but whether he or she is capable of making a choice at all.

More recently, the case of Hannah Jones led to widespread discussion of the older child, capacity and healthcare choices. Hannah, aged 13, had developed a heart defect as a result of treatment for leukaemia. The clinical team recommended a heart transplant. Hannah refused the transplant saying that she wished to be left alone to die in peace at home. Hannah's parents supported her decision to refuse the transplant. Her refusal of the transplant was legally challenged and child protection procedures were initiated. Eventually the NHS Trust abandoned legal proceedings at the High Court and Hannah's refusal was respected. Subsequently, Hannah changed her mind and had the heart transplant at the age of 14.

---

[69] *Re E* [1993] 1 FLR 386 and *Re S* [1994] 2 FLR 1065.

[70] *Re E op cit.*

[71] See [1994] 2 FLR 1065, 1075.

[72] *South Glamorgan CC v B* [1993] 1 FLR 574.

In each of these cases, minors were judged against the *Gillick* criteria irrespective of the fact that they were refusing rather than consenting to treatment. That is noteworthy because there have been judicial attempts to distinguish between consent to, and refusal of, treatment and to limit the application of the *Gillick* test to the former situation. Specifically, the case of *Re W*[73] decided that whilst a *Gillick* competent child could not have their right to choose treatment overridden, the same child could have their right to *refuse* treatment so usurped. It is a decision that sits extremely uneasily with the ethos of the *Gillick* decision (indeed Lord Scarman noted that a legally mature minor was able to take over parental power both to approve *and to decline* treatment). However, efforts to distinguish between consent and refusal pre-date both the Human Rights Act 1998 and the Mental Capacity Act 2005. Once a child reaches the age of 16, the Mental Capacity Act 2005 states that he or she should be treated as an adult save for the purposes of making an Advance Decision and appointing a Lasting Power of Attorney (LPA).

Consent and confidentiality

Once a minor has been judged to have capacity, he or she should be afforded the same rights of confidentiality as an adult; a principle that was affirmed in the case brought by Mrs Susan Axon[74] (discussed in Chapter 5). The difficulty arises when faced with a minor whom one does not believe to be *Gillick* competent; should a doctor in these circumstances protect that child's confidentiality? Does the doctor in this situation have a duty to protect a possibly vulnerable child and convey significant information to a parent? If a child comes to see a doctor with an expectation that such consultations are 'secret', is an obligation of confidence created by that expectation? As discussed in Chapter 5, confidentiality is essential to trusting therapeutic relationships and is highly valued by teenagers who may be intimidated by, or fearful of, the prospect of seeking medical advice.

The default position should be that consultations between doctors and teenage patients are confidential. In rare circumstances where a doctor is sufficiently concerned about an adolescent patient that he

---

[73] [1992] 4 All ER 627.

[74] *R (on the application of Axon) v Secretary of State for Health* [2006] EWHC.

or she needs to share information, that concern should be explained to the patient and permission sought with an explanation about what information will be disclosed, why, how and to whom. If an adolescent continues to refuse permission to share confidential information and there is a risk of harm (eg where there is abuse and/or a safeguarding issue), the information can be shared appropriately with an explanation that the serious risk of harm and legal obligations require disclosure on a 'need to know' basis.

Paediatric ethics and medical students

Paediatrics is, as students quickly learn, a different world. Children are not mini-adults and the biomedical and clinical sciences are sufficiently distinct as to demand new knowledge and skills to be mastered. The ethico-legal context too is distinct. For medical students to gain experience of working with young children, the consent of parents must be sought. The principles of seeking such consent are identical to those that apply to seeking an adult's consent. However, there are two important points to consider. First, consent from a proxy, even a parent, depends on another's judgement about whether a child really is happy for a medical student to observe and participate in a visit to clinic. Secondly, consideration of best interests in a child extends beyond the history and examination. Students have to be prepared to play, listen, wait and interact with their paediatric patients – medicine is but a part of what it means to attend to a child's best interests.

Paediatrics can be difficult experience for medical students. Observing suffering and death in children is, for many, harder to bear than previous experiences in adult medicine. The bravery of many paediatric patients can be inspiring and poignant in equal measure. Such emotions are natural and part of good paediatric care. 'Care' does not come without empathy and compassion. Take time to talk about your experiences with those you trust; an experienced mentor can be particularly valuable. Accompanying people at the darkest times of their lives is never easy but it is an integral part of medicine. It is not shameful, unusual or weak to feel sadness, distress or even fear – it is what will make you a committed and conscientious doctor. Learning to manage those emotions so that you neither deny nor are overwhelmed by your feelings is part of your training. Don't feel you have to do so alone; there are many who have felt as you do and there is a variety of sources of support and guidance. Do be kind to yourself and seek help if you feel overwhelmed.

Remember that paediatrics covers the full spectrum of ages. Take the time to see as many paediatric patients and types of services as you can. It may be tempting, but don't just confine your paediatric experience to the babies and toddlers who may be more naturally appealing to you than the towering teenage boy; they both matter and deserve your time, attention and willingness to learn.

Core Concepts: Paediatric Ethics and the Law

Where a child is too young to make his or her own decisions, someone with 'parental responsibility' will be asked to give consent and make healthcare choices on behalf of the child.
Parents usually share parental responsibility.
Unmarried fathers used to have to apply for parental responsibility but the law has changed and marital status no longer affects the allocation of parental responsibility.
The freedom of those with parental responsibility to make decisions on behalf of children is not unlimited: any decisions must be in the child's best interests.
Unilateral consent ie the agreement of one person with parental responsibility suffices legally but presents an ethical dilemma for clinical teams.
'Best interests' is a concept that incorporates, but is not entirely comprised of, best medical interests. It is informed by the concept of 'welfare' as described in the Children Act 1989.
Ethical practice requires clinicians to consider not only the clinical interests of the child but his or her social and emotional interests.
Where parents and clinicians disagree about what is in a child's best interests, the courts should be consulted for advice.
Whether a child is able to consent or not, the ethical concept of 'assent' can be useful as a reminder to involve children wherever possible in their care and to prioritise relationships between staff and families.

When considering whether older children have capacity to make their own healthcare decisions, doctors should use the criteria established in the *Gillick* case. Although the case concerned contraception, its judgment applies to all decisions relating to capacity and minors.
As with adults, capacity fluctuates and adolescents may be able to make some decisions but not others.
Where an apparently capacitous adolescent refuses treatment, the courts have overridden that refusal and drawn a (controversial) distinction between consent to, and refusal of, medical care.
Those aged 16 and 17 should, by virtue of the Mental Capacity Act 2005, be treated as adults.
An adolescent who has capacity by virtue of the *Gillick* criteria is as entitled to confidentiality as an adult; a position that was confirmed in the *Axon* case.

Assessments: Paediatric Ethics in practice

1.   Assessing an adolescent's capacity in A&E

> **Sample OSCE station**
>
> Lizzie Payne is a fourteen-year-old girl who has come unaccompanied to the Accident and Emergency Department (A&E). You are on a placement shadowing a junior doctor, Dr Campbell. Dr Campbell asks Lizzie why she has come to A&E. Lizzie explains that she *'got carried away'* with her boyfriend last night and didn't *'use anything'*. Dr Campbell establishes that Lizzie has had sexual intercourse within the last 48 hours and did not use any contraception. Lizzie asks for *'the tablet you can take afterwards to stop pregnancy'*.

Guidance notes

*   Lizzie should be invited to explain why she has come to A&E in her own words and her age confirmed in a way that is non-judgemental. Allowing Lizzie time to share her expectations and understanding of sexual health is essential not only to gain her trust but also to offer her appropriately relevant information at the right level of detail. You have to assess what Lizzie understands about sexual health and contraception,

including post-coital contraception. Lizzie appears to have reasonable base line knowledge of sexual health and contraception but by taking your lead from the words she uses, ie what she means by *'getting carried away'* and *'not using anything'*, the conversation is likely to be both easier and more effective.

- When assessing *Gillick* competence, the task is to translate the legal criteria into an empathic and supportive consultation. In addition, to exploring what Lizzie understands, the *Gillick* judgment requires doctors to ask about the possible involvement of parents and the consequences of not prescribing contraception: a task that can seem suddenly daunting when considered for the first time in an OSCE! You might find phrases such as *'have you thought about telling your mum or dad?'*, *'is there an adult family member to whom you could talk?'* and *'if I weren't able to help you today, what do you think might happen?'* useful in exploring whether parents can be involved in Lizzie's choices best interests.

- Whenever you are talking to Lizzie you should verify her understanding, check pace, be alert to her emotions, respond empathically where appropriate and invite questions. If Lizzie is *Gillick* competent, it is appropriate to discuss future contraceptive options with her and perhaps suggest places where confidential sexual health advice and treatment can be obtained.

2.   Confidentiality and minors

Sample OSCE station

Katherine Walter, aged 44, attends her GP's surgery. You are on your community health placement. Mrs Walter tells Dr Marsh, her GP, that she is very concerned about her elder daughter Zoe. Zoe is 15, and she is becoming something of a rebel. She is often in trouble at school and is always reluctant to do her homework. Mrs Walter explains that Zoe stays out late and *'refuses to talk about where she spends most of her time'*, although she know that her daughter has a boyfriend – Jack – of whom she disapproves. Mrs Walter says that she is particularly worried that Zoe may become pregnant and that she is losing sleep because of worry. Mrs Walter asks Dr Marsh whether Zoe has been prescribed the oral contraceptive pill.

Guidance notes

- If Zoe is *Gillick* competent, she is as entitled to confidentiality as any other patient (as confirmed by the *Axon* case). Whilst Mrs Walter is obviously anxious and needs her GP's support, Dr Marsh must not reveal Zoe's medical details to her mother. There is nothing to suggest that there is a public interest risk within the terms of *W v Egdell* or that Dr Marsh has Zoe's permission to discuss her care with her mother. The scenario requires Dr Marsh to explain that confidentiality cannot be breached without the patient's permission and also to handle a difficult situation.

- Dr Marsh might begin by verifying whether Mrs Walter is alone and if her daughter is aware of her visit. There is a fine line between exploring why Mrs Walter's daughter isn't talking to talk to her mother and making uninformed judgements about their relationship. Ways of discussing Zoe's reluctance to talk to her mother might include phrases such as *'You are obviously and understandably very worried. Does your daughter know how concerned you are?'* or *'it sounds as though it is a particularly difficult situation for you because Zoe won't talk to you. Do you have any thoughts about why that might be?'*

- Dr Marsh has to tell Mrs Walter something that she does not want to hear ie that confidentiality cannot be broken even though she is Zoe's mother. Mrs Walter may respond with frustration and become more upset, possibly even angry. This scenario is simple in terms of ethico-legal content but not in terms of the communication challenges. Dr Marsh may feel frustrated and even upset but it is important that these feelings are not conveyed to Mrs Walter either verbally or nonverbally. Dr Marsh might assure Mrs Walter that as her GP, she is available to support her through this difficult time and explore whether Mrs Walter has friends or family who may be sources of support

- At the end of the consultation, Dr Marsh may want to reiterate regret that she was unable to help Mrs Walter as she asked. However, an appropriate closure would be to summarise the possibilities for encouraging a discussion between her and Zoe, reminding her of ways the practice may be able to contribute to supporting them both as Zoe grows up.

3. Criteria for *Gillick* competence

Sample MCQ

A child may be described as *Gillick* competent if:

(a) The child is over 16 years
(b) The child is growing normally
(c) The child consents to medical treatment
(d) The child understands the nature of the intended medical treatment
(e) The child agrees to discuss treatment with his/her parents

Answer: d

---

4. The aim of the Children Act 1989

Sample MCQ

The *Children Act 1989* has one overall aim, best expressed as follows:

(a) Parents know what is best for their children
(b) The child's welfare is the paramount consideration
(c) All children are entitled to full education
(d) Children should never be harmed
(e) Protection plans should apply to all children

Answer: b

---

5. *Gillick* competence in clinical practice

Sample EMI

When answering the questions below, please choose the most appropriate answer from the statements in the box below that reflect the rules about children and consent to medical treatment:

(a)   Child is under 16 but is sufficiently mature and intelligent and can understand the proposed treatment, therefore can consent

(b)   Child is under 16 but has insufficient maturity and intelligence, does not understand the proposed treatment, therefore cannot consent and refusal should be overruled

(c)   Child is under 16 but insufficiently mature and intelligent, and has insufficient understanding, so cannot consent

(d)   Child is under 16, sufficiently mature and intelligent, with sufficient understanding but refusing treatment, therefore refusal should be upheld

(e)   Child is under 16, sufficiently mature and intelligent, with sufficient understanding but refusing treatment, therefore refusal should be overruled

(f)   Child is under 18, with sufficient understanding but refusing treatment, therefore refusal should be upheld

(g)   Child is under 18, with sufficient understanding but refusing treatment, therefore refusal should be overruled

(h)   Child is under 18, with sufficient understanding and can consent

(i)   Child is under 18, without sufficient understanding but refusing treatment, therefore refusal should be overruled

(i)   Rajan is 8 years old and attends a dermatology clinic regularly for the treatment of eczema. Rajan says that he does not want any more topical steroids, as it 'takes ages'. His parents are keen to continue the treatment because they understand that without the steroidal cream, the condition will get worse, not better. Should Rajan's refusal be upheld? (Select the most appropriate statement)

Answer: b

(ii)   Fred is 13 years old. He asks his GP, Dr Manzi, if he can take part in a research trial looking at headaches in school aged children. He has heard that his friend has registered on the trial and has been given a free iPhone to record his headaches. Fred has been asking his parents for an iPhone, but with no success. Dr Manzi is concerned that Fred doesn't have enough understanding of what's involved. Should Fred's consent be respected? (Select the most appropriate statement)

Answer: c

(iii)   Danielle is 15 years old and requests oral contraception from her GP, Dr Saunders. After a full discussion, Dr Saunders believes that Danielle is aware of what she is seeking, the consequences of underage sexual activity, the risks of getting pregnant and that she and her 16 year old partner need to use a condom to protect them both from sexually transmitted diseases. Should her consent be respected? (Select the most appropriate statement)

Answer: a

Chapter 7

A Meeting of Minds: Mental Health Ethics

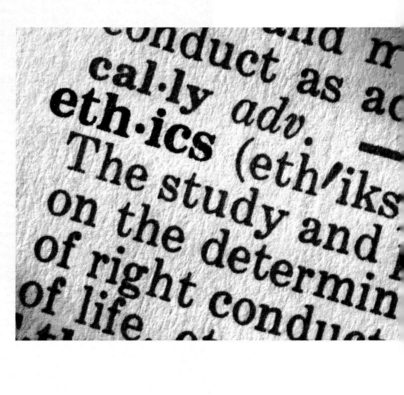

A Meeting of Minds: Mental Health Ethics

Introduction

The law relating to mental health is quite rightly of interest to ethicists and clinicians alike. It is an acknowledgement of the unique legal status of psychiatric illness. The consequences of restricting or removing someone's freedom cannot be overstated. The diagnosis and treatment of people who may have mental illness, the relationship between capacity and mental disorder, the maintenance of confidentiality and the balance between serving the patient and protecting others are all issues that are considered in this chapter.

The mental health legislation

Mental Health law regulates the provision of psychiatric services. The legislation consists of the Mental Health Act 1983, as amended by the Mental Health Act 2007. The statutes set out the circumstances under which patients may be detained for assessment[75] and treatment of a mental disorder. The Mental Health Act, and the accompanying Code of Practice, are lengthy documents and can be daunting. The legislation has both civil and criminal elements. At undergraduate level it is sufficient to know about the most commonly-used civil powers. This chapter describes the main provisions and powers under the legislation at an appropriate level of detail for non-specialists and medical students.

'Mental disorder' for the purposes of the Mental Health Act

The law applies to people who have a 'mental disorder'. A mental disorder is a broad category that encompasses a wide range of mental health problems ranging from schizophrenia to anxiety disorders. People with drug and/or alcohol dependence and addiction cannot be treated under the Mental Health legislation unless the substance abuse co-exists with another mental disorder.[76]

---

[75] Often described as being 'sectioned' ie to exercise the powers provided by a specific section of the Mental Health Act.
[76] Sometimes termed 'dual diagnosis'.

Addiction and dependence alone do not constitute a mental disorder for the purposes of the legislation.

Assessment and treatment under the Mental Health Act

It is important to note that the underlying premise of the legislation and Code of Practice is that admission should be voluntary rather than compulsory with alternatives to admission being considered wherever possible. For many, the most significant aspect of the legislation concerns the powers for compulsion[77] ie detaining patients without their consent for assessment and/or treatment. In practical terms, it estimated that compulsorily detained patients constitute about a quarter of people being treated as inpatients by mental health services. Where a person has a mental disorder such that assessment and/or treatment are indicated, compulsory admission may be considered if detention would be in the interests of the patient[78] and/or to protect others. The legislation requires that, in non-emergency situations, three people are required to admit a patient compulsorily, namely an Approved Mental Health Professional (AMHP)[79] or 'nearest relative'[80] who generally makes the application and two doctors (one of whom should normally be a specialist).

The key provisions for compulsory detention and the treatment of formal patients in hospital are shown in the box below.

> **Section 2:** an application for assessment may be made by a nearest relative or approved mental health professional. This section allows a patient to be compulsorily admitted for a period of up to 28 days, for assessment purposes. The admission must be approved by two doctors (one of whom must be a specialist in mental health).

---

[77] The definition of treatment was changed by the Mental Health Act 2007 from being likely 'to alleviate or prevent deterioration' to simply 'appropriate treatment' which should actually be available rather than being available in theory.

[78] The patient's interests encompass his or her health and safety.

[79] Approved Mental Health Professionals were one of the changes brought about by the Mental Health Act 2007 and replaced the role of the Approved Social Worker.

[80] The nearest relative is defined in law and, following amendment by the Mental Health Act 2007, includes and formally recognises civil partners.

Treatment for the mental disorder may be given without consent during the period of detention. Detention under section 2 cannot be renewed but may be transferred to a Section 3 order.

Section 3: an application for admission may be made by a nearest relative or approved mental health professional. The application must be supported by two doctors, one of whom must be a recognised specialist. Detention can be for a period of six months with the possibility of renewal. Treatment for the mental disorder may be given without consent during the period of detention; and

Section 4: an application for assessment may be made in an emergency with the support of one medical practitioner (who need not be a recognised specialist, although, if possible, he or she should have knowledge of the patient). The situation should be an emergency such that delay would be undesirable. Detention is permissible for up to 72 hours, during which time detention can be converted to a Section 2 order with the support of a second practitioner. No treatment may be given without consent.

Section 5: can be applied to prevent a voluntary patient from leaving the hospital where it is not possible to use sections 2–4. A report is required setting out how the criteria are met and why voluntary status is no longer appropriate. The maximum length of time for which a patient can be detained under Section 5 is 72 hours.

Sections 135 and 136: permit a person with, or appearing to have, a mental disorder to be removed to a place of safety for a maximum period of 72 hours.

In addition to the provisions that relate to compulsory hospital assessment and treatment, the Mental Health Act 2007 introduced 'Community Treatment Orders' which may be considered for patients who have been detained via the longer sections of the Mental Health Act. The orders set out specific conditions eg taking medication or attending therapy that a person will be required to meet post-discharge. The orders can be made for a period of six months initially and can be renewed thereafter. There are no powers to treat a person against his or her wishes in the community, rather the order provides for the patient's return to hospital if he or she is not fulfilling the discharge conditions.

Electroconvulsive therapy (ECT) is treated as distinct under the mental health legislation and cannot be given without consent for patients who have capacity, even if they are being held on a compulsory treatment section. If a patient gives consent to ECT, it must be recorded separately. If a patient with capacity refuses ECT, that refusal must be respected. Where someone lacks capacity and the clinical team believes that ECT is indicated, it can only be given if a Second Opinion Appointed Doctor (SOAD)[81] agrees that it is in the patient's best interests. People are also able to make an advance decision at a point when they have capacity refusing ECT in future.

Safeguards and the mental health legislation

There are a number of safeguards that exist to promote and protect the rights of those who are subject to the mental health legislation. People who are compulsorily admitted should be given information about their rights on admission. Mental Health tribunals[82] review decisions taken under the legislation and legal advice and representation is available to everyone, including those unable to pay.[83] In addition, patients are entitled to the services of an Independent Mental Health Advocate who exist to support an individual's interests and preferences.

Capacity, choice and treatment not covered by the Mental Health Act

The Mental Health Act only applies to the assessment and treatment of a mental disorder. For other healthcare, patients who are detained under the Mental Health legislation are like anyone else ie their capacity must be assessed using the criteria set out by the Mental Capacity Act 2005 (discussed at length in Chapter 3). For example, if a patient were being held under section 3 of the Mental Health Act for treatment of schizophrenia and developed a respiratory infection, his capacity to consent to treatment for the infection should be assessed as it would be for any other patient because the clinical team is only empowered to treat his mental disorder ie his schizophrenia. Put another way, simply because a patient

---

[81] An independent psychiatrist appointed by the Care Quality Commission and working as part of a dedicated service.
[82] The rules about how and when patients can appeal to Mental Health Tribunals vary depending on the provision under which a patient is being detained.
[83] Legal Aid funds legal advice and representation in such cases.

has a mental disorder it does not mean that he or she lacks the capacity to make *any* kind of decision about treatment.

In the late 1990s there were a number of significant cases concerning a patient's capacity and medical treatment under the Mental Health Act that caused concern and much comment. For example, the case of *Thameside and Glossop Acute Services Trust v CH* involved the court accepting that a caesarean section should be considered 'treatment for a mental disorder', namely the patient's paranoid schizophrenia. The rationale was that the patient's mental condition would deteriorate if she were to have a stillbirth and that she could resume drug therapy for the treatment of her paranoid schizophrenia once she was no longer pregnant. The court's reasoning can be, and was, questioned. First, medication could be resumed whether the patient ceased to be pregnant following a live *or* a stillbirth. Secondly, the degree of permissible force that could be used in a woman's 'best interests' remained unidentified. Finally, it is a somewhat strangulated interpretation to describe a caesarean section as 'treatment for a mental disorder'. This case can be read alongside the case of Ms S[84] which was discussed in Chapter 5 and confirmed that the Mental Health Act does not provide for compulsory treatment of a physical condition.

Another scenario that most doctors will, at some stage, encounter is that of the patient[85] who has self-harmed and is ambivalent about, or even refusing, treatment. How should you approach such a patient? A natural response is to ask whether the patient has a mental disorder and, in some cases, it will be appropriate to assess and treat a patient because he or she has a mental disorder. However, merely because someone has self-harmed it cannot be assumed that he or she has a mental disorder. Adult patients who do not have a mental disorder and have self-harmed should, like anyone else, be presumed to have capacity and an assessment is only required if there is legitimate cause to question the person's capacity. If an assessment of capacity is required, it should be made with reference to the criteria set out in the Mental Capacity Act 2005

---

[84] *St George's Healthcare NHS Trust v S ; R v Collins and others, ex parte S* [1998] 3 All ER 673.

[85] Self harm is believed to be one of the top five causes of acute medical admissions in the UK; see *Better Services for People Who Self-Harm: Quality Standards for Health Care Professionals*. London: Royal College of Psychiatrists, 2006.

that are discussed in Chapter 3. If the patient has capacity, consent that is informed, voluntary and continuing should be sought.

Staff may feel frustrated, helpless or even angry when working with someone who has self-harmed. Yet it is essential to remember the practical points that can enhance the assessment of capacity and create a supportive and reassuring environment. Remember that capacity can fluctuate and the team should work together to maximise and regularly review a patient's capacity. If a junior doctor working in A&E is unsure of his or her ability to assess capacity properly, a senior colleague or a psychiatrist should be consulted. If the patient has capacity and refuses treatment, he or she should be asked to sign a written statement to the effect that he or she has made an informed decision and is acting against medical advice. The patient should be advised of crisis or support facilities and reminded that he or she can return at any point (although, for example, in the case of a paracetamol overdose[86] there is a finite amount of time within which liver failure can be prevented and many patients will not realise this). If the patient is unwilling to sign a statement that refusal should be noted and witnessed by a second member of staff. Many doctors are concerned that if they respect a patient's capacitous decision to refuse medical treatment and the patient subsequently dies, an action might be brought on behalf of the patient's estate for negligent advice. However, if the patient was appropriately and honestly informed about the consequences of refusing treatment, no such action is likely to succeed. However, the low probability of a legal action is of little comfort to many doctors who argue that the unnecessary death of a patient is difficult to bear, even if the death was of an autonomous and informed patient.

If a patient lacks capacity, seeking consent is futile from a legal perspective. However, it might still be said to be sound ethical practice to explain the intended treatment to a conscious but incapacitated patient. Where a patient obviously lacks capacity (eg if he or she is unconscious) and in the absence of a valid advance decision or lawful proxy, emergency treatment can be given on the basis of necessity to serve the patient's best interests. The team

---

[86] Paracetamol is one of the most common types of drugs used by patients who self-harm.

should establish what treatment is necessary to avert an emergency and that such treatment is in the patient's best interests. The relative legal clarity does not mean that there are no ethical questions to be addressed. First, if a patient has self-harmed, it could be argued that the patient has attempted to assert his autonomy and decided to end his life. Might it be morally equivalent to an advance decision? If so, to treat the patient on the grounds that he is (conveniently) unconscious and that this is therefore legally permissible could be seen as unjustifiable interference with a patient's autonomy. Whether one accepts such an argument depends on whether one believes that a patient who deliberately harms himself is making an autonomous statement of intent with respect to his life.

Whose disorder is it anyway? Feminist ethics and eating disorders

Eating disorders warrant specific attention for two reasons. First, they offer a pertinent context in which to consider an influential area of ethical theory, namely feminist ethics. Secondly, eating disorders cases have resulted in judgments that have shaped mental health law and its implementation.

Feminist ethics offers a particular lens through which to consider eating disorders. Although the numbers of men diagnosed with eating disorders has increased in the last decade[87], it remains the case that most of those who present with an eating disorder are female.[88] Furthermore, many commentators argue that the majority of women have a poor body image and a significant number have an unhealthy relationship with food, even if they do not have a diagnosed eating disorder.[89]

---

[87] Indeed, some specialists are concerned that men with eating disorders are under-diagnosed and poorly treated because clinicians expect eating disorders to occur only in female patients.

[88] Females are commonly estimated to be ten times more likely to have an eating disorder than males.

[89] Orbach, S. *Fat is a Feminist Issue*. London: Arrow Books Ltd, 1979; *On Eating*. London: Penguin Books Ltd, 2002; *Bodies*. London: Profile Books Ltd, 2009; Chernin, K. The Hungry Self: Women, Eating and Identity. London: Harper Perennial, 1994; Wolf, N. *The Beauty Myth: How Images of Beauty Are Used Against Women*. London: Vintage Books, 1998.

Why do feminist ethics offer a valuable perspective for those seeking to understand eating disorders? First, the feminist approach argues that insufficient attention has been paid to the particular concerns, pressures and experiences of women in healthcare. Some suggest that there is disproportionate emphasis on risk and harm to others in psychiatry which overlooks the distress of women who are not a risk to anyone but themselves.[90] Secondly, feminist accounts of society highlight the ways in which women are expected to behave, and even conform, which have inevitable implications for women's mental health. Medicine, like all organised activities, reflects the economic, political and social context in which it occurs. As that context is gendered, so too are disease and healthcare. The premise of feminist ethics is that the doctor-patient relationship cannot be understood in isolation from gender roles. It is only by deconstructing and challenging the inherently paternalistic and powerful nature of medicine that truly ethical healthcare can emerge.[91]

Although there were influential women writing in the eighteenth and nineteenth centuries[92], feminist bioethics gathered momentum against the background of feminism as a political movement in the 1960s and 1970s. Feminists began to question the paternalistic nature of healthcare and the ways in which doctors perceived health, disease and patients. In 1972, Phyllis Chesler published a book that has become a classic text.[93] Chesler argued that society characterises the female role as conciliatory, emotional, sensitive and domestic. Chesler suggested that when women either adopt the female role in a way that is perceived to be excessive or reject the female role in a way that is seen to be aggressive they risk being labelled as 'mad'. Chesler's theory was picked up by Broverman *et al.* who, in a much cited study, asked male and female clinicians first to describe 'healthy' male and female adult behaviour and then to define healthy adult behaviour.[94] The majority of respondents

---

[90] *Fair Deal for Mental Health*. London: Royal College of Psychiatrists, 2008.

[91] Although feminist bioethics is a broad category, encompassing a wide range of views about priorities, analytic tools and conclusions covering most areas of healthcare and medicine.

[92] For example, Mary Wollstonecraft and Catherine Beecher.

[93] Chesler, P. *Women and Madness*. New York: Doubleday, 1972.

[94] Broverman, I. K., Broverman, D. M., Clarkson, F. F., Rosenkrantz, P. S. and Vogel, S. R. Sex Role Stereotypes and Clinical Judgements of Mental Health. *Journal of Clinical Psychology* 34 (1973) 1–7.

equated the behaviour of a healthy male with that of a healthy adult. Do those arguments have relevance today? Many writers suggest that those changes that have occurred in the respective positions and roles of men and women in twenty-first century society are overstated. For example, Lucy Johnstone[95] has argued that women continue to exist 'in a society in which being female means you are more likely to find yourself struggling with various situations which are known to be linked to mental health problems'.[96]

A feminist perspective on eating disorders suggests that the 'pathology' is an exaggerated reaction to the anxiety and unhappiness most women have about their bodies.[97] To quote Lucy Johnstone again, it is not simply societal ideals of body shape that influence anorexia but also the 'conflict between following the traditional and the newer but equally daunting expectations of women . . . that can be summarised as be thin, but feed others; be educated, but sacrifice your training in order to nurture others; be mother and career person, in short be superwoman'.[98] For feminist bioethicists, the connection between eating disorders and morality is clear. It is not only that you are considered beautiful, acceptable and successful by being slim, but also that there is moral virtue in being slim, ie women are self-controlled, strong and diligent if they manage their food intake and exercise sufficiently to remain slim.

Ethics and eating disorders in practice

Even if you are not persuaded by a feminist perspective on eating disorders, there are multiple dilemmas with which to grapple when considering patients with eating disorders. There is the perennial question of resource allocation: the Royal College of Psychiatrists has suggested that eating disorder services are at risk of becoming the 'Cinderella' of mental health provision.[99] Resources to treat eating disorders include staff time, expertise

---

[95] Johnstone, L. *Users and Abusers of Psychiatry* (2nd ed.) London: Routledge, 2000.

[96] At p. 104.

[97] Lawrence, M. *Fed Up and Hungry*. London: The Women's Press, 1987; Dally, P., Gomez, J. *Anorexia and Obesity: A Sense of Proportion*. London: Faber and Faber, 1991.

[98] At p. 109.

[99] *Fair Deal for Mental Health*. London: Royal College of Psychiatrists, 2008.

and, inevitably, facilities and money; all of which are in short and variable supply. Secondly, the question of what constitutes 'success' in the treatment of eating disorders and how that success is achieved is complex and contested. If management of eating disorders focuses on the presenting symptom(s), ie in the case of anorexia, a successful outcome may be framed in terms of weight gained. Yet ends may not necessarily justify means and there may be ethical concerns about the methods of treatment. Whilst systems of incentives, loss of privileges such as privacy and even force-feeding might increase a patient's weight, such an approach may also have significant implications for that person's faith and trust in healthcare professionals and fail to address the underlying distress that led to disordered eating in the first instance.

Clearly, it could be argued that there is a greater benefit to be gained (ie the ability to live) from the relative loss to the patient (ie the humiliation and discomfort of treatment) and therefore such treatment is ethical. However, as Johnstone points out, the evidence suggests that 'benefits' gained by such treatment methods are questionable because 'since, the underlying issues are not resolved, anorexics often lose weight again as soon as they are discharged, and may spend months or years being shuttled in and out of hospital to be fattened up and released again'.[100] It is suggested that such treatment could only be considered ethical if, at the very minimum, it occurs in the context of treatment that seeks to address the underlying issues to which Johnstone refers. However, even if excellent treatment is offered, should anorexic patients retain the right to refuse such treatment? Brumberg argues that 'anorexia nervosa is a freely chosen method of communicating and asserting power – in essence, an exercise in free will'.[101] Do you agree with Brumberg? Is it possible to be autonomously anorexic?

An alternative approach to the question of whether it is ethical to treat patients who have anorexia compulsorily is to consider the effect of non-voluntary admission and treatment on the therapeutic relationship. Jacinta Tan's work[102] has provided valuable insights

---

[100] Op cit at p 113.

[101] Brumberg, J. *Fasting Girls: The Emergence of Anorexia Nervosa as a Modern Disease.* Harvard University Press, 1988 at page 37.

[102] Jacinta Tan has created an excellent website containing summaries of her work and links to her publications. It is available at www.psychiatricethics.org.uk

into, and an empirical perspective on, the ways in which both patients and professionals view compulsory treatment and its influence on trust, the clinical relationship and long-term outcomes.

Eating disorders and the law

The use of the Mental Health Act for the detention of patients with eating disorders is complex and sometimes controversial. Anorexia nervosa is a mental disorder and patients can be detained compulsorily under the legislation. The more challenging questions concern the extent of appropriate treatment and the possible place of advance decisions. Can force-feeding and the treatment of the physical effects of anorexia nervosa constitute treatment for a mental disorder under s 63 of the Act? The question was considered by the courts in two cases: *Riverside Health NHS Trust v Fox*[103] and *B v Croydon AHA*.[104] In the first case, Ms Fox was a 37-year-old woman with anorexia nervosa, who was detained under section 3 of the Mental Health Act. Riverside Health NHS Trust sought a declaration that force feeding would be medical treatment under section 63 of the Mental Health Act. The Judge concluded that no other treatment could be offered to Ms Fox until she gained weight steadily and that therefore forced feeding constituted medical treatment for her mental disorder. The second case of *B v Croydon AHA* was more complicated. It concerned a woman, known as B, who did not have anorexia nervosa. B was detained under section 3 for treatment of a borderline personality disorder coupled with post-traumatic stress disorder. The proposed treatment was to be psychotherapeutic psychoanalysis. However, B had also stopped eating. The court was asked whether feeding by naso-gastric tube constituted lawful treatment for a mental disorder. The court held that the law must be interpreted sufficiently broadly to include 'ancillary acts' such as force feeding. Thus, if a patient has been diagnosed as suffering from a mental disorder that warrants detention under the Mental Health Act, feeding against the expressed wishes of the patient will constitute a treatment for the mental disorder and be lawful.

In common with all psychiatric care, compulsion should be used only as a last resort and when other options have been considered.

---

[103] [1994] 1 FLR 614.
[104] [1994] 2 WLR 294; see also the earlier case of *Re KB* (1994) 19 BMLR 144.

Voluntary treatment is to be preferred wherever possible and a multidisciplinary approach is recommended. Even where compulsory detention and treatment are employed, they should endure only for the minimum period and be subject to regular review.

Drug and alcohol dependency

The Mental Health Act does not allow for compulsory treatment via 'sectioning' for people whose sole diagnosis is drug or alcohol dependency. It may be the case that drug or alcohol dependency co-exists with another mental disorder (so-called 'dual diagnosis') in which case the Mental Health legislation may be relevant, but if someone has no other mental disorder other than a dependency on drugs or alcohol the Mental Health Act cannot be used.

Patients who have drug or alcohol problems raise several ethico-legal considerations, namely:

- Notions of harm – what constitutes benefit and risk in the context of treating dependency?
- Conceptualisation of responsibility – what effect does an individual's dependency have on autonomy and responsibility?
- Stereotyping and marginalisation – drug dependent people are frequently represented negatively both outside and within the healthcare professions.
- Utilitarianism – how can society best be served in treating and supporting people who are dependent on drugs and alcohol?
- Limited expertise and resources – the provision of services in the field of drug and alcohol dependency remains variable.
- Access to general services – justice and equity demands that all people, including those with drug and alcohol dependence, should have access to general healthcare.
- The regulation and classification of drugs, including the prescribing of controlled drugs.
- Confidentiality, data handling and information sharing, including working with the police.

At the time of writing, there are too few specialist services in the UK to meet the demand for treatment. It has been suggested that all medical students and doctors should receive dedicated training given the prevalence of drug and alcohol dependence in the UK. The aim of such training would be to increase knowledge, skills and confidence. At a minimum, all doctors should be able to provide general medical care to people who have drug and alcohol problems and be alert to the possibility that a patient is abusing drugs or alcohol whilst avoiding stereotyping – a requirement that is in keeping with General Medical Council's statement in *Good Medical Practice* that '*you must treat your patients with respect whatever their lifestyle choices*'.[105] Perceptions of people who are dependent on drugs and/or alcohol are often negative, with such patients being represented as devious, manipulative, violent, difficult and hopeless. Such perceptions coupled with concerns about pressures of time and limited expertise can lead to the marginalisation of people who have drug and alcohol problems and make accessing effective care extremely difficult. Andrew Dicker has argued that failing those who are dependent on drugs and alcohol is to fail society of a benefit.[106]

The classification and regulation of drugs is contained within Schedule 2 of the Misuse of Drugs Act 1971. The law has been regularly amended since it came into force to reflect changes in drug availability and the relative risks posed by different substances that are described as 'controlled drugs'. Broadly speaking, there are three categories of drug classification, namely Classes A, B and C – alcohol and tobacco are not covered by the legislation despite, as critics note, causing more health problems and premature deaths than illegal drug use. Class A is the category containing the most harmful substances including diamorphine, morphine, cocaine, methadone, methamphetamine, crack, LSD, ecstasy and any class B drug prepared for injection. Class B substances include amphetamines, barbiturates, codeine and cannabis. Under the Labour government in 2004, cannabis was reduced to the status of a Class C drug but, following concerns about its use and effects, it has since been restored to Class B status. Class C substances include anabolic steroids, benzodiazepines and growth hormone. The classification of drugs has recently been the subject of review and media campaigning calling for the regulation of substances

---

[105] *Good Medical Practice*. London: GMC, 2006.
[106] Dicker, A. GPs and Junkies. *BMJ* 1998; 317: 892.

such as mephedrone and related cathinones (which are now Class B drugs).

There are specific responsibilities for doctors prescribing controlled drugs. That process was closely scrutinised and reviewed following the case of Dr Harold Shipman. Some clinicians (and therefore students), particularly those not working regularly with drug dependent patients, are confused about the duty of confidentiality in respect of misuse of drugs. There was previously a legal duty on doctors to notify the Home Office under the Misuse of Drugs Act 1971 of drug abusing patients. However, that duty no longer exists in England and Wales. Instead, prescribers of controlled drugs are expected to return forms (either electronically or in hard copy) that contribute to the local or national drug misuse database. Otherwise, the duty of confidentiality to a drug abusing patient is the same as for any other patient ie it can be qualified by (i) the patient's consent; (ii) the patient's best interests where it is impracticable or impossible to seek consent; and (iii) where there is a serious risk of physical harm to an identifiable person or persons. There will, of course, be local protocols regarding the storage, prescribing and documenting of controlled drug provision.

Mental health ethics and medical students

Like paediatrics, mental health services can seem a different world to medical students. The approach of psychiatry is in stark contrast to much of what students have previously experienced. Dispensing with the well-honed clinical skills and history-taking approach of physical medicine can be intimidating or exhilarating depending on your perspective.

The first observation that many students make is about the ways in which care is given. The importance of the multidisciplinary team is evident on psychiatry placements. Students express surprise about the extent of consultation and multidisciplinary involvement in decisions. Other systemic surprises that students often discuss include the format and duration of ward rounds, the extent to which individuals are involved in their care and the negotiation of health and social care provision.

For some students, psychiatry can be a difficult placement. Working in mental health services may raise intensely personal questions about mental health or emotional wellbeing. It is important to be alert to such effects and to seek support early.

For other students, it is the negotiation of professional boundaries that can be challenging. Boundaries are commonly considered with reference to sexual transgressions and often explicitly discussed in relation to psychiatric care (in reality, they are as important in physical medicine as in mental health services). The concept of boundaries has been variously described but all interpretations encapsulate the notion of the limits that exist (physical, behavioural and emotional) to ensure a safe and effective therapeutic relationship. Boundaries are the fence within which a secure, clearly delineated professional space is created and maintained.

Whilst sexual boundary violations do, regrettably, occur in healthcare,[107] the broader issue of maintaining healthy professional boundaries is an integral part of professionalism. Sexual boundary violations are usually preceded by slips in boundaries spanning time, and many healthcare professionals will never transgress sexually but do have difficulty maintaining boundaries in their relationships with others. Self-disclosure, differential availability, attention or allocation of resource, mixing personal and professional contact, gifts,[108] emotional involvement, financial transactions, time, 'rule-bending' and 'making exceptions' can all indicate that boundaries are becoming blurred. Moreover, pushing, crossing and violating boundaries can come from any direction ie a patient may try to push the boundary with the clinician or medical student. However, the onus is on the healthcare professional to maintain boundaries.

A useful distinction drawn by Coe and Hiltz[109] is between boundary crossings (in which harm may not necessarily occur) and boundary violations (in which harm does occur).[110] What then makes a medical

---

[107] Council for Healthcare Regulatory Excellence. *Clear Boundaries Report: 2007* available at www.chre.org.uk

[108] Bowman, D. (2007) Probity and Presents: Ethical Perspectives on Gifts from Patients. *Management in Practice* 2007; 10: September/October; 27–29.

[109] Coe, J., Hiltz, L. (2009) *Handling Dilemmas and Lapses: Boundaries with Patients.* Presentation at the NCAS National Conference, London: 2 March 2009.

[110] See also Norris, D.M. Gutheil, T. G., Strasburger, L. H. (2003) This Couldn't Happen to Me: Boundary Problems and Misconduct in the Psychotherapy Relationship. *Psychiatr Serv* 2003; 54: 517–522.

student or clinician more or less likely to push or cross boundaries? Research has demonstrated that the following variables make a clinician more susceptible to crossing or violating boundaries:

- Poor setting of limits
- A personal crisis, particularly in relationships
- Idealisation of, or identification with, a 'special' patient
- Illness, isolation or other personal vulnerability
- Lack of awareness or denial of the importance of boundaries
- Excessive self-disclosure to patients
- Confidential 'off the record' conversations
- Extended/additional appointments or rescheduling to the end of the day
- Contact outside appointments

One of the most effective ways of checking over-involvement or ambiguous boundaries is regular discussion with experienced clinicians often via the multidisciplinary team meeting where consistency, normative negotiation and patient interests can be openly explored.

Finally, the detention and compulsory treatment of people under the Mental Health Act can be difficult for students to understand and accept. Most students have been trained to believe that autonomy, self-determination and the expression of free will are integral to healthcare. It can be difficult to meet people who are being held and treated against their wishes. Adapting to the notion of compulsory treatment takes time and it might be helpful if you talk to experienced psychiatrists, family members of those who have been detained and, of course, the patients themselves. As people recover, they will often speak positively about the use of the Mental Health legislation as part of the treatment process and acknowledge that without it, they would not have sought or received treatment. That is not to suggest an uncritical approach to the use of the Mental Health Act is recommended. On the contrary, the challenges of developing an effective therapeutic relationship in psychiatry demands that the best and most experienced psychiatrists remain reflective and humble about the nature of modern psychiatry throughout their careers. It is a state to which all students should aspire.

Core Concepts: Mental Health Ethics and the Law

Mental health ethics and law should be understood by all medical students and clinicians; people with mental health problems are not confided to the psychiatric setting.
The Mental Health Act 1983 was significantly amended by the Mental Health Act 2007. It, and the accompanying Code of Practice, provide the legal framework in which psychiatric services are provided.
There is provision in the Mental Health Act to detain people against their wishes for assessment and/or treatment ie 'sectioning' in colloquial terms. Specific safeguards apply to all people detained compulsorily under the law. Where possible, voluntary admission is preferred over compulsory admission.
A person may only be treated for a mental disorder under the law and not for physical conditions. However, force-feeding a person who is detained under the Mental Health Act constitutes an 'ancillary act' ie it is sufficiently related to the treatment of the mental disorder, and is therefore lawful.
Feminist ethics offer an interesting theoretical perspective on the prevalence, experience and treatment of eating disorders in Western societies.
Addiction to, and dependency on, drugs and alcohol are exempt from the Mental Health Act unless they co-exist with another mental disorder for which compulsory detention would be justified.

Assessment: Mental Health Ethics in practice

1.   Mental health ethics

Sample SBA

Roger, 57, with a history of recurrent schizophrenic disorder presents to A&E in a profoundly psychotic state. He has auditory hallucinations and is evidently paranoid. He is not capacitous. A decision is made to admit him to hospital under the *Mental Health Act 2007* as he will not voluntarily co-operate and his health is at risk. Which ethical precept underlies this decision?

(a)   Strong paternalism
(b)   Weak paternalism
(c)   Respect for autonomy
(d)   Doctrine of Double Effect
(e)   The slippery slope argument

Answer: b

2.   Capacity and treatment

Maria attends A&E. Maria appears uncommunicative, pale and distressed. Maria's mother tells you that she has had to *'force Maria to come, literally drag her into the car and all the time she was kicking and screaming.'* Maria refuses to tell you why her mother felt it necessary to bring her to A&E. However, Maria's mother tells you that her daughter *'has taken three packets of paracetamol tablets and a few of my Temazepam tablets that I take to help me sleep'*. The protocol for treating patients who have taken an overdose of paracetamol is gastric lavage and charcoal therapy.

(a)   How would you determine whether Maria is capacitous to consent to treatment?

(b)   If Maria has capacity but refuses treatment, what would you do and why? Please explain the relevance of the Mental Health Act and common law in your answer.

(c)   If Maria had presented at a very low weight, having been diagnosed with anorexia nervosa, would the Mental Health Act have allowed the medical team to treat her by feeding her without her consent?

Guidance notes

Part (a)   If Maria is under the age of 16, the *Gillick* criteria should be used to determine whether she can understand the treatment options sufficiently to make her own choices about treatment. If she is over 16, she is presumed to have capacity. If her capacity is in doubt, criteria in the Mental Capacity Act 2005 should be used to make an assessment, ie can she (i) understand what she is told; (ii) remember what she has been told; and (iii) weigh up information to reach a considered decision that iv) she can communicate? The assessment should be carried out in a way that maximises the chance of her having capacity.

Part (b)   If a mental disorder or illness is suspected, a psychiatrist should be called to carry out a mental health assessment. The doctor must ensure that Maria is adequately informed about the consequences of her refusal (presenting the likely events in a neutral and supportive manner). It should be made clear that treatment options continue to be available even if she leaves the hospital and subsequently changes her mind. It is useful to remember that other members of staff or family and friends might be better placed to explore Maria's refusal of treatment with her. If she continues to refuse treatment, advice should be sought from a senior colleague. Her refusal of treatment should be fully documented and she should be asked to sign a document acknowledging that she is making an informed refusal of treatment. If she refuses to sign the document, it should be recorded in the notes.

Part (c) Section 63 of the Mental Health Act 1983 provides for compulsory treatment for a mental disorder including ancillary acts. There has been some legal debate about whether gastric lavage and charcoal therapy constitutes an ancillary act and it would be preferable to obtain consent if possible. The forced feeding of anorexic patients does constitute 'treatment for a mental disorder' which was specifically considered in two cases, namely *KB and Riverside Mental Health Trust v Fox* and *B v Croydon AHA (applying the judgment in KB)*. These cases have established that forced feeding of anorexic patients constitutes ancillary acts that are necessary for treatment of the mental disorder and are therefore lawful under the MHA 1983. It is essential not only that the treatment is necessary, but that it is also in her best interests (the determination of which can be difficult in many circumstances but especially in an emergency situation such as this). If Maria is unable to consent to, or refuse, treatment herself, the therapy given must be limited to that which is required to avert the immediate emergency (which must be interpreted conservatively).

Some ethicists might argue that Maria, having deliberately harmed herself, has made an effective refusal of life-saving treatment and that this should be respected as an extension of the principle of patient autonomy and self-determination. However, this is not a universal perspective and most ethicists would argue that the conclusion that a patient has taken an autonomous action by harming herself is an assumption that should be challenged (particularly on the basis of some data from the psychiatric literature on motives and self-harm). In the absence of clearer evidence (eg an appropriately specific advance decision) emergency treatment should be given to avert the acute episode.

3. Mental health law

Sample SAQ

Mr White is 38 years old and attends Dr Haq's GP surgery. Mr White has a history of schizophrenia and appears unwell to Dr Haq, telling him the television is watching him and his neighbours are following him home. On discussion, Mr White is not willing to be admitted to hospital for assessment by the psychiatric team. Dr Haq decides that, given the deterioration, Mr White should be compulsorily admitted under the Mental Health Act 1983, as amended by the Mental Health Act 2007.

(a) Explain how the different provisions in the Mental Health Act sections 2–4 allow for compulsory admission.

(b) Name four key changes to mental health legislation introduced by the Mental Health Act 2007.

Guidance notes

Part (a)   Section 2 allows for 28 days compulsory detention for assessment, with an application made by an approved mental health professional and which must be supported by two doctors (one of whom should be an approved specialist). The patient should be suffering from a mental disorder warranting admission and should be detained in the interests of his own health or those of others. Most forms of treatment can be given without consent during the period of detention apart from ECT. Section 3 allows for a six-month compulsory detention period (which is reviewable). An application can be made by a relative or an approved mental health professional and should be supported by two doctors. The patient should be believed to be suffering from a mental disorder. Like an admission under section 2, most forms of treatment, aside from ECT, can be given under this provision. Section 4 allows for emergency detention for a maximum period of 72 hours for immediate assessment (not treatment). The grounds for emergency detention are the same as for section 2 but, in addition, detention should be required on the basis of 'urgent necessity'. The application should be made by one doctor who need not be an approved specialist. The section can be converted into an ordinary section 2 admission with the support of a second medical opinion within the 72 hour period.

Part (b)   The Mental Health Act 2007 was an important piece of amending legislation. Amongst its effects were the:

- Introduction of a single definition of mental disorder
- Requirement that appropriate treatment be available if the patient is detained
- Introduction of supervised community treatment orders
- Expansion of professional roles including the replacement of the Approved Social Worker role with that of the Approved Mental Health Professional
- Distinct status of ECT
- Redefinition of the roles of the nearest relative and an acknowledgment of civil partnerships
- Introduction of Independent Mental Health Advocates
- Change to the name and function of the review tribunals
- Removal of 'sexual deviancy' from the category of excluded sole causes

Chapter 8

I Blame My Parents: Genethics

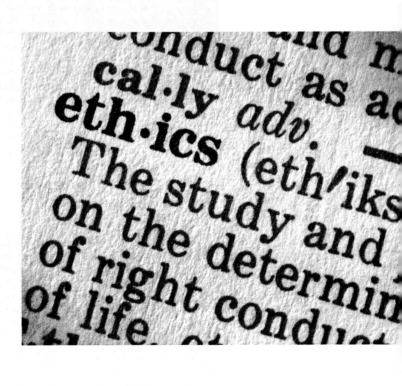

I Blame My Parents: Genethics

Introduction

Genethics describes the study of the moral dimensions of medicine that involves genetic information. It is a broad and growing field which is complex and incorporates a range of genetic issues ranging from cloning to pre-implantation genetic diagnosis and from stem cell research and therapy to testing for late-onset genetic diseases. The Human Genetics Commission existed until recently to advise on the social, ethical and legal implications of genetics. Unlike the Human Fertilisation and Embryology Authority (discussed in Chapter 5), the Human Genetics Commission was an advisory organisation rather than a regulator, comprising members from a range of backgrounds.[111] Following the review of government bodies by the UK government, a proposal was made in 2010 to abolish the Human Genetics Commission.

This chapter explores some of the most common ethico-legal issues that occur in the field of genethics. Although most medical students will spend limited time with clinical genetics services, it is an area that often forces a second look at the 'first principles' and assumptions that underpin much of Western bioethics. For example, the emphasis on autonomy and individual rights becomes more difficult when considering that one person's genetic diagnosis may have significant implications for other family members.

The nature of genetic information

Genetic information is often considered particularly significant. It is the foundation of our identities and remains constant throughout life. The decisions that might be taken on the basis of genetic information are sometimes a particular source of ethical concern. Specifically, the spectre of eugenics lurks. Eugenics is the enhancement of the human race via genetic manipulation and/or selective breeding. Unfortunately, there have been well-documented examples of eugenics as policy, the most well-known example being the Nazi Party's policy. Even where outright eugenics is not a concern, many worry that by enabling people to make genetic choices using methods

---

[111] www.hgc.gov.uk

such as screening and pre-implantation genetic diagnosis, we are creating a society that, if not discriminatory towards those with disabilities and impairments, is less tolerant, less inclusive and less diverse. It is suggested that by selecting for health, we marginalise the sick and that by choosing those without impairment, we are more likely to exclude those with impairments. Some suggest that as the range of people visible in society diminishes so too does our collective understanding of difference.

The counter argument is that efforts to screen for, and potentially eliminate, genetic disease does not logically (or practically) commit us to disvaluing those who have disease or disabilities. Modern medicine has traditionally combined the treatment of disease and its symptom burden with attempts to eliminate the same disease. For example, society's considerable research efforts to eradicate cancer do not equate to disregarding those who have cancer. Others argue that genetic information provides people with choices and that knowledge facilitates autonomy by enabling individuals to make informed decisions. As discussed in the section on pre-implantation genetic diagnosis in Chapter 5, questions remain about the nature of the knowledge and information on which significant decisions will be based. For example, a clinician working in a medical context with patients who have spinal muscular atrophy may have a very different perspective from individuals who have spinal muscular atrophy.[112] Medical knowledge is not the only or even the best way of 'knowing' about a particular condition. Genetic information is but one piece of a complex and multifactorial jigsaw. Human beings are more than their chromosomes and DNA: it is people who make decisions about genetics and that must not be forgotten.

Genetics before birth: saviour siblings

As discussed in Chapter 5, the availability of assisted reproduction techniques such as IVF has the potential to help not only couples who are unable to conceive naturally, but also those who wish to create and select an embryo because there is a particular genetic disease within the family eg where there is a young child with a

---

[112] The value of challenging perceptions of disability is central to a project called 'Dining with a Difference' which invites senior staff from both the public and private sectors to a dinner hosted by people with disabilities (www.diningwithadifference.com)

condition such as Diamond-Blackfan Anaemia. Diamond-Blackfan Anaemia requires complex treatment involving blood transfusions and medication. Unfortunately, the effectiveness of treatment is variable and limited; in most cases, the excess iron will eventually cause organ damage and shorten life. Given the intensive nature of treatment and the curtailed live expectancy, the best option for people with Diamond-Blackfan Anaemia is a bone marrow transplant.

A bone marrow donor can either be an unrelated or a related donor. The creation of a sibling who could be a potential donor for the sick child is likely to lead to the best outcome and is less risky than donation by an unrelated donor. Assisted reproduction techniques have made it possible for families to create and select embryos that are healthy and could act as a related donor for an existing child who is sick: a so-called 'saviour sibling'.

Initially, the Human Fertilisation and Embryology Authority was willing only to allow families to screen out disease but not to deliberately seek a match with a living child. It was an approach that curiously acknowledged that disease should be prevented in a future person yet also simultaneously seemed to deny possible treatment for the same disease in an existing person. The rationale was that screening out disease in an embryo was to prevent suffering in an embryo itself, whereas screening for a match was specifically done to reduce or end suffering in another child but it would also potentially cause harm to the person whom the embryo may become – gathering stem cells is often described as 'harmless' but marrow transplants do carry risks.

In ethical terms, the question of the saviour sibling often focuses on means and ends. Could all children be said to be means to their parents' ends to some extent? There are multiple reasons why people have children and we rarely interrogate parental motive when individuals conceive without assistance. Is there a moral difference between choice via pre-implantation genetic diagnosis and chance ie natural conception resulting in a match? Prior to the availability of reproductive techniques, some families with a sick child had many children in the hope that one of the siblings might be a suitable donor. Such questions informed the debate and eventually the HFEA agreed to license IVF and pre-implantation genetic diagnosis to create a potential donor for an existing child with a genetic condition.

Since that decision by the HFEA there have been several families who have used IVF and pre-implantation genetic diagnosis to create a child that is a match for a sick sibling. Some of these families have described their experiences in the media and their stories are thought-provoking and touching. Beyond the individual accounts, the Human Genetics Commission has recommended that so-called 'saviour siblings' and their welfare should be monitored with a view to understanding the longer term wellbeing and development of these children and their families.

Genetic testing

It is increasingly possible for individuals to be tested for genetic conditions. The basic principles of seeking and obtaining consent apply to such testing and most clinical services have well-developed systems to support people through the process of genetic testing. Particular questions often arise about the timing of a genetic test, its potential effects and the implications both for the individual tested and others. Once a test is done it cannot be 'undone' with concomitant implications for autonomy, choice, privacy and confidentiality. The ethical issues warrant particular attention when a test is proposed for someone who is unable to choose for him or herself, and whose life may be irrevocably altered by testing eg children or those who lack capacity to consent to a genetic test. Much work has been done in an effort to establish basic principles that should inform ethical practice[113] in genetic testing irrespective of the clinical context. The rationale for general principles is that patients and families should experience an equitable service with minimal scope for significant variation.

It is worth noting that just as patients are not obliged to undergo genetic screening, there is no 'right' to genetic testing or screening if it is not indicated; the rationale being that no patient has the right to request or even demand any medical investigation or treatment. However, the increasing availability of genetic testing kits over the

---

[113] For a critical analysis of the 'special' ethical status of clinical genetics see Lewens, T. (2004) What is Genethics? *J Med Ethics* 2004; 30: 326–328.

counter and, perhaps more worryingly, online makes genetic testing more accessible than ever leading the Human Genetics Commission to produce specific guidelines for 'direct-to-consumer' testing kits. If a doctor refuses to perform a genetic test that is requested by a patient, he or she must consider whether it would unreasonable or illogical in the eyes of others to refuse. If so, the doctor could be vulnerable to a claim of negligence. If a screening test gives a false negative result, an action for damages may only be brought if it can be shown that the test was performed negligently.[114]

Weighing the risks and benefits of genetic testing

In genetics, different types of benefits and harms have to be weighed to reach an ethical conclusion. For example, the benefits of genetic testing may include: increased knowledge; development of treatments; reduced uncertainty; alertness; early intervention when symptoms develop; truthfulness; transparency; and access to effective screening, while harms may incorporate: labelling; stigma; breaches of confidence; burdensome knowledge; psychological distress;[115] discrimination;[116] and even mental illness. These variables are difficult to weigh for adults who have capacity to act autonomously, but are still more challenging when considering whether the welfare and best interests of a person who cannot give consent are served by genetic testing.

In balancing risks and harms, the clinical condition for which the test is being conducted is inevitably relevant. There is an enormous range of types of testing which yield different information of variable utility.[117] Genetic testing *per se* is neither inherently moral nor immoral. The matter of whether a person is symptomatic; if there is treatment and/or ameliorating support available for a condition; the likely time of onset of a disease; the impact of the condition on

---

[114] *Rance v Mid-Downs AHA* [1991] 1 All ER 801.

[115] For an analysis of the ways in which 'psychological harm' is invoked in decisions about genetic testing, see Malpas, P. Predictive Genetic Testing of Children for Adult-onset Diseases and Psychological Harm. *J Med Ethics* 2008; 34: 275–278.

[116] The potential for discrimination based on genetic information is explicitly prohibited by law in some jurisdictions eg the Genetic Information Non-discrimination Act of 2008 is now part of US law.

[117] For an excellent review of the types, purposes and effects of genetic testing see Burke, W. Genetic Testing. *N Engl J. Med.* 2002; 347(23): 1867–1872.

life and function; and its scope to affect other family members and / or future children all inform whether a test should be conducted. Even if testing is deemed appropriate, all of those involved should remember that information can be burdensome, particularly if it is given inappropriately or without regard to emotional stability and support. There is consensus that information should be shared carefully and gently over a period of time in the context of trusting relationships. The ethical acceptability of genetic testing depends on the honest fostering of, and respect for, autonomy to facilitate informed choice[118] and decision-making.[119]

Genetic testing of those who lack capacity: ethical perspectives

There are particular ethical considerations when offering genetic testing to those who lack the capacity to make a choice for themselves. For example, when exploring whether genetic testing on children is appropriate, the UK Clinical Genetics Society[120] has proposed that there are core ethical principles to consider. Although the principles have been the subject of debate[121,122], they provide a useful starting point when considering genetic testing for anyone who is unable to consent to, or refuse, a treatment. The principles are:

- Genetic testing should never been seen as 'routine'.
- Subject to the limitations of the law, parents or persons with parental responsibility may make an informed choice whether to have a child tested for child-onset conditions but only subject to the legal limits of parental consent, ie only if it is demonstrably in the child's best interests is testing likely to be appropriate.

---

[118] Andorno, R. The Right Not To Know: An Autonomy Based Approach. *J Med Ethics* 2004; 30: 435–440.
[119] McGuffin P., Owen M. J., O'Donovan M. C., Thapar A. and Gottesman I. (1994) *Seminars in Psychiatric Genetics (College Seminar Series)*. London: RCP Gaskell.
[120] *The Genetic Testing of Children: Report of a Working Party of the Clinical Genetics Society*, op cit.
[121] *Response to the Clinical Genetics' Society Report: 'The Genetic Testing of Children'*. Genetics Interest Group (1995).
[122] Michie, S., Martineau, T. M. Response to GIG's Response to the UK Clinical Genetics Society Report 'The Genetic Testing of Children'. *J Med Genet* 1995; 32(10): 838.

- Following genetic counselling, parents may wish to make an informed choice about whether a child should be tested for carrier status. Ideally such testing will take place when the child is capable of being involved in the decision.
- Children should not generally be tested for adult-onset conditions for which there are no pre-symptomatic treatments and, in any event, where adult-onset disease testing is contemplated, genetic counselling should be available.
- The principles described above should apply equally to children who are being considered for adoption or those in care.

In providing genetic testing to anyone who lacks capacity, the task is to establish whether such testing is in the individual's best interests. Genetic testing should be undertaken for no reason other than that it is in the person's interests – the quest for information or the alleviation of anxiety about someone's genetic status are not sufficient justification to perform a genetic test. If there is no immediate benefit to the individual and it is possible that damage such as labelling, stigma and psychological harm may ensue, then it is more difficult to make the case for testing. The UK Clinical Genetics Society guidance on pre-symptomatic testing advises that such testing should not usually be conducted unless there are exceptional circumstances.

It is well-documented that 'best interests' extend beyond best *medical* interests. Testing, even where a person is not symptomatic, can be useful if it allows for access to support; planning for optimal health and social care services; preparatory and open discussion of the future; and for the family or carers to organise their lives to support the individual in future. Even where testing is conducted on those who lack the capacity to consent, it is important, as in any area of clinical practice, to ensure appropriate information is shared with the individual explaining the nature of the test and the implications of its results.

The challenge of determining a person's best interests may be further complicated by medical uncertainty. For example, it may be unclear or unknown if the condition for which a test is being considered would benefit from treatment either now or in the future. Indeed, such uncertainty may be cited as a rationale for research so that people known to have a particular condition, as a result of genetic testing, can be monitored as part of research activity. In such a situation, the ethical guidance is unequivocal: even if collective biomedical knowledge would be enhanced, the psycho-social implications of testing must be formally evaluated. Furthermore, even where a test is diagnostic of a specific condition, there may, indeed probably will, be a wide range in the symptom or disability burden – people with identical diagnoses may have radically different experiences.

The courts have indicated that, wherever possible, people should be given the opportunity to make decisions for themselves. In cases involving a child, it is desirable to wait until he or she is likely to be *Gillick* competent (see Chapter 6).[123] However, such an approach is predicated on the assumption that a child will develop sufficiently to have capacity, which may not be the case if the condition in question is linked to learning disabilities. If a decision is made to defer testing until a person has capacity, plans should always be in place for timely and accurate counselling in advance of testing and active follow-up post testing. Where someone does not have capacity, it is the Mental Capacity Act 2005 (see Chapter 3), in conjunction with the specific principles relevant to genetic testing that are described above, which should inform the decision whether to proceed with genetic testing.

Sharing genetic information

Genetic testing challenges traditional notions of confidentiality in that genes are shared with relatives, and information that is revealed by a genetic test on one person can contain information that is relevant to others. Testing one member of a family may have significant implications for the medical status and wellbeing of

---

[123] Genetic testing of adolescents has been seen as an area worthy of special ethical consideration, the rationale being that genetic information may become more significant when a minor becomes sexually active that. However, in common with the functional criteria used in assessing the extent to which an adolescent can make decisions about healthcare in general, age is but one criterion considered by geneticists who, in a recent survey of European practitioners, cited cognitive, sexual and emotional maturity and available support as crucial to determining whether an adolescent can choose to have a genetic test; see Borry, P., Stultiens, L., Goffin, T., Nys, H. and Dierick, K. Minors and Informed Consent in Carrier Testing: A Survey of European Clinical Geneticists. *J Med Ethics* 2008; 34: 370–374).

other family members. The implications for others of a genetic test (and any ensuing diagnostic label), and the information revealed therein should be carefully considered. However, the model on which clinical genetics works is based on the principles found in medicine at large. Individuals have to give consent to their own genetic testing assuming they have the capacity to do so. If testing is being conducted for the purpose of assisting a third party, that should be explicitly clear as part of the consent process.

Sometimes genetic testing may be undertaken because an individual wants to contribute to an understanding of his or her family's health and illness. Often clinical genetics services will work with families to explore the options available and to consider the implications, both individual and collective, of testing. However, sometimes, patients seeking testing may not wish other members of the family to know about their decision. In such situations, the first principles approach is helpful: the rare situations in which a breach of confidence might be considered are likely to be those where there is a risk of harm, or at least, a loss of benefit (in the case of treatable conditions). The disclosure of genetic information may, the GMC has said, warrant disclosure particularly when a clinician has a responsibility to more than one person eg where a GP is doctor to several members of the same family. As with disclosure of any confidential information, it is important to recognise that any decision to reveal medical data to a third party should not be taken lightly and that the entitlement to share confidential information in certain circumstances does not amount to a duty to do so. However, it is possible that a breach of confidentiality can be justified in a *minority* of cases where it would be in the interests of another person to receive genetic information that the patient does not wish to disclose. The Joint Commission on Medical Genetics has existing guidance on consent and confidentiality that is helpful and clear. Those guidelines are scheduled to be revised for the publication of a second edition in late 2011 and it is worth looking out for the updated guidance.[124]

---

[124] Available from www.bshg.org.uk which is a rich resource for those interested in clinical genetics.

The other issue that can sometimes arise in relation to genetic information is the disclosure of that information to third party organisations such as employers and, more commonly, insurance companies. There is a parallel with HIV testing in that when testing first became available some insurance companies required people who had been tested for HIV to disclose that they had sought an HIV test, irrespective of the result of the test or the reason for seeking an HIV testing. More alarming still, sometimes sexual orientation or even types of employment were used as proxies for HIV risk in the context of insurance applications. Concerns were raised vociferously about privacy, stigma and discrimination. Eventually, the Association of British Insurers worked in conjunction with clinicians, advocacy groups and the insurance industry to produce best practice guidance on HIV testing and the provision of insurance.[125] Like HIV testing, there is a specific Code of Practice[126] published by the Association of British Insurers which comprehensively addresses the issues in relation to disclosure of confidential genetic information and the provision of insurance. The Human Genetics Commission also has a working group with a brief to monitor genetics and insurance. The guidance provides greater detail than most medical students would require or wish to read, but it is worth a look to see both the sorts of issues that arise in relation to genetic information and insurance, and how concerns about privacy and discrimination have been addressed by the industry in consultation with key stakeholders.

Conclusion

Genetic testing presents particular ethical challenges that have been the subject of careful consideration by cross-disciplinary groups and useful national guidance. Genetic testing should be considered with reference to benefits; both in the immediate and longer term whilst also acknowledging that evaluation of possible benefit is an uncertain endeavour. In clinical genetics, the consequentialist approach to ethics is particularly visible because, in general, a distinction is drawn between symptomatic and pre-symptomatic testing and the likelihood of an effective intervention. However,

---

[125] *Statement of Best Practice on HIV and Insurance*. London: Association of British Insurers, 2008 (due for revision in 2011). Available at www.abi.org.uk
[126] Code of Practice for Genetic Tests. London: Association of British Insurers, 2008.

it would be a mistake to think of genetics as solely dependent on a consequentialist analysis: questions and matters of principle in relation to truth-telling, candour and trust are common themes in clinical genetics. Another, perhaps less common way, to approach ethics in clinical genetics is to consider what a virtuous clinical geneticist might be like: what are the traits or characteristics that he or she would demonstrate in daily practice? Would those virtues differ from those expected from any doctor? If so, how and why?

In many ways, it is important not to conceptualise genetics as too different or particularly irrespective of the neat nomenclature of 'genethics'. The fundamentals of sound ethical practice and analysis apply as much in clinical genetics as they do to other areas of medicine. There may be particular types of information that should be considered when seeking consent, but the component parts of consent remain unaltered. Likewise, there may be considerations that are specific to genetic information, but the notion of confidentiality being central to a trusting therapeutic relationship, and disclosure of information being limited to situations where there is a reasonable risk of harm, are universally applicable in medicine. An awareness of the specific context in which clinical genetics is practised coupled with a sound grasp of the basic building blocks of ethico-legal knowledge and skills are likely to stand any student, future geneticist or not, in good stead.

 # Core Concepts: Genethics

Genethics is the term used to describe the moral dimensions of medicine involving genetic information.
The Human Genetics Commission formerly existed to advise on the ethical and social implications of genetic progress but its abolition was proposed by the government in 2010.
Genetics causes moral disquiet for some because of its associations with eugenics and discrimination against those who have genetic diseases and disabilities.
For others, providing genetic information facilitates choice and informed decision-making and can co-exist alongside support and treatment for those with genetic diseases.

The use of IVF and pre-implantation genetic diagnosis to both screen out and select embryos that could be donors for sick children, so-called 'saviour siblings', has been authorised by the HFEA.

The debate about saviour siblings often pivots on whether children are being created as means to an end ie the treatment of an existing child. Others suggest that all families have children for a range of reasons and that saviour siblings can enjoy a loving family environment.

There is no obligation to undergo genetic testing nor can someone demand a genetic test that is not indicated.

There are particular ethical considerations when people use direct-to-consumer testing kits that do not allow for pre-test counselling, support and follow-up.

Genetic testing is neither inherently moral nor immoral. Its purpose and implications should be considered with reference to the basic principles of consent and confidentiality.

Where a person lacks capacity to consent to a genetic test, it should only be conducted where there is a benefit to the individual concerned and where it can be shown that benefit is in the person's best interests.

Assessment: Genethics in practice

1. Screening for bowel cancer and a patient's request

Sample OSCE station

Mrs Stone, age 42, attends a hospital outpatient clinic for investigation of lower abdominal discomfort and continuing bowel symptoms. She discloses early in the consultation that her mother died from bowel cancer and she is 'very worried' about the possibility that she has bowel cancer. Mrs Stone has done some reading on the internet, and she knows that the NHS bowel cancer screening programme is routinely available to those aged 60–69. People aged over 70 can also ask to participate in the programme. Mrs Stone wishes to discuss whether she should be screened for bowel cancer even though she is considerably younger than the age at which the NHS programme applies. You have been asked to talk to Mrs Stone about her concerns before she sees the consultant. You will be asked to summarise your discussion and to identify the key ethico-legal issues relating to Mrs Stone's concerns at the end of the station.

Guidance notes

- After introductions, allow Mrs Stone to explain, in her own words and time, her concerns about her symptoms in general, and bowel cancer, in particular. Careful and active listening will allow Mrs Stone to convey most accurately what she both understands about bowel cancer screening and her priorities for the consultation.

- For consent to screening procedures to be meaningful, counselling must consist of more than simply quoting statistics on risk, sensitivity and specificity. But how much more is required? Doctors are bound by the GMC to disclose information that they believe any reasonable person in the patient's position would require for an informed choice. Mrs Stone is an anxious patient who has first-hand experience of a relative with bowel cancer and she has also done some reading online. It is reasonable to expect that she is keen to discuss what she knows and to find out more.

- It is essential to be clear about the scope of screening for abnormality. As such, to complete this station, you need to know something about how screening works, its effectiveness at detecting disease, the rates of identifying bowel cancer amongst those who have been screened and the range of results/treatment pathways. Depending on the stage in your training, this might be information that is supplied to you as part of the station or you might be expected to have sufficient understanding yourself to provide Mrs Stone with what she is seeking.

- Mrs Stone is considerably younger than the people targeted by the NHS screening programme. She seems to perceive an increased risk because of her mother's medical history and it may be helpful to acknowledge that understanding of the genetic component of bowel cancer is increasing.[127] However, it is important not to substitute an empathic response to Mrs Stone's concerns with a lecture on genetics.

---

[127] For a summary of the literature on genetics and bowel cancer, see http://info. cancerresearchuk.org/cancerstats/types/bowel/molecularbiologyandgenetics

- The question of choice following screening can be ethico-legally complex. Once a patient agrees to undergo most 'routine' screening, there is a potential chain of further investigations. If Mrs Stone is recommended to have an invasive test as a result of screening, in what sense is her choice to undergo the invasive test 'free'? The way in which this issue is usually conceptualised is as what might be called 'contingent autonomy' ie if Mrs Stone is properly counselled when deciding whether or not to have screening, she will be encouraged to consider what choices he would prefer to make if further investigations and/or treatment are indicated. This so-called 'contingent autonomy' emphasises the importance of effective pre-screening consultations whilst not, of course, removing the need for Mrs Stone to give valid consent to any future treatment.

- For consent to screening to be valid and in accordance with best practice, the following points might be discussed:

    - Screening has been shown to reduce the mortality rate in patients with bowel cancer[128] because it offers the possibility of earlier, and therefore more effective, intervention and treatment when the disease is not symptomatic.

    - However, screening does not necessarily provide certainty. Indeed it may exacerbate anxiety by revealing to the patient what can best be described as 'partial knowledge'. When screening for bowel cancer, polyps may be detected which are not cancer but have the potential to develop into cancer later in life. Honesty about uncertainty is essential. For example, as well as the normal/abnormal result from bowel screening, approximately 4 patients in 100 will have ambiguous test results.[129] The manner in which these probabilities are communicated is crucial.

---

[128] Cochrane Database of Systemic Reviews (2006) *Screening for Colorectal Cancer using the Faecal Occult Blood Test: An Update.*
[129] See www.cancerscreening.nhs.uk/bowel

- Screening may lead to further investigations and interventions however 'routine' eg a colonoscopy and/or the removal of polyps.

- Screening for bowel cancer is only one part of investigating Mrs Stone's symptoms although it is the aspect that she has highlighted as her priority, but the screening decision should be contextualised by summarising the next steps available to her. It is unlikely to be a decision that Mrs Stone makes immediately and candidates should explicitly invite her to think about the possibilities and perhaps point her to further resources in advance of a follow-up consultation. Even if Mrs Stone eventually decides that she does not wish to pursue screening, she should be able to make that decision following a dialogue with clinicians that enable her to leave feeling more informed about her options. As a medical student, it is important to emphasise that you will be feeding back to the consultant and that she will have the opportunity to talk to the consultant herself before she makes any decisions.

- There is a lot of complex information to discuss with Mrs Stone (who we can assume is already anxious). It is essential therefore to pace the discussion as is remaining alert to verbal and nonverbal cues. Information should be offered in discrete chunks, checking for understanding and leaving time for the patient to take in what is being said and ask questions.

- This is a challenging scenario and it may be that you are unable to answer all Mrs Stone's questions, in which case an honest expression of uncertainty and an offer to find out more is the best option.

Chapter 9

Death, Distress and Decisions: End of Life

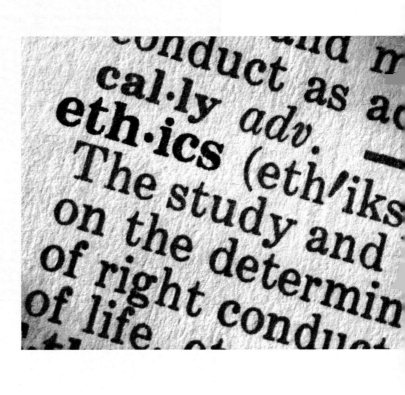

Death, Distress and Decisions: End of Life

Introduction

Clinical practice at the end of life raises numerous ethico-legal issues that most students will encounter not only in their teaching and clinical placements but also by simply opening a newspaper or listening to the news. Questions regarding the ways in which people are treated at the end of life, the acceptability or otherwise of assisted dying and the work of organisations such as Dignitas in Switzerland are a constant presence in the professional and mainstream media.[130] This chapter will consider the key issues that arise at the end of life including:

- Decision-making, autonomy and responsibility at the end of life: who decides what happens to a person at the end of life? What is the relative status of preferences expressed by a patient, his or her family or a doctor? What are the effects of an advance decision or Lasting Power of Attorney?
- Notions of quality of life and futility: should a clinical team consider a person's quality of life in making treatment decisions? What does futility mean? What happens if there is disagreement about treatment?
- The law: what is the legal position regarding assisted dying?
- Specific decision points: when is it appropriate to discuss resuscitation with a patient and/or his or her family members? Who decides when it is right to move from active to palliative treatment?

First, it is worth clarifying the terminology that is used (sometimes differently and confusingly) when discussing the end of life. Common terms and their meanings are set out in the box below.

---

[130] See, for example, the BBC documentary *Choosing to Die* that was presented by Sir Terry Pratchett (13 June 2011) in which he followed two men who was seeking the assistance of the Dignitas organisation to end their lives.

> **Active euthanasia**
> An act that contributes to death
>
> **Physician assisted suicide, assisted dying or assisted suicide**
> Types of active euthanasia in which someone helps another to die
>
> **Passive euthanasia**
> An omission that contributes to death
>
> **Suicide**
> Causing one's own death; assisted suicide: contributing to another's death by act
>
> **Active euthanasia, physician assisted suicide, assisted dying and assisted suicide are currently illegal in UK, passive euthanasia and suicide are not.**

Decision-making, autonomy and responsibility at the end of life

Much of this book has emphasised the importance of patient autonomy and choice. The facilitation of, and response to, people's preferences and wishes are central to ethical practice. However, for some, it is unacceptable that at the end of life people remain unable to make choices or, more specifically, one particular choice, namely to die. In the UK, assisted dying is unlawful and, as such, if someone no longer wishes to live with the symptoms of serious disease, doctors (and those who are not doctors) are unable to accede to requests for help in ending life even if it is the person's expressed wish.

Many people at the end of life experience pain and it is often the management of such pain that illuminates the boundaries of lawful practice and highlights the ethical issues for healthcare professionals working with people at the end of life. Most clinicians would accept that it is their duty to alleviate pain so far as possible – and, in many cases, effective pain-control can be achieved. In such cases, clinicians balance the potential risks of pain alleviation (eg respiratory depression and dependency) against the benefits. However, there are patients for whom analgesia provides only partial or limited relief and who may believe that it is in their best interests is for clinicians to support and even assist them in ending their lives. If someone is apparently clear and sure that the ultimate benefit is the complete end of pain and therefore life, should what appears to be an expression of autonomy and a desire for self-determination be respected? And, if one accepts that autonomy is key that may mean accepting that people are free to make the 'wrong' decision or a mistake, even at the end of life. It isn't possible to equate autonomy with a certain decision that will never be regretted.

For some ethicists, such as Professor Len Doyal, respecting an individual's choice to die is not only ethically desirable but congruent with a doctor's discretion to withdraw treatment and can be in a person's best interests.[131] Professor Doyal has gone further and argued that involuntary euthanasia may be in the best interests and respect the dignity of those who are unable to express a choice.[132] In contrast, there are ethicists who argue that autonomy is not an unfettered freedom; life has moral status and death is not something that can be requested or even demanded. The notion of apparently 'free choices' is contestable on the basis that we are all inevitably influenced by society, the effects of our illness on our families and the quality of information we receive which has led some to argue that autonomy is an illusory concept. As such, it is suggested by some that society should protect vulnerable people from seeking death because they feel they ought to, rather than as an active choice. Whatever one feels about assisted dying, it is worth considering the influences that might be shaping a person's decision-making just as one would in any other area of clinical practice. Such consideration translates into practical steps like alleviating pain; discussing what is known and not known about a patient's future experience in accessible and realistic terms; exploring the patient's relationships with family and friends and understanding how these inform decision-making; and allowing time and the opportunity for questions, changes of mind and inconsistent responses in what is likely to be a non-acute, ongoing decision-making process.

A number of claims have been made for the effects of permitting assisted dying. The so-called 'slippery slope' argument is also

---

[131] Doyal, L., Doyal, L. Why Active Euthanasia and Physician-Assisted Suicide Should Be Legalised. *BMJ* 2001; 323: 1079–1080.

[132] Doyal, L. Dignity in Dying Should Include the Legalisation of Non-Voluntary Euthanasia. *Clinical Ethics* 2006; 1(2): 65–67.

frequently considered by both supporters and opponents of euthanasia. Professor John Keown, an ethicist who has consistently argued against euthanasia, suggests that the experience of the Netherlands (where voluntary euthanasia has been decriminalised) is that permitting patients to end their lives has resulted in a slippery slope in which control is variable and the vulnerable feel pressure to consider euthanasia as part of end-of-life care.[133] The high-profile American ethicist, Ezekiel Emanuel,[134] cites empirical data to argue that permitting assisted dying does not enhance the quality of care at the end of life and may even compromise standards. In contrast, others argue that despite the decriminalisation of euthanasia in the Netherlands, palliative care provision and the trust between doctors and patients have been enhanced rather than diminished.[135] One of the most significant reviews of the empirical data of the last two decades in the Netherlands suggests that there has not been a 'slippery slope' effect with the majority of cases being effectively regulated and conducted within the law, although the authors note that there is a minority of situations in which the legal criteria of reporting are not followed.[136]

Acts and omissions

There are several key concepts that inform the ethical analysis of ending life. The first is the contested distinction between acts and omissions.[137] For some an omission, ie the withholding of a

---

[133] Kweon, J. Euthanasia in the Netherlands: Sliding Down the Slippery Slope? Notre Dame Journal of Law, Ethics and Public Policy 1995; 9(2): 407–448; Keown, J. *Euthanasia, Ethics and Public Policy*. Cambridge: Cambridge University Press, 2002.

[134] Emanuel, E. Euthanasia: Where the Netherlands Leads Will the World Follow? *BMJ* 2001; 322: 1376–1377.

[135] Georges. J.J., Onwuteaka-Philipsen, B. D., Van Der Heide, A., Van Der Wal, G., Van Der Maas, P.J. Physicians' Opinions on Palliative Care and Euthanasia in the Netherlands. *Journal of Palliative Medicine* 2006; 9(5): 1137–1144; Gordijn, B., Janssens, R. Euthanasia and Palliative Care in the Netherlands: An Analysis of the Latest Developments. *Healthcare Analysis 2004*; 12(3): 195–207.

[136] Rietjens,J.A.C., Van der Maas, P.J., Onwuteaka-Philipsen, B.D., Van Delden, J.J.M., and van der Heide, A. Two Decades of Research on Euthanasia from the Netherlands: What Have We Learned and What Questions Remain? *Journal of Bioethical Enquiry 2009*; 6(3): 271–283.

[137] Mohindra, R. Positing a Difference Between Acts and Omissions: The Principle of Justice, Rachels' Cases and Moral Weakness. *J Med Ethics* 2009; 35: 293–299.

medical intervention is morally distinct from an act ie carrying out a medical intervention. For those who argue for the moral distinction between an act and an omission, active and passive euthanasia can and should be ethically distinguished.[138] Even if the consequence of both an act and omission is the death of a patient, it is argued that passive and active behaviour are morally distinct. There is, for some commentators and many clinicians, an essential difference between killing and 'letting [someone] die'.[139] Put in practical terms, it is the perceived moral difference between withdrawing ventilation from a terminally sick patient and giving that patient a fatal injection.

Many ethicists challenge the significance of any possible distinction between acts and omissions. For some, even if there is a sustainable distinction, it is not a persuasive basis for the moral analysis of euthanasia, where notions of agency and responsibility are important rather than a focus on active and passive causation.[140] Interestingly, whilst many ethicists believe that the argument that there is a crucial moral difference between acts and omissions is not persuasive, for many clinicians (who are, after all, the ones likely to be making and implementing decisions at the end of life) the distinction between acts and omissions is both important and convincing.[141] It is unlikely, perhaps even undesirable, that students will be sure of what they feel about acts and omissions. That does not matter. As Tony Hope observes,[142] the potential for distinguishing acts and omissions is *'one of those simple, complex ideas'* that preoccupy philosophers for their entire careers. However, it is important to be aware that it is a distinction commonly invoked in discussions about the ethics of end-of-life care. Time spent reviewing personal intuitions in a structured way, with reference to the persuasiveness

---

[138] See, for example, Stauch, M. Causal Authorship and the Equality Principle: A Defence of the Acts and Omissions Distinction in Euthanasia. *J Med Ethics* 2000; 26: 237–241; McLachlan, H.V. The Ethics of Killing and Letting Die: Active and Passive Euthanasia. *J Med Ethics* 2008; 34: 636–638.

[139] Glover, J. *Causing Death and Saving Lives*. London: Penguin Books, 1977 at page 93 ff.

[140] Coggon, J. On Acts, Omissions and Responsibility. *J Med Ethics* 2008; 34: 576–579.

[141] Dickenson, D. Are Medical Ethicists Out of Touch? Practitioner Attitudes in the US and UK at the End of Life. *J Med Ethics* 2000; 26: 254–260.

[142] Hope, T. Acts and Omissions Revisited. *J Med Ethics* 2000; 26: 227–228.

or otherwise of distinguishing acts and omissions, is likely to be worthwhile.

The Doctrine of Double Effect

A second concept that has both ethical and legal significance at the end of life is the doctrine of double effect. Essentially, the doctrine of double effect is based on the principle that it is possible to distinguish between foresight and intention. While healthcare professionals are precluded, like anyone else, from intending to cause the death of a patient, it is, of course, perfectly permissible for healthcare professionals to want to alleviate their patients suffering by prescribing appropriate medication. As informed professionals, clinicians will know that such medication may have the foreseen effect of shortening the patient's life. Therefore the law applies the doctrine of double effect as a means of resolving this tension. In the context of the end of life, one might foresee that a particular analgesic, for example, has the potential to affect respiration but the intention is to alleviate pain. The drug has a 'double effect' and in medical law, it is the distinction between foresight and intention that constitutes the difference between a murder charge and lawful treatment. In short, a doctor who prescribes a drug with a double effect is deemed to have intended the benefits even whilst foreseeing the side effects. It is, of course, important that the drug chosen is appropriate for the circumstances and used proportionately to manage symptoms.

The rationale for the doctrine of double effect comprises four elements, namely:

1.   The act is good in itself eg to prescribe pain-relieving or suffering-alleviating medication;
2.   The primary and sole intention of the person acting is to bring about the positive effect(s) of the act eg the principal aim when prescribing analgesia is to alleviate a patient's pain;
3.   The positive effects of the act are not dependent upon any co-existing negative effects; and
4.   Any potential negative effects are outweighed by the potential positive effects eg the alleviation of pain is the priority and, as such, overrides any side effects from the medication prescribed.

A notable medical case that demonstrated the significance of the doctrine of double effect and its limits was that of *R v Cox*.[143] Dr Cox was a doctor who had been treating a patient, Mrs Lillian Boyes, for rheumatoid arthritis for approximately 13 years. Dr Cox knew both the patient and her family well. With the knowledge and support of her family, Mrs Boyes asked Dr Cox to end her life and therefore her suffering. Dr Cox administered a lethal dose of potassium chloride to Mrs Boyes. Suspicions were subsequently raised by a nurse and Dr Cox was charged with attempted murder. Students are often puzzled about why Dr Cox charged with attempted murder rather than murder. Dr Cox was charged with attempted murder, rather than murder, because it could not be shown that the injection had actually caused Mrs Boyes death because her body had been cremated. Dr Cox was convicted of attempted murder: the court held that potassium chloride does not have 'a double effect' and he must, therefore, be considered in law to have intended to cause the patient's death rather than alleviate her pain. In sentencing the doctor, the judge in the case, Ognall J expressed the view that the act of injecting Mrs Boyes with potassium chloride was a breach of an 'unequivocal duty' towards a patient. The judgment was approved in the later case of *Bland*[144] although, a number of the judges in the *Bland* case recognised the difficulty of distinguishing between withdrawing life sustaining treatment and taking steps to end the life of a patient. Dr Cox received a suspended prison sentence and a reprimand from the GMC. The decision to prosecute Dr Cox was much criticised.[145] However, in law, it did not matter that Dr Cox acted at Mrs Boyes' request and with her family's support.

When thinking about both the case of Dr Cox and your own views on end of life care, you might find it helpful to consider the following questions:

• Mrs Boyes had asked Dr Cox to help her die – is this a request a doctor can ever fulfil?

---

[143] *R. v Cox* (1992) 12 BMLR 38.

[144] Airedale NHS Trust v Bland [1993] AC 789.

[145] See for example Helme, J., Padfield, A. Safeguarding Euthanasia. 142 *NLJ* 1992; 1335 in which the authors declared the decision to prosecute Dr Cox 'disproportionate' to any wrong committed by the defendant.

- Is there a moral distinction to be drawn between patients with chronic illnesses who may be suffering great pain, such as Mrs Boyes, and patients who are terminally ill (who may also be in great pain)?
- If pain is an overwhelming factor and the permanent alleviation of pain is the expressed wish of the patient, what role does the doctor have in caring for the patient?

Suffering and futility

There are other concepts that you will encounter in relation to debates about care at the end of life, such as the nature of the intervention or treatment ie seeking to distinguish between ordinary and extraordinary acts[146] on the basis that whilst there is a duty to preserve life by standard means, there is no obligation to do everything possible, especially if to do so would be excessively burdensome. Even if one accepts that it is possible to draw such a distinction, why is there moral difference in the nature of the treatment itself? Life-sustaining treatment can be routine(eg nutrition and hydration) or highly specialised and technically advanced. Yet the distinction continues to have relevance, as discussed in the section on advance decisions below.

The notion of extraordinary care often informs the concept of futility ie treatment where there is no meaningful prospect of improvement or recovery. It is an approach that looks to the outcome, or rather predicted outcome, to determine the moral worth or otherwise of an intervention. The term 'futile' is often used even when treatment may achieve some goals. Fundamentally, then, futility must be defined relative to the outcome that we seek to achieve eg if the outcome/goal is complete health, then treatment is often futile. If the intended outcome or goal of treatment is the prolongation of life for a few hours or day, then intervening may not be futile at all.

Perhaps predictably, the challenge about *who* should define 'futility' and *how* complicates such an approach. After all, all medical treatment is ultimately futile because all human beings ultimately die. Futility

---

[146] This was considered in the case of *Burke, R. (On the Application Of) v General Medical Council and Others* [2005] EWCA 1003.

may be interpreted quite differently by clinical staff and patients. For example, one might take a quantitative approach eg where 100 patients have this condition, only 1 will breathe independently again. Alternatively, it might be interpreted qualitatively eg an individual may be willing to undergo interventionist treatment repeatedly because this individual thinks 'I value even the remote chance that I am the 1 in 100 who breathes independently and there are other things in my life that make me want to pursue every option until the last'.

Resuscitation decisions will often invoke, either implicitly or explicitly the notion of futility without necessarily involving the patient. Indeed, so commonly is the concept of futility invoked to inform ethico-legal decision-making in resuscitation (cardiopulmonary resuscitation or CPR) practice, that it has led to a quasi-bioethical movement named the 'Futilitarians'.[147] The primary benefit of CPR is that it gives a chance of extending life. However, the survival rates are low; much lower than might be expected based on the ways in which resuscitation is often portrayed in medical dramas. CPR is also invasive and carries risks; following a partially successful resuscitation attempt, these may include rib or sternal fractures, hepatic or splenic rupture, brain damage following hypoxia and long-term admission to intensive care.

The principles that apply to resuscitation decisions are the same as for any other form of treatment. If the patient has capacity, CPR should be discussed honestly in the context of the patient's particular condition. The relationship of CPR to other treatments such as hydration and analgesia should be considered and discussed. It is important to be clear that even if a patient is 'not for resuscitation', the clinical team will do all that can be done to ensure he or she remains comfortable. DNAR does not equate to no care at all. Occasionally, if the clinical team (led by consultant-level expertise) believes that CPR would not be successful, and the patient does not raise the issue of resuscitation, it may not be necessary to discuss DNAR status. However, information should not be withheld from patients just because it is difficult to discuss or feels uncomfortable. Direct questions must be answered honestly

---

[147] A label that has been adapted from a philosophical school formally known as 'Futilitarianism' which proposes that all human endeavour is ultimately futile.

and there should be careful justification if it is concluded that a patient who has capacity should not be involved in discussions. Remember that patients are entitled to see their medical records, which could mean that someone learning of their resuscitation status in a way that is unexpected and upsetting, which is likely to compromise trust and the therapeutic relationship. The perceptions of patients, clinicians and families about the value of resuscitation can differ widely and lead to misunderstanding. A crucial part of ethical practice in the context of resuscitation is therefore to explore existing understanding and be honest about both what is known and unknown with regard to the patient and the disease process.

When a patient lacks capacity, it may be that someone has been granted Lasting Power of Attorney (LPA) or that there is a valid advance decision that makes reference to CPR. If so, decisions should be made with reference to either the person who has LPA or the content of the advance decision. Where there is neither LPA nor a valid advance decision, decisions about a patient's resuscitation status should be made on the basis of best interests. It may be that there is a family member or third party who can advocate the patient and help inform the deliberations of what is in his or her best interests. End of life choices and decisions are difficult and can result in conflict within the team or with the patient and/or his or her family. There may be assumptions, misunderstandings and expectations that have not been articulated or heard. Ethical practice means one should aim to elucidate and explore the perceptions of everyone involves and facilitate the honest exchange of beliefs. Specific questions to ask might include: are the family unrealistically optimistic? Has the clinical team offered a clear and accessible account of the patient's care to date? Who might be able to offer the patient and his or her family support at a difficult time in their lives? Can the clinical team explain what a 'good death' might mean?

Even if decisions regarding a patient's resuscitation status are made relatively easily with no disagreement, practical difficulties can still affect the implementation of the decision. What can medical students and doctors in training do to maximise the effectiveness of decision-making about resuscitation? First, it is important to be aware of the relevant guidelines, both national and local, on CPR.

Secondly, seize the opportunity to develop and practise the skills involved in having difficult conversations with patients and/or their families: resuscitation is an emotional and sensitive subject to discuss. Where discussion about resuscitation has happened, it is vital to share that conversation with senior staff and to document that discussion in the notes, in addition to completing the required paperwork (eg many NHS Trusts have a specific form[148] for DNAR orders). There is a scenario involving resuscitation decision-making at the end of this chapter which picks up many of the points discussed in this section of the chapter.

Who decides at the end of life?

The question of who decides what happens at the end of life does not differ from the basic principles that apply to any other clinical encounter. As such, if a person has capacity, it is for him or her to choose what treatment they wish to accept. The limitations on choice are that a person cannot demand care that is not deemed to be in his or best interests and no one can request euthanasia. Most decisions are therefore made by a process of discussion and negotiation over a period of time. The different stages of decision-making at the end of life are explored in more detail later in this chapter in the section on palliative care.

Where a person lacks the capacity to make a decision about his or her own care, there are a number of possibilities. There may be a valid advance decision or LPA (the criteria for validity for both advance decisions and LPA are to be found in Chapter 3). An advance decision is likely to give the clinical team an indication of the patient's wishes and, if it has been well-drafted, may refer to particular considerations such as resuscitation status. If someone has been granted LPA, that person will be able to make decisions on behalf of the incapacitous patient.

If there is neither an advance decision nor a LPA in place, the clinical team must act in the patient's best interests. Best interests is more than merely best *medical* interests and clinical teams may seek to get a sense of the person from talking to family members,

---

[148] The United Kingdom Resuscitation Council recommends the use of a model form. It is available at: www.resus.org.uk/pages/DNARrstd.htm

friends and carers. Ultimately, in the absence of a valid LPA, third parties should inform and advise the clinical team about the patient's likely wishes and preferences, but decisions will be made by a doctor (usually the consultant) who is required to act in the patient's best interests.

End-of-life decisions and the law

Assisted dying is illegal in the UK as illustrated by the case of *R v Cox*. However, withholding or withdrawing treatment may be lawful in the UK because it is not deemed to be in the patient's best interests either to begin or continue treatment, or because the patient refuses treatment. The importance of the patient's wishes at the end of life as in any other clinical situation was confirmed in the case of Ms B.[149] The case was curious because Ms B, as a capacitous patient, was entitled to ask for the withdrawal of treatment and it remains unclear why it proceeded to court. Ms B was paralysed following two haemorrhages into her spinal cord and dependent on a ventilator. Ms B no longer wished to continue being artificially ventilated and requested that ventilation should be withdrawn. The question determined by the court was whether she had capacity to make such a decision. Dame Elizabeth Butler-Sloss, the judge in the case, visited Ms B on an intensive care unit and concluded that she did have capacity. The Ms B case is a good example of how basic principles apply at the end of life. As readers will know well by now, a person with capacity is entitled to refuse treatment even where that refusal results death. Ms B would not have been able to request that someone assist her in dying or give her lethal treatment, but she could refuse life-preserving ventilation so long as she had the capacity to make a choice.

There have been notable legal cases concerning the clinical discretion doctors have when deciding whether to withhold or withdraw treatment, namely those actions involving Tony Bland[150] and Leslie Burke. The cases demonstrate the distinction between and insisting on or demanding treatment, and refusing available treatment or expressing preference between clinical indicated options. The *Bland* decision represented a landmark in medical law.

---

[149] *B v An NHS Trust* [2002] EWHC 429 Fam.
[150] *Airedale NHS Trust v Bland* [1993] 1 All ER 821, HL.

The case concerned Tony Bland who was in a persistent vegetative state following severe brain injury in the Hillsborough Stadium disaster. The hospital brought an action, with the support of Tony Bland's parents, to withdraw life-sustaining treatment. The case eventually progressed to the House of Lords where the Law Lords authorised the withdrawal of treatment, including artificial hydration and nutrition, from Tony Bland. In contrast to the case of Tony Bland, Leslie Burke's action was concerned with the continuation of treatment. Leslie Burke has cerebellar ataxia (also known as Friedreich's ataxia), a degenerative neurological condition that at some point is likely to make it difficult or impossible for Mr Burke to convey his wishes to the clinical team. Mr Burke was concerned that the guidance issued from the General Medical Council[151] on withholding and withdrawing treatment allowed for clinical discretion on the part of doctors to decide whether beginning or maintaining treatment was in a patient's best interests. Mr Burke sought judicial review of the GMC guidance, arguing that the right to life enshrined in the Human Rights Act 1998 demanded that the professional guidelines should be redrafted. At first instance, the court supported Mr Burke. However, following an appeal by the GMC, the Court of Appeal supported the GMC guidance and rejected Mr Burke's arguments. Mr Burke sought to appeal to the House of Lords but it refused to hear the case. In 2006, Mr Burke lodged an appeal with the European Court of Human Rights which was unsuccessful. It remains the position that doctors are entitled to withhold and withdraw treatment when the situation is considered futile, provided they do so within the law and existing professional guidance.

There have been a series of cases where individuals have sought clarification and guidance regarding the involvement of others at the end of life. First, there was the case of Diane Pretty[152] who sought either exemption from criminalisation or a guaranteed pardon for her husband if he were to assist her in committing suicide. Ms Pretty had motor neurone disease and she was fearful of a prolonged death in which she would experience suffocation

---

[151] *Withholding and Withdrawing Life Prolonging Treatments: Good Practice and Decision Making.* London: GMC, 2002. This guidance has been replaced by *Treatment and Care towards the End of Life: Good Practice in Decision Making.* London: GMC, 2010.
[152] *R. (Pretty) v DPP* [2001] UK HL 61.

and asphyxiation. Using the Human Rights Act 1998, Diane Pretty argued that she had a right to die and that, as her disease prevented her from committing suicide without the assistance of her husband, the Director of Public Prosecutions should guarantee that either her husband would not be prosecuted or that, if he were to be prosecuted, he would be pardoned. The case progressed through the British court system and eventually reached the European Court of Human Rights which rejected Diane Pretty's claim that the European Convention on Human Rights provided for a right to die. Diane Pretty died in 2002 from motor neurone disease.

More recently, Debbie Purdy's case[153] has been considered. Ms Purdy has progressive multiple sclerosis and she, like Diane Pretty, was concerned that if her husband were to assist her death by whatever means (including arranging for her to travel to Dignitas in Switzerland) he might be prosecuted and convicted. Ms Purdy sought guidance from the Director of Public Prosecutions in relation to the criteria that would be applied when considering whether to prosecute someone who had helped another person take steps to end his or her life. The case differed from Diane Pretty's in that Debbie Purdy was seeking guidance about the discretion the DPP has when deciding whether to prosecute someone, whereas Diane Pretty was seeking a definitive statement that her husband would be not prosecuted at all or, if he were to be prosecuted, that he would be guaranteed to receive a pardon. As a result of the House of Lords decision in the Purdy case, the Director of Public Prosecutions issued interim guidance that was subject to a consultation period followed, in February 2010, by the publication of final guidance.

The guidance lists the factors that will weigh either in favour of, or against, prosecution whilst emphasising that each case will be treated on its own merits. It is important to stress that the guidance issued following Debbie Purdy's action does not change the law: assisted dying remains illegal. However, there is now greater clarity about how the Director of Public Prosecutions will reach a decision about whether to prosecute someone who has assisted another in dying. The factors weighing *in favour* of prosecution are summarised below.

---

[153] *R. (Purdy) v DPP* [2009] UK HL 45.

Characteristics of the diseased	Characteristics of the person accused of assisting
Under 18 years of age or an adult who lacked capacity	Not solely motivated by compas-sion
Did not know the person who assisted	Pressured the deceased or did not prevent others from pressurising the deceased into dying
No or insufficient evidence of voluntary, clear, settled and informed choice	Worked in an environment where people can commit suicide
Did not seek assisted suicide or could have committed suicide without help	Was acting in his or her capacity as a health or social care professional

Thus, the DPP guidance is clear: doctors are a special category and must not act in a professional capacity to assist the death of a patient. Nonetheless, the status of those who accompany a person to another jurisdiction where assisted dying is legal remains uncertain. In 2009, Lord Falconer and Baroness Jay proposed an amendment to the Coroners and Justice Bill that would have permitted people to help someone with a terminal illness travel to a country where assisted dying is lawful. The amendment was defeated by 194 votes to 141 in the House of Lords.

Attempts to change the law on assisted dying continue. One of the most noteworthy efforts to amend the law was made by Lord Joffe in the form of his Bill, 'Assisted Dying for the Terminally Ill' which went through several iterations but would have allowed physician-assisted suicide for those who were terminally ill. In 2006, the Bill was defeated on its second reading in the House of Lords by 148 votes to 100 after a lengthy passage through parliament. Campaign groups exist on both sides of the debate and it is a topic that is unlikely to fade from the public and professional agendas.

Activities: End-of-Life in practice

Case Study

Dr Linden is caring for Mrs Roberts who has bone cancer. She is in tremendous pain and he prescribes opiate analgesia in increasing doses. Mrs Roberts dies of respiratory complications from the high doses of analgesia. Dr Linden is not prosecuted.

Case Study

Mrs Roberts becomes increasingly distressed by her pain and declining condition. Mrs Roberts begins to become disorientated and confused. Mr Roberts decides on impulse to give his wife an overdose of prescribed and over-the-counter medication mixed with a large quantity of alcohol. Mr Roberts is subsequently arrested.

Questions

(i)   Why was Dr Linden not prosecuted?

(ii)   Under what circumstances might Dr Linden have been prosecuted?

(iii) What is the legal distinction between the cases?

(iv)   What factors in the second case weigh in favour of the prosecution of Mr Roberts?

(v)   Has Mr Roberts done anything that is *morally* different from Dr Linden?

(vi)   What ethical and legal issues do you think you will find difficult in caring for patients in great pain?

Ethico-legal perspectives on palliative care

Why does palliative care warrant a distinct section in a chapter concerned with the end of life? The model of palliative care is quite different from the traditional biomedical model in which curative treatment (or at least effective improvement) is the principal goal. The ideological shift from cure to care inevitably reframes the ethical issues. Moral and legal questions occur at all stages of palliative care. This section of the chapter discusses some of the ethical issues that arise as a patient moves through the palliative care process[154] using case studies to illustrate the ethico-legal points to consider.

Referral to palliative care

Decisions about when to cease 'treatment' and to begin palliation can cause moral dilemmas for both patients and healthcare professionals. Respect for, and the fostering of, patient autonomy demand that

---

[154] For those interested in the patient perspective of palliative care, see Lawton, J. *The Dying Process: Patients' Experiences of Palliative Care*. London: Routledge, 2000.

the decision whether or not to begin palliation must be an honest and negotiated process between the patient and all members of the healthcare team. These negotiations should, of course, reflect the moral equivalence of each party in the interaction notwithstanding the difference in power between patient and healthcare professional. Healthcare professionals may themselves feel anxious, and be reluctant to accept that the time has come to move from cure to a model of care with which they may be far less comfortable and for which their training has not necessarily equipped them. These issues are raised in the following case study.

Case Study

Mr Maxwell is a thirty-year-old man with haemophilia. He was diagnosed as HIV positive fifteen years ago following a blood transfusion. Mr Maxwell developed AIDS five years ago and he has not responded to medication. Mr Maxwell has become very depressed and keeps telling his GP that he *'just wants everything to be over. The combination of haemophilia and AIDS means I'm never going to enjoy a fulfilling life, doesn't it?'* Mr Maxwell's medical team are keen to recruit him to a trial of a new drug that shows promise in treating even well-established AIDS, however, Mr Maxwell refuses to discuss the trial and asks that *'if you can't put me out of my misery, at least spare me the medical heroics'*. Mr Maxwell's GP, Dr Feinstein, recommends that Mr Maxwell should be transferred to a hospice, but the medical team are extremely unhappy about the proposed transfer believing that Mr Maxwell has *'a reasonably optimistic prognosis if developments in HIV pharmacology live up to their promise'*. In the interim, Mr Maxwell contracts pneumococcal pneumonia. What treatment (if any) should be offered to Mr Maxwell?

Mr Maxwell's case illustrates the conflicts that can arise when a patient refuses treatment for reasons that are perceived to be clinically ill-founded. However, a patient is likely to take into account more than simply the available clinical evidence when making decisions about future treatment and interventions. Do the medical team have an ethical duty to acknowledge that whilst the clinical evidence may suggest treatment should continue, Mr Maxwell (as an autonomous adult) is entitled to weigh the clinical evidence low down in his priorities when making a decision about his future care?

In one paper[155] exploring and comparing patients' and oncologists' reactions to refusals of treatment for cancer, the authors suggest that clinicians have an ethical duty to take a broader approach to treatment decisions than simply weighing the medical pros and cons of possible interventions. Patients, the authors suggest, must be seen *in context* because it is the patient's particular social context that is frequently determinative in the decision whether or not to accept further treatment (even when such treatment appears likely to be clinically successful).

It might be argued that Mr Maxwell's decision-making is potentially impaired by his depression. Certainly there is considerable evidence to suggest that patients with both chronic and terminal illnesses become depressed. Further, it is recommended that the patient's clinical depression must not be seen simply as an inevitable sadness arising from their circumstances. Where clinical depression in the terminally or chronically ill patient is diagnosed it should be treated accordingly, perhaps in conjunction with a psychiatrist.[156] However, the test for determining whether Mr Maxwell has the capacity to make an autonomous decision about his future treatment is no different from that used for any other patient.

If you need to remind yourself, the detailed discussion of capacity and its assessment is to be found in Chapter 3. In brief, if Mr Maxwell is able to comprehend and retain information about the treatment options and he is able to weigh that information up to reach a considered decision that he can communicate, then he has capacity to refuse treatment. If Mr Maxwell is conscious during his pneumonia, the use of antibiotics should be discussed with him and, if he makes an informed refusal of further intervention, his choice should be respected. If Mr Maxwell falls into unconsciousness before such a conversation can take place, the team will need to consider the wishes that he expressed prior to developing pneumonia. Mr Maxwell's words refer to '*medical heroics*'. Would the use of antibiotics be within the category of '*heroics*'? This situation demonstrates the immense difficulty that there can be in interpreting a patient's statements about future treatment. It is, of course, desirable that a

---

[155] Huijer, M., van Leeuwen, E. Personal Values and Cancer Treatment Refusal. *J Med Ethics* 2000; 26: 358–62.
[156] Kaye, P. *Decision Making in Palliative Care*. Northampton: EPL Publications, at pp. 95 ff.

calm and focused discussion about possible future interventions takes place between the healthcare team and the patient, but the realities of pressure in the NHS make such conversations increasingly difficult. Furthermore, it is always difficult to fully consider the entire range of potential developments and to require healthcare workers to do so would be to demand a wholly unreasonable level of 'crystal ball gazing'. If Mr Maxwell has appointed a LPA or has a valid advance decision, what happens next should reflect his wishes as expressed by either his proxy or the advance decision (see Chapter 3 for the details of both processes). If, however, there is neither a LPA nor an advance decision, the team will have to agree on what it means to act in Mr Maxwell's best interests based on what is known about his illness and previously expressed views. It is a difficult call and one cannot say with certainty what would be the 'right' course of action. However, it is important that whatever the conclusion, it can be justified and explained with reference to Mr Maxwell's previously articulated perspective and a definition of best interests that goes beyond the medical.

The patient and clinician in palliative care

The biomedical model of diagnosing and treating disease is reinterpreted in palliative care where the primary aim is the alleviation of suffering from a holistic perspective, and the focus is more likely to be on maximising quality, rather than quantity, of life. To understand what is meant by maximising quality of life, the patient and, if appropriate, the patient's carers must be involved in decision-making. There is an emphasis on advanced care planning in palliative care as a means of fulfilling patient's wishes when the patient's capacity may be impaired. The role of the multidisciplinary team is crucial in effecting the best possible quality (rather than quantity) of life for as Patricia Webb says 'patients may be suffering an unresolved past, an unsatisfactory present and a lost future'.[157]

Kenneth Calman[158] has argued that the amelioration of quality of life is inextricably linked to reducing the dissatisfaction that may

---

[157] Webb, P. (ed.) *Ethical Issues in Palliative Care: Reflections and Considerations.* Altrincham: Hochland and Hochland Ltd, 2000 at p. 27.

[158] Calman, K. Quality of Life in Cancer Patients: A Hypothesis. *J Med Ethics* 1984; 10: 124–7.

exist between what the patient hopes and expectation of life are and what the reality is. As such, telling the truth and fostering autonomy are essential to ethical palliative care. The sensitive and holistic management of chronic illness and dying are the aims of palliation. The medicalisation of death and dying means clinicians have a particular role in explaining what a non-medicalised death is likely to mean. However, as the case of Mr Hascombe (below) illustrates, the broad aims of palliative care, particularly when considered in the context of a stretched National Health Service, can create significant ethical dilemmas when deciding on treatment.

Case Study

Mr Hascombe is a 52-year-old man who has an advanced cerebral tumour, the symptoms of which cause him to be aggressive, distressed and disorientated for increasing periods of the day and night (although on occasion, he is calm if not completely lucid). Mr Hascombe is a patient on the general medical ward of a district hospital because there is no local hospice or specialised unit. Dr Khan would like to give Mr Hascombe Midazolam to sedate him and *give him some relief from his symptoms*. Nurse Malleson objects because *we might say that it is for Mr Hascombe's benefit but we really want him to take the Midazolam for our convenience*. Can Mr Hascombe consent to taking Midazolam? If he cannot consent to taking Midazolam, would Dr Khan be justified in giving it to Mr Hascombe anyway?

Mr Hascombe is unlikely to have capacity to consent to taking the Midazolam because, at this stage in his illness, he is insufficiently lucid to comprehend, retain and weigh up information about his treatment. Therefore, Mr Hascombe must be treated in his 'best interests'; is it in his best interests to leave him in an agitated, aggressive and distressed state on a busy ward? It would perhaps be a less difficult question to answer if Mr Hascombe did not have moments of calm. However, the case study states that these moments of calm fall short of lucidity, and it could be argued that it is morally justifiable to give Midazolam because the benefits to be gained from not using Midazolam to sedate Mr Hascombe are likely to be slight when compared to the benefits likely to follow from sedating Harry. Downie and Randall have argued[159] that where

---

[159] Randall, F., Downie, R. S. *Palliative Care Ethics: A Companion for All Specialties.* (2nd ed.) Oxford: Oxford University Press, 1999 at pp. 189 ff.

the behaviour of patients with dementia or confusion *'is threatening if not actually violent… it seems morally justifiable to sedate the confused patient as much as it is necessary to protect others from distress… In a more common example, we accept that confused patients who keep others awake at night should be sedated, whether they like it or not!'*

While it is possible to argue that there is a moral case for sedating Mr Hascombe with Midazolam because it is not in *his* best interests to be distressed and aggressive is on a busy ward, it is less easy to see the moral justification for sedating noisy and confused patients solely because they disturb other patients or even the clinical team. Presumably, the rationale for sedation is that the behaviour of the confused and noisy patient is adversely affecting the wellbeing of other patients to whom the healthcare team owes a duty. However, if this were accepted as a moral justification for sedating patients without consent, then perhaps newborn babies on the postnatal ward should be routinely sedated to prevent nocturnal crying disturbing post partum mothers?

Palliative care and relatives or carers

Palliative care focuses not only the needs of the patient, but also on the needs and concerns of the patient's family, carers and friends. For some patients though, the involvement of their family may add a further pressure to their lives. Palliative care may provide an opportunity for patients to reconcile and resolve personal and familial conflicts and tensions. However, if fostering and respecting autonomy is the pre-eminent ethical principle of palliative care, patients should not be compelled to accept well-meaning opportunities for reconciliation. In the case study below, the conflicts that may arise between the patient and his or her relatives are illustrated.

Case Study

Ms Launer, aged 36, is an unmarried woman who has advanced, primary progressive multiple sclerosis. She has been admitted to a hospice where she has been a patient on an intermittent basis for the last three years. Dr Wieden, the consultant, advises her that the MS is affecting her vital organs to such an extent that *'this time will be different from your previous stays with us'*. Ms Launer asks Dr Wieden whether he thinks she will die and when. Dr Wieden explains that he does expect her to die within the next eight weeks. Ms Launer asks Dr Wieden to tell his team that no one must reveal the likely imminence of her death to her mother whom she describes as *fragile and difficult*. Ms Launer explains that as long as her mother thinks that her daughter is in the hospice for respite care like her previous admissions, *'things will be okay between us, but if she knows I'm going to die she'll make my last few weeks a complete misery'*. Ms Launer's mother visits the hospice most days. What, if anything, should the palliative care team tell Ms Launer's mother about her daughter's condition?

This case illustrates how moral dilemmas about truth-telling may resonate even if all the obvious seductions to collusion, eg withholding the true diagnosis or prognosis from the patient, have been avoided. Ms Launer has made a clear and direct request that information about the severity of her condition remains confidential. She has also expressed a fear that if her mother knows the truth about her condition, psychological harm and emotional distress will ensue as a consequence of the disclosure. Ms Launer has capacity and therefore she is able to choose not to disclose the severity of her condition to her mother. If a clinician were not to respect Ms Launer's request, he or she would be riding roughshod over an autonomous and explicit request from a patient. Ms Launer's decision may not seem desirable or sensible to those caring for her, but it is a capacitous decision and, as such, should be respected. However, the palliative care team may want to explore with Ms Launer what she would like them to say to her mother if she asks questions when she visits her daughter. If there is regular, non-judgemental and supportive discussion between Ms Launer and the clinical team, she may feel that her decision is not irrevocable and the door is left open to change.

Palliative care and teamwork

A poorly functioning team in which rivalry and power struggles dominate the agenda will hinder the achievement of the ethical aims of palliation.[160] It is, as Jeffrey says,[161] important not only

---

[160] Ingham, J., Coyle, N. *'Teamwork in End of Life Care'* in Clark, D., Hockley, J., Ahmedzai, S. *New Themes in Palliative Care*. Buckingham: Open University Press, 1997.

[161] Jeffrey, D. *'Care Versus Cure'* in Webb, P. (ed.) *Ethical Issues in Palliative Care: Reflections and Considerations*. Altrincham: Hochland and Hochland Ltd, 2000 at p. 24.

to acknowledge and respect the autonomy of the patient but also the professional autonomy of other members of the healthcare team. It has frequently been suggested that the rest of healthcare could learn valuable lessons from the philosophy of holistic care that underpins palliative care. There is debate about the aims of palliative care and what each professional group contributes to those aims. Randall and Downie distinguish between the task of achieving a 'medical good' and the extrinsic aims of palliative care (ie the dealing with psychological or emotional distress). Randall and Downie maintain the distinction between the knowledge-based component of palliative care, and the wisdom-based component of palliative care in which psychological or spiritual needs are the focus because they wish *'to prevent the concept of palliative care becoming so wide that no training would qualify a person to undertake it, and no treatment could count as adequate'*.[162] It is the combined efforts of the diverse members of the palliative care team that results in a shared holistic aim. Functional teams meet and share their perspectives and knowledge, not to 'convert' others, but to contribute to the best quality of holistic care.

The diverse perspectives and experiences that can be such an asset within a functioning palliative care team can also create tensions and disagreements about the optimum way(s) in which to treat patients. The following case study illustrates the differences of opinion that can arise.

Case Study

Fenella Atkinson is eighteen years old and has leukaemia. She was diagnosed two years ago and has been looked after by the paediatric oncology and haematology teams at her local hospital. Initially, Fenella's leukaemia was treated aggressively with chemotherapy and she underwent a bone marrow transplant (her sister, Louisa, acted as the donor). However, six months ago the leukaemia returned and Fenella is adamant that she does not want any more treatment. Fenella's parents are desperate for *'all the stops to be pulled out'* for their daughter. Fenella asks that there be a meeting between the palliative care, oncology and haematology teams. There is considerable disagreement not only between the teams, but also within the teams themselves. Several

---

[162] Randall, F., Downie, R. S. *Palliative Care Ethics: A Companion for All Specialties.* (2nd ed.) Oxford: Oxford University Press, 1999 at p. 20.

members of staff suggest that Fenella is *'understandably scared of the traumatic treatment programme she'd have to go through again'*. A couple of nurses express the view that they would *'find it immensely difficult to care for such a young girl who need not necessarily die if only we could persuade her to give the chemo another try'*. What is the best outcome for Fenella? How can the teams work together to achieve your preferred outcome?

Fenella Atkinson has reached the age of majority. Had the facts in the case study arisen before she reached the age of eighteen, the palliative care team would have had to consider whether Fenella was *Gillick* competent (discussed at length in Chapter 5). As Fenella is eighteen years old, her capacity is presumed as for any other adult. Fenella must be informed about the implications of her refusal and she should be encouraged (but not pressured) to discuss her response to the information with her parents and the healthcare teams. There is an inevitable tension between, on the one hand, exploring the reasons for Fenella's refusal which is ethical practice, and on the other hand, subjecting Fenella's reasons and values to some sort of 'quality assessment' which is far from ethical practice. Fenella should know that her decision is not irrevocable, but as time passes it will be increasingly difficult to stop the progression of her disease. However distressing Fenella's choice may be for her parents, and however uneasy Fenella's position may make some of the healthcare team feel, if she has made an informed, voluntary and continuing decision to refuse treatment, respect for that decision must be ethical practice.

Dilemmas at the end of palliative care

As patients approach death, their needs and the needs of their family and carers will alter. The changing situation requires that ethical and moral issues are revisited and reconsidered. The case study below demonstrates how difficult it can be to support both the patient and the family as death approaches.

Case Study

Mrs Krowoski has ovarian cancer with metastatic disease of the bone and brain. She is being cared for at home by the community palliative care team. She has repeatedly asked 'to die in my own home'. Mrs Krowoski is one of the minority of patients in whom only partial pain control can be achieved. She develops a gastrointestinal obstruction and becomes distressed by the pain. Her husband, Mr Krowoski, is finding it increasingly difficult to care for his wife at home and their children are upset to see what their mother is enduring. Mr Krowoski pleads with the palliative care team to admit his wife to the hospice. The team discusses admission with Mrs Krowoski, but she is adamant she wants to remain at home. To whom do the palliative care team owe their primary duty? Should Mrs Krowoski be transferred from her home to the hospice?

Mrs Krowoski is the patient. However, there would be few teams who would not frame their duties to Mrs Krowoski without reference to her familial context. Mrs Krowoski clearly wishes to remain at home and for many people, home is the best place in which to receive palliative care. However, in some cases, particularly those involving patients like Mrs Krowoski for whom pain is not well-controlled; the burden of care (and attendant distress) that falls to the family is significant. Can Mr and Mrs Krowoski's perspectives be resolved?

One obvious, practical approach to this case may be to involve the services of a Macmillan nurse or similar support, who could provide greater home-based care. However, the resource implications of such a solution are significant and in many areas, such round-the-clock services will simply not be available.[163] There may be other sources of practical help that will enable Mr Krowoski to cope with his wife's needs and these should be explored. Communication and the negotiation of priorities at what is a time of heightened emotion and distress is essential. This is a situation in which the combined efforts of different members of the team, perhaps each focusing on a different aspect of the family's needs, may allow each party in the case to manage their distress and anxiety. It is unclear

---

[163] Indeed, a report published in June 2011 revealed considerable inequities, described as 'stunning' in the availability and provision of palliative care services in the United Kingdom; see *Palliative Care Funding Review: Final Report* – available at http://palliativecarefunding.org.uk [accessed 1 July 2011].

from the facts of the case study whether Mr and Mrs Krowoski have discussed their feelings with each other and this may be a conversation that could be facilitated by the palliative care team. The support of the palliative care team could be invaluable in helping the couple to communicate honestly with each other.

However, if Mr and Mrs Krowoski continue to disagree about where she should receive care in the final days of her life, to whom do the palliative care team owe their primary duty? Mrs Krowoski is the patient and the person with whom the team have the most direct therapeutic relationship. The autonomy and preferences of the patient are the team's primary concern. However, the situation has changed for Mrs Krowoski and in order for her to make a truly autonomous decision about her care, the palliative team should honestly discuss with her the medical advantages of admitting her to a specialist environment, and the implications of her refusal to be transferred. Randall and Downie argue that in cases such as these, it for the patients and their relatives to resolve the conflicts together. This is true, but the palliative care team has an important role in facilitating the process of reaching an agreement. It is perhaps because palliative care teams are so successful in this role that, as Randall and Downie comment, *'fortunately, in a climate of open discussion with willingness to review the decision it is very rare for an amicable solution not to be found'.*[164]

Conclusion

The available literature on ethics at the end of life and euthanasia is vast and encompasses philosophical analyses, legal critiques, policy proposals, empirical studies and theological perspectives. Medical students neither could nor should become familiar with the range of work that exists on the subject of euthanasia. However, it is helpful to understand the key issues that recur in debates and discussions about euthanasia and to consider one's own position in the context of the ethical frameworks or principles that you bring to your learning and future practice. It may be that you have a faith-based posi tion or a strong intuition about end-of-life care and euthanasia. Take the time to reflect on where your views come from and how someone who disagrees with you might

---

[164] Randall, F., Downie, R. S. *Palliative Care Ethics: A Companion for All Specialties.* (2nd ed.) Oxford: Oxford University Press, 1999 at p. 56.

challenge your opinions. At some stage in your medical school training, you will meet people who are dying, and their families. Revisit your own feelings in the light of those experiences: what would it mean to provide effective care to that person at the end of his or her life? Finally, some practising doctors will be open to discussing their own perspectives with you, perhaps as part of a mentoring relationship. Such conversations can be invaluable and are always memorable.

 # Core Concepts: End of Life

Basic principles apply at the end of life eg patients who have capacity should be involved in decision-making.
Where a patient lacks capacity, there may be a valid advance decision or third party appointed via the Lasting Power of Attorney provision to inform decision-making.
For some, the freedom to choose when and how one dies is an expression of autonomy and should be permitted in law.
For others, to permit assisted dying would be to begin a slippery slope in which individuals, particularly those who are older, sick or have disabilities, might feel obliged to end their lives prematurely.
The distinction between acts and omissions is often part of moral debates about end of life care ie the difference between giving a lethal injection (an act) and not ventilating a terminally ill patient (an omission). The distinction finds translation in the law and professional guidance on withholding and withdrawing treatment.
The case of Tony Bland confirmed that where a patient is in a persistent vegetative state, and unlikely to make any meaningful recovery, a court can authorise withdrawal of treatment.
The doctrine of double effect applies where a clinician appropriately prescribes treatment with the primary intention of alleviating suffering but also foresees that the treatment may have secondary effects.
R v Cox was a case in which the doctrine of double effect did not apply because Cox gave the patient an injection of potassium chloride which is not used to treat rheumatoid arthritis and is commonly believed not to have a double effect.

Following the case of Debbie Purdy, the Director of Public Prosecutions issued new guidance in which he set out the factors that would influence the decision whether or not to prosecute someone who assisted in another's death. However, it remains illegal to assist another person to die.

The debate about changing the law on assisted dying continues with passionate arguments from campaigners on both sides.

End of life and medical students

Seeing patients at the end of life can evoke strong and mixed emotions. The first time that you encounter someone dying or witness a death is memorable and can be distressing. Many people go into medicine if not to cure, then to improve health or quality of life. To meet people to whom medicine can apparently offer little is a stark and sometimes unwelcome reminder that medicine is limited. For some students the visible evidence of medicine's limitations is frightening and upsetting; it may challenge what one thought about the value of medicine and working as a doctor. For other students, particularly those who are fortunate to witness high quality clinical care at the end of life, the experience of seeing staff support a patient in achieving a 'good death' can be revelatory, comforting and even uplifting.

End-of-life care prompts strong emotions and it is important not to diminish or deny those feelings. Learning to accept loss and death is part of becoming a doctor. To feel sadness and regret is a sign of empathy and compassion. However, for some, the distress may become more significant and debilitating perhaps because the death of a patient has been a reminder of personal loss, suffering or bereavement. A wise and supportive mentor or tutor can be a source of help if you should find yourself struggling with the emotions you feel. For a small number, it can be useful to talk to a counsellor about the emotions evoked by end of life care. The important message is not to be alone or to struggle on without seeking support.

Many students (and practising clinicians) will have strongly-held personal views about the acceptability or otherwise of assisted dying. Indeed, one of the most recent campaign groups to argue for changing the law to permit assisted dying largely comprises healthcare professionals,[165] and there are groups of clinicians who offer a different perspective on the issues.[166] In teaching sessions it is common for discussions, while courteous, to become intense and animated. It is not problematic to have feelings about end-of-life care in general, and the specific questions relating to assisted dying. Indeed, it may be inevitable or even desirable. However, it is important to be aware of one's own values, beliefs and preferences and have insight into how these might inform one's professional practice. In some ways, the fact that assisted dying remains illegal limits the extent to which the personal potentially conflicts with the professional, yet for some students, the day-to-day care of people at the end of life can raise fundamental questions about the value of life, the nature of personhood and the purpose of medicine and healthcare. Taking the time to explore, in a safe environment, the ways in which your own experiences and beliefs might shape the ways in which you perceive and respond to clinical situations is time well spent.

Assessments: End-of-Life in practice

There are some sample questions that relate to end of life issues in Chapter 2. This section contains some more examples of both written questions and OSCE stations that relate to end of life decision-making.

1. Relatives and resuscitation

> You are working on a general medical firm at a large hospital. You have been looking after Harry Quast, aged 76, who has had congestive heart failure for three years. Mr Quast was originally admitted with pulmonary oedema to the Intensive Care Unit (ICU) where he was intubated and ventilated. On the second day in the ICU, Mr Quast had ventricular fibrillation from which he was successfully resuscitated. Mr Quast is now on a general medical ward, and he is alert and aware. Susie Mantini, the patient's daughter, regularly visits her father on the ward. Mrs Mantini has asked if she can *'have a private word'* with you.

---

[165] Healthcare Professionals for Assisted Dying (HPAD); see www.hpad.org.uk
[166] See, for example, the Christian Medical Fellowship: www.cmf.org.uk

Mrs Mantini tells you that she has been watching her father become *'ever sicker'* and *'less able to cope to the point where he really has no life at all'.* She tells you that when her father was in ICU, she saw him having ventricular fibrillation and heard the resuscitation from outside the cubicle. Mrs Mantini feels that the resuscitation was *'brutal, shocking and demeaning'.* Mrs Mantini asks whether *'it would be possible to decide Dad shouldn't be resuscitated in case it happens again'.* Mrs Mantini stresses that she is *'really grateful for everything you're doing for Dad, but it can't be right to stick needles and tubes in him to bring him back to a life barely worth living',* adding *'he's had a good life, and I don't want to prolong his suffering'.*

Please discuss Mrs Mantini's request.

Guidance notes

The scenario requires a sound knowledge of decision-making with regard to resuscitation and DNAR orders. It is an area of clinical practice that can be confusing and as a student on the wards you may see wide variation in practice. What follows is a description of optimal practice regarding resuscitation decision-making.

- DNAR orders are overseen by the consultant in charge of a patient's care but should involve the multidisciplinary team and if, as is the case with Mr Quast, the patient has capacity, the patient himself and anyone whom the patient nominates. Indeed the UK Resuscitation Council recommends that the agreement of every member of the clinical team should be verified if possible and advises that, in the event of doubt, further senior clinical advice should be sought.
- It is important to discuss DNAR decision-making openly and honestly, being clear about what is factually true and what is uncertain, and without assumption. Remember what you, as a medical student, understand about resuscitation is not necessarily known by Mr Quast and his daughter.
- Mrs Manitini is likely to be frightened, tired and upset at what has happened to her father. However, she is not the patient – Mr Quast is – and it is essential to remember that throughout this challenging discussion.

- You are going to have to tell Mrs Mantini that you are unable to discuss her father's care without his express permission ie this is a scenario where you will have to demonstrate empathy for her whilst remaining firm about the boundaries of clinical confidentiality. For further information on confidentiality see Chapter 3.
- You are likely to have to respond calmly in the face of emotion. Mrs Mantini will probably express frustration and even anger. However, although you cannot discuss her capacitous father's care with her in detail, you are able to both listen to, and acknowledge the legitimacy of, her distress, concerns and anxieties.
- Mr Quast is, we can reasonably assume, capacitous. Despite being seriously ill a few days previously, he is alert and aware of what is happening to him. As such, Mr Quast is entitled to make his own choices about his care and to decide who, if anyone, he wishes to involve.
- The first task therefore is to explain clearly and sensitively to Mrs Mantini that you are unable to discuss her father without his permission. It is important to remember that there is a difference between simply telling Mrs Mantini that you cannot give her any information, and *explaining* kindly and courteously why you are not able to talk to her about her father, eg you should explain to Mrs Mantini how and why healthcare decisions about capacitous adults are made when considering resuscitation status. It is possible to have a general discussion with Mrs Mantini about her concerns whilst remaining alert to verbal and nonverbal cues without breaching her father's confidentiality or promising a DNAR order will be made.
- A DNAR order cannot be made simply because Mrs Mantini has asked for it. Mrs Mantini may ask whether you would be willing to make such a decision and *'not tell'* her father – the answer should be that DNAR orders cannot be made without a patient's knowledge on the basis of a family member's request.
- In this case, if Mr Quast is capacitous, it is for him to reflect on whether and when he believes that resuscitation would be too burdensome or deleterious to his dignity. His resuscitation status should be discussed with him sensitively and clearly, avoiding euphemisms

('we wondered if you wanted any heroics?', 'do you want us to pull out the stops?' etc).[167] He may or may not wish to involve his daughter in these discussions.

- It may be possible to facilitate a discussion between Mrs Mantini and Mr Quast, but proceed with caution as it is Mr Quast's decision whether or not to share information with his daughter because he is the capacitous patient.
- Avoid making judgemental comments about either Mr Quast's quality of life or Mrs Mantini's perception of her father's quality of life. All resuscitation decision-making should be predicated on an individual assessment of each patient with opportunities for discussion and review.
- Aim to maintain an organised, calm and empathic approach throughout.

2. **Decisions at the end of life**

Sample EMI

Mr Hailsham, who has is 65 and has severe Parkinson's disease, develops a life-threatening pneumonia in a UK hospital. He has told medical staff that he does not want any more attempts at cardiopulmonary resuscitation. Mr Hailsham develops respiratory failure and deteriorates. When he relapses into unconsciousness, his family insists that treatment continues. Dr Mahmood decides to ventilate Mr Hailsham.

EMI: Questions

When answering questions (i)–(iii) below, choose the most appropriate answer from the list that follows:

A   The doctor has acted correctly.
B   The family are entitled to consent to the ventilation of this incapacitated patient.
C   The patient is entitled to ask the medical team not to resuscitate him again.
D   The doctor's behaviour is paternalistic.

---

[167] Ebrahim, S. Do Not Resuscitate Decisions: Flogging Dead Horses or A Dignified Death? *BMJ* 2000; 320: 1155–1156.

E The doctor need not obey the patient's wishes as it is not written down.

F The doctor's behaviour is beneficent.

G Patients over the age of 65 are not able to decide whether or not they wish to be resuscitated; it is a decision for the healthcare team

H No one is legally allowed to consent for another adult, but relatives might represent or advocate the patient's views to the healthcare team.

I Patients have to express their wishes about resuscitation explicitly otherwise it is up to the doctor to decide.

J Patients can nominate a proxy via the LPA process to act on their behalf in healthcare decision-making if they become incapacitated.

EMI: Answers

(i) Which statement below describes the role a capacitous patient has in resuscitation decision-making?

Answer: Statement C

(ii) Which statement reflects the ethical model the doctor is adopting by ventilating the patient?

Answer: Statement D

(iii) Which statement describes the position of relatives in respect of decision-making?

Answer: Statement J

3. **Resuscitation decisions**

Sample SAQ

You are working on a general medical firm and the consultant, Dr Walton, explains that all NHS Trusts are now obliged to have guidelines on issuing DNAR orders. Dr Walton says that he tends to consider DNAR orders where he believes treatment to be futile.

(a) Suggest five points that should be included in guidance on issuing DNAR orders. (5 marks)

(b) Suggest five difficulties that can occur in practice even guidance on issuing DNAR orders exists (5 marks)

(c) What does 'futile' mean? (3 marks)

Guidance notes

Part (a)   The United Kingdom Resuscitation Council lists the following as key points for inclusion in all Trust 'not for CPR' guidelines:

- It is important to involve capacitous patients in decisions.
- When a patient lacks capacity, staff should consider whether there is a) a valid advance decision that refers to the patient's preferences about resuscitation or b) someone who has lasting power of attorney.
- In the absence of either a valid advance decision or lasting power of attorney, relatives might be asked to represent the wishes of the patient. It should be made clear to relatives in such a situation that they are not being asked to determine the outcome but to advocate the wishes of an incapacitous patient.
- Communication, explanation and documentation are essential at all stages in the resuscitation decision-making process.
- Trusts must have resuscitation guidelines that adheres to the United Kingdom Resuscitation Council policy and should be updated in accordance with changes to the national policy.
- Consultants should be responsible for DNAR decisions.
- Decisions must be reviewed frequently.
- Children should be treated as a separate category when taking 'not for CPR' decisions.

Part (b)   The difficulties that can occur in respect of DNAR orders irrespective of the existence of guidance include:

- Awareness of guidelines may be extremely low.
- Discussion of DNAR status with patients may be ethically desirable but difficult to implement in practice.

- Involvement of a senior colleague may not be practical in an emergency situation or at certain times of day/night resulting in sub-optimal decisions.
- Discussions may take place but not be adequately documented or communicated to other members of the healthcare team.
- Guidelines may encourage conflation of judgements about 'quality of life' and the meaning of 'clinical futility'.
- The role of relatives or other parties close to the patient may not be well-understood.
- Valid advance decisions remain relatively rare and continue to be poorly-understood by healthcare staff
- LPA can be perceived as burdensome and staff may avoid engaging honestly with the person who holds LPA.
- Where there is neither a valid advance decision nor someone with LPA, DNAR orders have to be made on the basis of best interests, which can be difficult to evaluate accurately eg the term 'best interests' can be used without reference to legal concept of 'best interests' nor the GMC guidance on the determination of best interests.
- It should be understood and made clear that ongoing therapies should not cease as a result of DNAR status eg pain relief, hydration etc
- Guidelines do not address other difficult dilemmas that may surround resuscitation eg should relatives witness resuscitation attempts?
- Guidelines should be accompanied by education and support for staff who may not be skilled or confident in implementing guidelines.

Part (c)   The meaning of futility:
- Clinical futility has a specific meaning in ethical literature; namely, that there is an

extremely high probability that the patient's quality of life is demonstrably so very poor as not to be commensurate with the extreme pain, suffering or distress (physical or emotional) being experienced and therefore attempts to prolong the patient's life cannot be justified.

- It is frequently invoked to support decisions to withdraw treatment or make DNAR orders. There is inevitably an element of value judgement in reaching such a determination and where a patient has capacity it is desirable to discuss the patient's perception of his or her own quality of life.
- Where a patient tells clinicians that his or her quality of life does not fall within the definition, it is more difficult to make a legitimate case for futility.

4. Palliative care

Sample SAQ

Pamina Desai is a 65-year-old woman who has lung cancer. She is extremely unwell and in considerable pain. Dr Taylor, Pamina's oncologist, suggests that she might benefit from referral to the palliative care team.

(a) What ethical issues should be considered when referring a patient to palliative care? (3 marks)

Pamina finds the palliative care team extremely helpful. As she becomes sicker, Pamina becomes an inpatient at the hospice. Pamina's sister visits from her home in France. Pamina tells the clinical team that she does not want to see her sister and explains that they have been estranged for many years. Pamina tells the consultant in charge of the palliative care team, Dr Kitching, that she does not want him to tell her sister anything about her condition.

(b) How should the clinical team at the hospice respond to Pamina's refusal to see her sister? (2 marks)

Guidance notes

Part (a)   What ethical issues should be considered when referring a patient to palliative care?

- Clinicians need to be able to explain the reality of a non-medicalised death and this may not be a skill for which individual experience or training has necessarily prepared them.
- Provision of palliative care services remains inconsistent nationally and the resource implications of such inconsistency may inform referral decisions in such a way as to be ethically questionable, and this compromises the clinician's role as 'advocate' for a patient's individual needs.
- The timing of the referral is not only important from the perspective of maximising autonomy but also affects the extent to which palliation is likely to be in the patient's best interests ie it should occur at the point at which the patient is likely to achieve maximum benefit.

Part (b)   How should the palliative care team respond to Pamina's refusal to see her estranged sister or to allow anyone to talk to her sister about her care?

- If Pamina has capacity as set out in the Mental Capacity Act 2005 (ie she can comprehend, retain and weigh up information so as to make a decision that she can communicate), she is entitled to the same level of confidentiality and choice about all aspects of her care as any other capacitous adult.

- No one can oblige Pamina to see her sister or to give permission for information about her medical care to be shared with her sister.

5. Assisted dying

Sample SAQ

Mrs Rita Prior has severe rheumatoid arthritis. Mrs Prior approaches her consultant, Dr Lee, and tells him that she *'couldn't bear much more pain in the future'*. She asks whether there is anything *'you could do, Dr Lee, to put me out of my misery if it comes to it? I really wouldn't want to go on'*. Dr Lee is alarmed by Mrs Prior's request and recalls the well-known case of Dr Cox in which a doctor responded unlawfully when managing a patient's pain as a result of rheumatoid arthritis.

(a) In the case of *R. v Cox*, how did Dr Cox, the doctor concerned, respond to his patient, Mrs Lillian Boyes?

(1 mark)

(b) Of what offence was Dr Cox convicted? (1 mark)

(c) Why did the fact that Dr Cox's intentions were kindly not affect the outcome of the case? (2 marks)

(d) Explain what is meant by the doctrine of double effect.

(3 marks)

(e) Why do you think the 'doctrine of double effect' defence was not accepted in the case of *R v Cox*? (1 mark)

(f) Suggest two ethical issues that a doctor should consider when treating a patient in chronic pain. (2 marks)

Guidance notes

Part (a)   How did Dr Cox respond to Mrs Boyes?

- Dr Cox administered a fatal dose of potassium chloride in response to repeated requests by the patient and her immediate family for him to assist her with her pain.

Part (b)   Of what offence was Dr Cox convicted?

- He was convicted of attempted murder (the patient's body had been cremated so it was not possible to prove causation and charge him with murder).

Part (c)   Why did the fact that Dr Cox's intentions were kindly not affect the outcome of the case?

- Because his actions constituted an intentional act with the aim of assisting Mrs Boyes death which is unlawful.

Part (d)   Explain what is meant by the 'doctrine of double effect'.

- The doctrine of double effect is the mechanism by which the criminal law distinguishes between intention and foresight.
- The name of the doctrine is a description of the dual consequences that may result from a particular type of treatment.
- Thus, in treating chronic pain, a doctor may foresee that a particular treatment will have potentially harmful consequences but his or her intention is not to harm, but is rather to alleviate pain. Therefore, his or her actions will not be culpable under the criminal law.

Part (e)   Why did the doctrine of double effect not apply in the case of *R. v Cox*?

- Because Dr Cox injected Ms Boyes with two ampoules of potassium chloride which was regarded by the majority of experts giving evidence at the trial as having no analgesic value.

Part (f)   Suggest two ethical issues that a doctor should consider when treating a patient in chronic pain.

- Any two of the following:
    - It may be difficult to respect patient autonomy if they wish to use unlawful methods of pain relief (eg illegal drugs)
    - The distinction between beneficence and non-maleficence can be unclear if analgesia has significant side effects

- The doctor may become involved in making subjective quality of life judgements
- Dependence on medication may become a problem which, in turn, affects the doctor's duty of care to his or her patient
- Properly informed consent may be overlooked or difficult to obtain in an encounter with a patient who is in chronic pain
- Doctors may find it difficult to be truthful with patients about the likely consequences of living with chronic pain
- Doctors may struggle with their duty of confidentiality if they believe a patient is finding it difficult to manage their pain

Chapter 10

Rights and Wrongs: Human Rights and Global Ethics

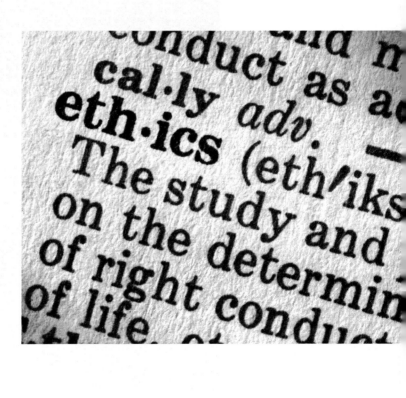

Rights and Wrongs: Human Rights and Global Ethics

Introduction

It is commonplace to hear people say that they *'know their rights'*. It is a lay expression but nonetheless reflects the status of a 'right' as a fundamental entitlement about which there can be no argument and that must not be denied. This chapter explores the place of rights in ethics and law and includes a brief overview of the statutory enactment of rights in the Human Rights Act 1998 which came into force at the start of the twenty-first century (1st October 2000).

The second part of the chapter focuses on global health and the attendant ethics. Most of the ethics and law that students training in the developed world experience during their training takes a domestic view of healthcare. For some, that is inevitable because the medical curriculum is crowded and the majority of students will go on to work in the particular environment of the NHS. However, increasingly it is seen as valuable for medical students to develop a global perspective on health and to develop in all future doctors an understanding of the wider context in which health, disease and clinical care are experienced by others. This chapter contains a section on electives overseas and some of the particular ethical questions that can arise in relation to medical student electives.

There is a natural link between human rights and global health. The rights to health, life, liberty and freedom from torture are all partially or completely unknown for people living in certain parts of the world. Whilst there have been high-profile cases involving questions of rights in the UK (and some of those are discussed in this chapter), it is undoubtedly the case that by taking a global perspective on health and healthcare, the importance of rights, both moral and legal, becomes clear and urgent.

Human rights and healthcare

The language of rights is not new; the Magna Carta, in the thirteenth century, referred to individual rights. In more recent times, it has been the traumatic legacy of war and conflict that has contributed to the development of human rights. Following the Second World War, the United Nations was created and the Universal Declaration of Human Rights was developed.[168] The United Nations continues to be a focus for the promotion and protection of human rights across the world, often concentrating its efforts on particular groups or situations according to priority. Within Europe, the establishment of the Council of Europe led to the development of the European Convention on Human Rights. Non-governmental organisations play a significant part in the enactment of human rights in particular areas of life. For example, in the area of health and healthcare, the World Health Organisation leads the way in disseminating an empirical account of global health inequalities and developing standards of care that promote and protect human rights across the world.[169] On the ground, organisations such as Médecins Sans Frontier, the Red Cross and Doctors of the World provide local aid and work to protect health often in situations of war, conflict or natural disaster.

Simply expressed, rights are fundamental and minimal entitlements. Human rights are protected via laws, treaties, covenants and agreements. Underpinning rights are values such as equality, dignity, freedom, respect and autonomy. The incorporation of the European Convention of Human Rights into national law in the form of the Human Rights Act 1998 (HRA 1998) marked a legal sea change in its introduction of a rights-based analysis of human activity. The HRA 1998 contains broad provisions that describe human rights in general terms. The box below describes the specific Articles of the HRA 1998.

---

[168] The Universal Declaration of Human Rights was developed at the same time as the National Health Service and the anniversary of both was marked by the Department of Health; see *Human Rights in Action* (2nd ed.) London: Department of Health, 2008.

[169] The World Health Organisation's Constitution states that *'the enjoyment of the highest attainable standard of health is one of the fundamental rights of every human being without distinction'*.

The Articles of the Human Rights Act 1998[170]

1.	Obligation to respect human rights
2.	Right to life
3.	Prohibition of torture
4.	Prohibition of slavery and forced labour
5.	Right to liberty and security
6.	Right to a fair trial
7.	No punishment without law
8.	Right to respect for private and family life
9.	Freedom of thought, conscience and religion
10.	Freedom of expression
11.	Freedom of assemble and association
12.	Right to marry and found a family
14.	Prohibition of discrimination

The articles within the HRA 1998 have different status. Articles 3 (prohibition of torture, inhuman or degrading treatment or punishment), 4 (prohibition of slavery and forced labour) and 7 (no punishment without law) are absolute rights from which no derogation is permitted. In contrast, articles 8–12 are qualified rights where derogation is permitted. Any derogation must be necessary in a democratic society, based in law, proportionate, consistent with the aims of the original European Convention on Human Rights and non-discriminatory. For all but the absolute rights, the HRA 1998 is interpreted in the context of existing legislation. If current law prevents a public body acting in accordance with the HRA 1998, the court has the power to declare the legislation to be 'incompatible' with the Act (but not to repeal or otherwise to set aside the offending statutory provision).

The provisions of the HRA 1998 apply to public bodies such as NHS Trusts. In practical terms, the Act's reach extends to clinicians working for a NHS Trust. There is considerable potential for human rights to influence clinical practice. Looking at the list of articles above, you will see the scope for a rights-based analysis of areas of practice. For example, the prohibition of discrimination precludes particular groups from being treated differently within

---

[170] Article 13, which provides for the right to secure an effective remedy from a national authority following a breach of rights, has been omitted because it has not been incorporated into the Human Rights Act 1998.

the NHS, for instance on the grounds of age or sexuality. The right to liberty may have implications for public health powers of detention. The right to a private and family life is relevant to confidentiality and the holding of clinical data. The right for life has formed the basis for a number of high-profile medical cases, some of which have already been discussed in this book.[171] Respect for human rights means protecting the most vulnerable which is essential to healthcare. Increasingly, regulators and those who review the quality of care that is provided in health and social care will consider the extent to which human rights are promoted and protected in their reports.

An area of clinical practice that illustrates the potential tensions between protecting human rights and the utilitarian principles on which the NHS operates is that of public health and communicable diseases. The traditional approach in Western medical ethics is to consider the moral issues attendant on an encounter between an individual clinician and patient. In general, ethico-legal duties, entitlements and dilemmas are understood to flow from a dyadic (and often one-off) encounter. It is perhaps not surprising that this particular model of the medical encounter has come to dominate given that medical training and the regulation of the profession by the GMC tend to emphasise the role of the doctor as an advocate for the individual patient. Alongside the normative framework of professional training and regulation sits the Human Rights Act 1998 which requires clinicians to think about individual freedoms. Yet, the problems posed by communicable diseases are significant. Urban areas in the UK have, in recent times, faced the challenges posed by an outbreak of tuberculosis. Internationally, the fight is even greater: the World Health Organisation (WHO) has described failings in tuberculosis control as 'a global emergency'. Adherence on the part of those who are diagnosed with tuberculosis is vital if relapse and the development of drug resistant disease are to be avoided. What powers should public health practitioners have in respect of patients who are smear-positive and are erratic about treatment regimes? Should public health practitioners have the power to compulsorily detain such patients and, if so, what are the implications for the human rights of those so detained?

---

[171] See the discussion of the cases involving Diane Pretty and Ms B in Chapter 8.

The moral rationale for compulsory detention is generally said to be the utilitarian argument that the effect of compulsory detention on individual autonomy is a smaller loss than the potential damage such an individual may cause to society if he or she is not detained. However, given that patients with TB are frequently already 'marginalised' within society, it has been suggested that such measures are indicative of discrimination which is, of course, explicitly prohibited under the Human Rights Act 1998. Richard Coker[172] has led the way in examining the tension between human rights and public health in his career. He argues[173] that ethical practice demands that clinically informed assessment of risk, which is based in evidence, and the exploration of less restrictive alternative approaches to adherence must precede any move towards compulsion. Approaches to TB and its treatment vary considerably depending on the jurisdiction. Famously, for example, the city of New York introduced legislation to authorise the compulsory detention and treatment of people with TB. Such approaches are rare in the UK; although there are powers of compulsion within the Public Health legislation, education and negotiation are the preferred ways of working for many clinicians. The medical anthropologist, Ian Harper, suggests that the discourse over the last decade has shifted from compulsion to patient-centred approaches to care,[174] a shift that is congruent with the change in conceptualising patient involvement with healthcare as adherence and concordance rather than compliance.

Inevitably, ethical questions and values underpin the response to non-adherent patients who have communicable diseases. For those who prioritise liberty, any infringement of a person's individual rights and freedoms is a significant matter that should be embarked

---

[172] See, for example, Coker, R.J. Communicable Health Disease Control and Contemporary Themes in Public Health Law. *Public Health* 2006; 120: Supplement 23–8; Coker, R. J., Thomas, M., Lock, K., Martyn, R. Detention and the Evolving Threat of Tuberculosis: Evidence, Ethics and Law. *The Journal of Law, Medicine and Ethics* 2007; 35(4): 609–615; Atun, R. A., MnKee, M., Coker, R. J., Gurol-Urganci, I. Health Systems' Responses to 25 Years of HIV in Europe: Inequalities Persist and Challenges Remain. *Health Policy* 2008; 86(2): 181–194.

[173] Coker, R.J. Tuberculosis, Non-Compliance and Detention for the Public Health. *J Med Ethics* 2000; 26: 157–159.

[174] Extreme Condition, Extreme Measures? Compliance, Drug Resistance and the Control of TB. *Anthropology & Medicine* 2010; 17(2): 201–214.

upon only when there is evidence to suggest that to detain and/ or treat people against their wishes is effective proportionate to the restriction imposed upon them. For others, the nature of the therapeutic relationship is one of trust and many of those who are most at risk of communicable diseases may be suspicious of authority figures already; any attempts at coercion inevitably compromises the trust between doctor and patient and is damaging, counterproductive and unacceptable. Many commentators note the socio-economic and political factors that shape the prevalence and experience of TB across the world, arguing that the risk discourse which dominates interventions, such as quarantine and compulsory testing and treatment, isolates the most vulnerable from the most globally advantaged taking a reductionist and constraining approach to the ethical questions that arise.[175] Those who prefer a more utilitarian or communitarian approach might argue that effective public health depends on a population perspective which may result in individual losses to freedom in the interests of the wider wellbeing of society. As Len Doyal notes, the question of what constitutes a sufficient 'interest' on the part of society is crucial when weighing the acceptability or otherwise of compulsory treatment. For example, Doyal argues that coercion and compulsion might be justifiable if a longer term and more disseminated benefit to society can be demonstrated that goes beyond the short-term benefits of limiting a local outbreak.[176] In thinking about your own perspective on the tension between individual human rights and public health, consider the case study below.

Case Study

There has been an outbreak of tuberculosis at a local hostel. The situation is being compounded by the non-adherence of the majority of the patients to the treatment regime. You have been asked to advise the hostel's medical team on strategies to improve adherence to the treatment that are ethically and legally sound. What strategies would you suggest and how would you support your approach?

---

[175] Stephenson, P.H, Woodward, E. *Tuberculosis and the Ethics of Global Health Care* in Loewen, G. (ed.) *Evaluating the Scholarly Achievement of Professor Elvi Whittaker: Essays in Philosophical Anthropology*. Lewiston, NY: Mallen Press, 2010.
[176] Doyal, L. Moral Problems in the Use of Coercion in Dealing with Non-Adherence in the Diagnosis and Treatment of TB. *Ann N Y Acad Sci* 2001; 953: 208–215.

Traditionally, practitioners working in public health were considered to work in an exceptional healthcare environment. Indeed, one commentator has likened the situation of the public health practitioner to that of a soldier fighting a war in which the '*usual rules and laws*' do not apply.[177] Military analogies aside, thinking about public health and human rights as enacted in the prevention and treatment of infectious disease is to reveal the inherent tensions, complexities and challenges of this particular area of ethico-legal practice. It is a field where theoretical approaches to ethics – rights, principles of autonomy, utilitarianism and communitarianism – collide and sometimes conflict. It is up to you how you respond to the ethical questions that arise, but these are questions that cannot be ignored.

Global health and ethics

There are many ways in which to consider medical ethics from a global perspective. Indeed, as with all the topics covered in this book, there are people who make a life's work of studying one or two aspects of what is discussed here. This section is intended to introduce the issues that fall within the broad heading of global health ethics, using some specific examples to illustrate the questions and analysis. As always, further reading and resources are included in the footnotes and the Appendix at the back of the book.

Cultural competence

A fundamental issue in global health and its attendant ethics involves understanding culture and its effects on the provision and experience of healthcare. For those who travel and work overseas, the notion of the culture shock will be familiar. Indeed, cultural change is one of the reasons why we travel. Cultural awareness and cultural sensitivity might therefore be considered two of the desirable characteristics or behaviours in medical students, doctors and others who go to work overseas; the virtues of global health practitioners if you like. It is worth taking a moment to think about what culture means. A working definition might be that culture describes a shared framework of values, beliefs, attitudes and

---

[177] Burr, C. 'The AIDS Exception: Privacy vs. Public Health' in Beauchamp, D., Steinbock, B. (Eds) *New Ethics for the Public's Health*. Oxford: Oxford University Press, 1999.

behaviour which inform how people live their lives. Often we only become aware of culture when it is new or different from that to which we are used. Culture not only influences the art, literature, food, political system and living arrangements of a society, it also influences health both in terms of the healthcare system and the health beliefs of those within the system. It is worth pausing for a moment to reflect on what constitutes your 'culture' and whether you have specific beliefs about health as a result.

There is a growing literature on how cultural differences and distinctiveness can influence the provision of healthcare. Remember that one does not need to travel to experience diverse cultural beliefs about health; most medical students and doctors encounter a range of cultures and pluralistic beliefs on a daily basis. Examples of the ways in which cross-cultural interactions between patients and clinicians can create ethical dilemmas include differences in belief about the extent to which bad news should be honestly disclosed; the ways in which symptoms, particularly in certain diseases, are interpreted; and the effect of patriarchal family dynamics on medical decision-making. One of the aims of medical education might be therefore to develop students and future doctors who are culturally competent. Cultural competence is defined by Carter as *'the ability of a healthcare provider to function effectively in the context of cultural differences with the clients he or she serves.*[178] However, Carter prefers the term 'cultural engagement' to the more common 'cultural competence' which, he argues, depends on a curious, respectful approach that neither stereotypes nor perceives culture as a 'problem' to be solved. For Michael Paasche-Orlow, cultural competence is *'A matter of basic ethics [...] culturally competent care is a moral good that emerges from an ethical commitment to patient autonomy and justice. [...] In this sense, cultural competence and Western medical ethics are largely mutually supportive movements.'*[179] Paasche-Orlow goes on to suggest that the culturally competent have three aims, namely to (i) acknowledge the significance of culture; (ii) demonstrate respect for culture; and (iii) minimise the negative consequences of cultural difference. Insoo Hyun[180] suggests that

---

[178] Carter, R. T. Back to the Future in Cultural Competence Training. *The Counselling Psychologist* 2001; 29: 787–789.

[179] Paasche-Orlow, M. The Ethics of Cultural Competence. *Acad Med* 2004; 79(4): 347–350.

[180] Hyun, I. Clinical Cultural Competence and the Threat of Ethical Relativism. *Cambridge Quarterly of Healthcare Ethics* 2008; 17(2): 154–163.

a healthcare professional, future or practising, must make three commitments namely to (i) accept the significance of cultural diversity; (ii) attend to the influence of culture on the healthcare experience; and (iii) work to develop practical interventions that are sensitive and responsive to cultural difference and its effect on health and illness.

Cultural relativism

There are practices which occur globally that are considered desirable in some societies and unethical in others; many of which raise questions about cultural relativism. Essentially, cultural relativism is predicated on the assertion that there are no moral absolutes and that our perceptions of what is right and wrong are based on social norms. Our ethical beliefs will therefore be subject to change and reinterpretation according to context, time, location and environment. In brief, a cultural relativist perspective asserts that we should be wary of, and avoid, making statements of absolute morality. Cultural relativism argues that, in the words of John Ladd, *'the moral rightness and wrongness of actions vary from society to society ... there are not absolute universal moral standards on all [humans] at all times.... whether or not it is right for an individual to act in a certain way depends on or is relative to the society to which he [or she] belongs.'*[181]

Cultural relativism itself can be divided into two categories: descriptive and prescriptive relativism. As you might expect, descriptive relativism describes an account of the empirical realities or facts of differing moral standards and beliefs. Prescriptive relativism denotes a claim that one ought not to apply the morality of one group to another. The claim of prescriptive relativism is, in itself, moral in character in that it asserts that it is wrong to judge the relative morality of different groups. As with most ethical theories, there are attractions in cultural relativism. A relativist perspective fits well with a global view of the world in which plurality, diversity and difference are not merely tolerated but celebrated. Relativism implies tolerance, liberalism and respect. Inherent in relativism is scepticism about universal truths and experiences and it is an approach that avoids privileging particular groups or nations.

---

[181] Ladd, J. *Ethical Relativism*. Belmont, CA: Wadsworth, 1973.

However, and again like most ethical theories and frameworks, there are difficulties with relativism: it can tend to assumptions that culture is homogenous and uniform within a particular society, and it may militate against constructive criticism and dialogue and perhaps sets up a false dichotomy, in which one is either relativist or absolutist, leading to stagnate ethical debate.[182]

Whether one is persuaded by cultural relativism as an approach, it has made a valuable contribution in responding to the questions of intercultural moral evaluation. Even if one ultimately rejects a relativist approach, by considering its claims one has to engage with important questions about how we can judge the ethical standards and actions of other people who do not share our cultural background. It is generally argued that cultural relativism and cultural competence are limited by ethical practice which has to be alert to pluralism, harm and legal boundaries whatever the location and social environment. Cultural variety is not inherently or always moral.

Female genital mutilation: an example

Female Genital Mutilation (FGM) refers to the partial or total removal of the external female genitalia. FGM is usually performed by a traditional practitioner without anaesthetic, sterile procedures or surgical instruments. Unfortunately, mortality and serious complications, both in the short and longer term, are common particularly when traditional FGM is practised. In 2010, there were estimated to be between 100 and 140 million girls and women worldwide who have undergone FGM.[183] Currently, there are estimated to be 2 million girls at risk of FGM. FGM is practised in 28 African countries, some parts of the Middle East and South Asia. The highest prevalence of FGM is in Djibouti, Guinea and Somalia where 98% of females experience FGM. In Eritrea, Somalia, Mali and Sudan, FGM is experienced by 90% of females. There have been some tentative calls for the medicalisation of the practice to minimise harm, but most human rights groups oppose medicalisation and call for a complete ban. In the UK, it is a criminal offence to

---

[182] See, for further analysis, Macklin, R. *Against Relativism: Cultural Diversity and the Search for Ethical Universals in Medicine*. Oxford: Oxford University Press, 2000.
[183] *Female Genital Mutilation: Fact Sheet No 241*. Geneva: World Health Organisation, February 2010.

participate in, to conspire, procure or facilitate FGM (see the Female Genital Mutilation Act 2003). The law has been extended to apply to UK nationals acting overseas.

FGM may be performed for a variety of reasons: psychosexual reasons (eg preservation of chastity); sociological reasons (eg identification with the cultural heritage and social cohesion); hygiene and aesthetic reasons; religious reasons (eg some communities believe that it is demanded by the Islamic faith, although the practice predates Islam); and mythical reasons (eg enhancement of fertility and promotion of child survival). The potential complications of FGM are considerable. Immediate complications from FGM include severe pain, shock, haemorrhage and infection, leading, in some cases, to death. Long-term complications from FGM include abscesses and fistulas leading to painful sexual intercourse and difficulties with childbirth. Indeed, there is an increased risk of maternal and child morbidity and mortality due to obstructed labour following FGM. As well as the serious physical sequelae, there may be psychological effects ranging from anxiety to severe depression.

Female Genital Mutilation is an example of a widespread practice that is particular to certain cultural groups and geographical location. It is considered not only to be morally unacceptable in the United Kingdom but also constitutes a criminal offence. What are your views about FGM? Do future doctors have a moral obligation to work to end the practice of FGM? Do future doctors have moral obligations to the women affected by FGM?

Global health in practice: the medical student elective

The elective is the point at which most medical students will think, in practice, about global health and its ethics. Most medical schools encourage students to travel and experience clinical work and healthcare in a different environment or country. There is an ethical dimension to each stage of the elective from planning[184] where to go to how you behave once you are there.

---

[184] *Medical Electives: A Guide to Planning it Right.* (BMA TV Podcast): Available at www.youtube.com/watch?v=izHzVotYaYs

First, where to go: potential destinations are not morally neutral and there are ethical questions to consider when you are thinking about where to visit. Factors such as the health, political and socio-economic status of the location and its people, and your own personal safety, are all relevant when deciding where you would like to go. Ideally, you will think beyond the few weeks or months of your visit and consider whether you are contributing to sustainable projects or helping to develop partnerships that will endure long after your elective finishes. Increasingly, medical schools are forming meaningful collaborations that are built on co-development, and that recognise that a stream of unsupervised medical students may not be in the interests of those living in resource-poor environments.

Secondly, it is useful to think about what you as an individual will bring to the elective. An elective can often be a wonderful opportunity to grow in confidence and have new experiences, but it is important to be realistic. Practical considerations like whether you can speak a language sufficiently well to function or are physically fit enough to manage the conditions in a demanding destination are often overlooked and can lead to a miserable time. Think about your responsibilities to those whom you will be living and working with, and take time to reflect honestly on your personal capabilities, limits, strengths, skills and vulnerabilities.

Once you have decided on a destination that you think would suit you, it is time to attend to details. What is the timing of your elective period? Will there be other students present and, if so, how many? Different seasons may make a visit more or less difficult or quiet. There may be prevailing external factors – conflict, political unrest or natural disasters – that might change between planning and undertaking your elective. Although your medical school is likely to set objectives for the elective period, it is worth considering your personal reasons for your choice of elective. It is likely that you have multiple aims for your elective including developing your clinical skills and knowledge, having a break from the daily routine, making professional connections and developing personally and / or professionally. How would you articulate your reasons for your elective and who should know about your motivations and intentions prior to your arrival?

Ideally before you arrive, you will have thought about what is likely to await you when you arrive at your destination. There should be a match between the skills and knowledge that will be expected of you and that which you have to offer. It is particularly important to think about the boundaries of what you can offer on elective and how you will act within those boundaries. By anticipating at least some of what might happen on elective you are better-placed to thrive and to respond when the unexpected does happen (as it surely will). It is natural to focus on your clinical skills when preparing for your elective, but the skill of saying '*no*' politely can be essential whilst you are on elective.[185] No matter what the local environment, you are representing your own Institution and should therefore always comply with the expectations of your medical school and the ethical standards expected of medical students training in your own country.[186] The British Medical Association has produced an excellent resource that covers the ethical and practical aspects of medical student electives and is highly recommended.[187]

The following two cases demonstrate some of the ethical challenges that can arise on medical student electives.

Case Study

Kasia is working in a large public hospital in a city in the US. Kasia feels she is gaining excellent clinical experience but she has felt uncomfortable about the ways in which some of the members of staff treat the patients (who are among the poorest and most marginalised in the country). One day, a homeless man arrives in crisis and despite resuscitation attempts, he dies. The resident in charge asks Kasia to '*have a go at intubating and get some practice*' on the deceased man. How should Kasia respond?

---

[185] Banatvala, N., Doyal, L. Knowing When to Say No on the Student Elective. *BMJ* 1998; 316: 1404–1405.

[186] Bowman, D. Ethical Debate: Students Whose Behaviour Causes Concern. *BMJ* 2008; 337: 2882.

[187] *Ethics and Medical Electives in Resource-Poor Countries: A Toolkit.* London: BMA, 2009. Also available at www.bma.org.uk/careers/medical_education/medicalelectivestoolkit.jsp

Kasia's experience is a reminder that ethical dilemmas do not just occur in Electives in resource-poor nations. Differences in systems can in themselves be a culture shock. Perhaps it is particularly shocking when there are significant differences in a country that feels familiar and where English is spoken: I recall a trip many years ago to New Haven, Connecticut, where I visited an open access health clinic for those without insurance, not far from the wealth of Yale University, and I was stunned by the experiences of those who could not afford healthcare in the US.

Aside from the shock of the new, or at least, the different, Kasia has been asked to do something that is not merely questionable, it is completely unacceptable. No student in the UK would accede to such a request (and hopefully, no student in the UK would be asked to do such a thing). In the UK, the norms of consent and permission extend beyond death as demonstrated by practice in relation to organ donation.[188] Respect for the deceased must trump any pressure she may feel from the Resident in Charge. It may not be easy to say 'no', but say 'no' Kasia must. The form of words is up to Kasia: some feel most comfortable invoking 'medical school rules' that preclude them from doing what has been suggested; others feel it is important to be honest about how uncomfortable they feel about the request and highlight the ethical implications of treating the newly-dead in such an instrumental way. However Kasia chooses to express herself, she has to draw a boundary, politely but firmly.

---

[188] For a comparative perspective on practice in the US, see Moore, G.P. Ethics Seminars: The Practice of Medical Procedures on Newly Dead Patients – Is Consent Warranted? *Acad Emerg Med* 2001; 8(4): 389–392; Berger, J., Rosner, F., Cassell, E. Ethics of Practising Medical Procedures on Newly Dead and Nearly Dead Patients. *J Gen Intern Med* 2002; 17(10): 774–778; Schmidt, T.A., Abbott, J.T., Geiderman, J.M. *et al.* Ethics Seminars: The Ethical Debate on Practising Procedures on the Newly Dead. *Acad Emerg Med* 2004; 11(9): 962–966; Iserson, K.V. Teaching Without Harming the Living: Performing Minimally Invasive Procedures on the Newly Dead. *J Health Care Law and Policy* 2005; 8(2): 216–231; Moore, D. Never Let Your Sense of Morals Keep You from Doing What's Right: Using Newly Dead Bodies as an Educational Resource. *Health Matrix* 2008; 18(1): 105–125.

Case Study

Marcus is working in a residential school for orphans in Swaziland. He is uncomfortable to see that physical punishment is commonplace, even routine. He observes children as young as five years old receiving corporal punishment. When he asks about the system, he is told by the headteacher that it is the *'only way to discipline'* the pupils and encouraged to participate. How should Marcus respond?

Like Kasia, Marcus has encountered difference that is shocking. Unlike Kasia, Marcus is not being asked directly to participate actively, but nonetheless by witnessing what is happening, Marcus is likely to feel complicit. Whilst it is unrealistic to think that Marcus, as a visiting medical student, can change practice, is there something that Marcus can do that means he is not merely a silent observer? This was the situation in which a former student of mine found himself and, after several email exchanges with me, he decided to broach the subject at the staff meeting. Courteously but clearly, the student named his discomfort. He honestly explained that he was surprised to find that corporal punishment was being used because his previous experience had been limited to British schools where such punishment was unlawful. The door had been opened to discussion and several members of staff were fascinated to know what sorts of techniques were used to discipline children in the UK and whether they were effective. The student was able to share ideas for alternatives and offered to get some resources for the members of staff who were particularly interested. A few days later, the student shared some materials from the Royal College of Psychiatrists on discipline and children which were so popular he asked for more to be sent to him on his Elective. As the student's elective finished, several senior members of staff were considering running a pilot of non-physical disciplinary techniques.

If Marcus too can be honest but respectful he may be able to start a discussion and explain that he is curious about, but discomforted by, the disciplinary approach because it is so different from that with which he is familiar. It is unlikely that he will revolutionise practice during his short Elective period, but he can do more than merely stand by. Marcus does not need to be aggressive, judgemental or critical, but neither does he need to be passive, unquestioning and accepting. It is his choice.

Core Concepts: Human Rights and Global Ethics

Human rights are fundamental entitlements that apply to every human being.
Following the end of the Second World War, the establishment of the United Nations led to a focus on human rights.
Human Rights are protect by treaties, covenants and laws (international, European and national).
The Human Rights Act 1998 incorporated the European Convention of Human Rights into UK law.
There are 14 Articles within the Human Rights Act 1998.[189]
Articles 3 (prohibition of torture, inhuman or degrading treatment or punishment), 4 (prohibition of slavery and forced labour) and 7 (no punishment without law) are absolute rights from which no derogation is permitted.
Articles 8–12 are qualified rights where derogation is permitted. Any derogation must be necessary in a democratic society, based in law, proportionate, consistent with the aims of the original European Convention on Human Rights and non-discriminatory.
For all but the absolute rights, the HRA 1998 is interpreted in the context of existing legislation.
The Human Rights Act has implications for a wide range of clinical activity and healthcare eg resource allocation, compulsory treatment, care at the end of life and confidentiality.
An area where there is an inherent tension between human rights and the interests of society is detention for the compulsory treatment of infectious disease.
A fundamental issue in global health and its attendant ethics involves understanding culture and its effects on the provision and experience of healthcare. Cultural competence refers to the ability of someone to work effectively in an environment of cultural difference, and to recognise and respond to the impact of that cultural difference whilst avoiding assumptions and stereotypes.

---

[189] Although Article 13, which provides for the right to secure an effective remedy from a national authority following a breach of rights, has been omitted because it has not been incorporated into the Human Rights Act 1998.

Cultural relativism is the position that morality is not universal but is necessarily determined by context and local social norms.

Medical students encounter global health ethics and cultural relativism in practice most often on their electives. Attention to the ethical dimensions of the Elective both prior to, and during, the Elective period is invaluable.

 # Assessment: Human Rights and Global Ethics

1. Human rights and global ethics

Sample SAQ

(a) What does it mean to say that someone has a 'human right'? **(2 marks)**

(b) Suggest four ways in which the Human Rights Act 1998 has implications for healthcare. **(4 marks)**

(c) Suggest two arguments in support of, and two arguments against, the compulsory detention and treatment of those with infectious diseases. **(4 marks)**

(d) What is cultural competence? **(2 marks)**

(e) Suggest two advantages and two limitations to cultural relativism. **(4 marks)**

(f) Suggest four ethical questions that should be considered by medical students in planning and participating in their electives. **(4 marks)**

Guidance notes

Part (a)   A human right describes an entitlement that is fundamental to all human beings irrespective of race, ethnicity, religion, gender or nationality. No one can compromise or remove another's human rights. Human rights are protected by treaties, covenants and laws. Human rights were a conceptual legacy of the Second World War following the establishment of the United Nations.

Part (b)   Although the Human Rights Act 1998 (which incorporated the European Convention on Human Rights) applies in its entirety to NHS Trusts as public bodies, there are particular provisions of the Act that have implications for healthcare, namely:

- Article 2 – The right to life: this provision has been cited in several high-profile medical cases including that of Diane Pretty and Ms B. It has implications for decisions about continuing and withholding or withdrawing treatment.

- Article 5 – The right to liberty: this provision has implications for situations in healthcare where compulsion may be used to detain, assess, examine or treat patients such as those with mental health disorders, infectious diseases or whose capacity is otherwise compromised.

- Article 8 – The right to respect for private and family life: this provision has implications for the management of clinical data and confidentiality in healthcare

- Article 14 – The right to prohibition of discrimination: this provision has implications for the allocation of resources and prevents particular groups, eg the elderly, from being treated differently or in a way that disadvantages them in comparison to the rest of the population.

Part (c)   Arguments for compulsion include:

- Those who prefer a more utilitarian or communitarian approach might argue that effective public health depends on a population perspective, which may result in individual losses to freedom in the interests of the wider wellbeing of society.

- As Len Doyal notes, the question of what constitutes a sufficient 'interest' on the part of society is crucial when weighing the acceptability or otherwise of compulsory treatment. For example, Doyal argues that coercion and compulsion might be justifiable if a longer term and more disseminated benefit to society can be demonstrated that goes beyond the short-term benefits of limiting a local outbreak.

Arguments against compulsion include:

- For those who prioritise liberty, any infringement of a person's individual rights and freedoms is a significant matter that should be embarked upon only when there is evidence to suggest that to detain and/or treat people against their wishes is effective and proportionate to the restriction imposed upon them.

- For others, the nature of the therapeutic relationship is one of trust and many of those who are most at risk of communicable diseases may be suspicious of authority figures already; any attempts at coercion inevitably compromises the trust between doctor and patient is damaging, counterproductive and unacceptable.

Part (d)   Cultural competence refers to the ability of someone to work effectively in an environment of cultural difference and to recognise and respond to the impact of that cultural difference whilst avoiding assumptions and stereotypes.

Part (e)   Advantages of cultural relativism include:

- Plurality, diversity and difference are not merely tolerated but celebrated. Relativism implies tolerance, liberalism and respect.

- Inherent in relativism is scepticism about universal truths and experiences and it is an approach that avoids privileging particular groups or nations.

Limitations of cultural relativism include:

- It can tend to assumptions that culture is homogenous and uniform within a particular society.
- It may militate against constructive criticism and dialogue, and perhaps sets up a false dichotomy in which one is either relativist or absolutist, leading to stagnant ethical debate.

Part (f)   Students planning and participating in their electives should consider:

- The moral status of the proposed destination eg pay attention to factors such as the health, political and socio-economic status of the location and its people.
- The sustainability or otherwise of participating in projects and / or whether it is possible to contribute to partnerships that will endure after the elective finishes. The timing of the elective might also be relevant.
- The particular aspects of living and working in a different culture where healthcare is organised and experienced differently. If going to a resource-poor environment, the BMA resource is useful as preparatory reading.
- The contribution of the student to the elective eg does he or she speak the language? What skills does the student have to offer and do those match expectations and / or need?
- The boundaries within which the student should work on the elective including how to respond when the unexpected happens.

Chapter 11

Fallibility, Being Human and Making Mistakes

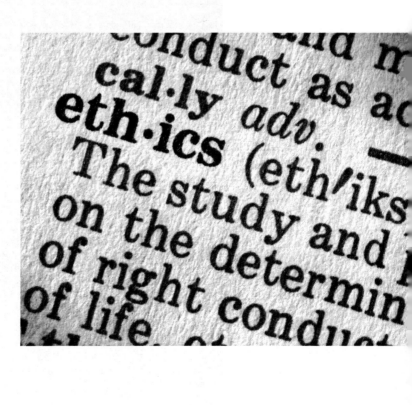

Fallibility, Being Human and Making Mistakes

Introduction

The issue of accountability in medicine has long been a vexed area. Following a series of high-profile scandals in which doctors were deemed to have erred and then covered up mistakes and in the wake of significant public inquiries[190], there has been a notable move over the last fifteen years towards a profession that is more open and accountable. There are multiple agencies that exist to review the 'quality' of healthcare, from the National Institute of Health and Clinical Excellence (NICE) to the Care Quality Commission (CQC). The maintenance and governance of professional standards is the responsibility of everyone working in the National Health Service, and the Public Interest Disclosure Act 1998 exists to provide statutory protection for those who wish to express formal concern about a colleague's performance. However, individual doctors and medical students still struggle when they have concerns about a colleague's fitness to practise or a peer's competence. This chapter examines the problems that can arise for students and doctors when assessing or questioning professional competence.

Who is competent?

It is perhaps unsurprising that it can be difficult to determine 'competence' in medicine. There has been significant research on this topic by, among many others, Marilyn Rosenthal[191] and she suggests several reasons for this difficulty. First, as in any profession, few doctors (if any) get through their careers without making a mistake (or several) which cannot and should not mean that they are labelled incompetent. Secondly, continuum and consistency in performance are vital when doctors are asked to judge their peers.

---

[190] The Kennedy Inquiry is probably the most well-known of these public inquiries. The Inquiry was chaired by Sir Ian Kennedy and investigated the provision of paediatric cardiac surgery services in Bristol during 1984–1995. See www.bristol-inquiry.org.uk where the Inquiry papers and Final Report are still available.

[191] See Rosenthal, M. *The Incompetent Doctor*. Buckingham: Open University Press, 1996; Lloyd-Bostock, S., Mulcahy, L. and Rosenthal, M. *Medical Mishaps: Pieces of the Puzzle*. Buckingham: Open University Press, 1999.

It is only after a certain number of mistakes that questions begin to be asked about competence. However, the judgement about competence is made more difficult by the fact that it is extremely hard to draw the boundary between the 'avoidable' and the 'unavoidable' mistake in a discipline as uncertain as medicine, Finally, doctors are trained to be aware of the fallibility of the human being and are perhaps more forgiving and 'loyal' than other professions when it comes to judging the actions of their colleagues. There is, Rosenthal suggests, a norm of non-criticism.

'Whistleblowing'

Given the atmosphere of loyalty and perhaps complicit silence that has been described repeatedly in the literature, and that many readers will recognise from their own training experiences, it is not surprising that the issue of whether, when and how to take action about a colleague who may be putting patients at risk is often avoided completely. The ethical position on the responsibility of a doctor to raise any concerns he or she has about a colleague is clear and unequivocal. The GMC states that doctors have a duty to report colleagues who are putting patients at risk.[192] The guide goes on to say that whilst doctors are expected to look after and care for each other, their first duty is to protect patients.

The Public Interest Disclosure Act 1998 offers a statutory framework within which protection is provided for those (in any profession) who have decided to disclose sensitive information about the performance of their colleagues. The statute states that it is a breach of employment legislation to penalise or dismiss an employee who makes a 'qualifying disclosure' under the Act.[193] However, as is so often the case, the law is a blunt instrument that offers general principles only. Thus, the mere existence of the Public Interest Disclosure Act 1998 is only useful when the difficult decision to speak out against a colleague has already been taken. The existence of the Act on the statute book is itself of no use in helping to determine whether, when or how one should act in the face of possible incompetence by a colleague, nor does it protect those

---

[192] *Good Medical Practice.* London: General Medical Council, 2006.
[193] See section 1 of the Public Interest Disclosure Act 1998.

who do choose to 'inform' on their colleagues from discomfort and isolation in the workplace.

Consider the case below which illustrates how difficult it can be to express concerns about a colleague, especially when that colleague is senior.

Case Study

Dr Prince has been a general practitioner for 15 years. He is well liked and respected by both patients and colleagues alike. For some time, however, he has appeared to be disorganised, behaved erratically and increasingly irritable in staff meetings. Dr Prince has made two potentially serious mistakes that were picked up by a local pharmacist and a hospital doctor. Dr Linton is the general practice trainee at Dr Prince's surgery and thinks that she has smelled alcohol on Dr Prince more than once. One day a patient tells Dr Linton that *'she likes Dr Prince but he's getting a bit too fond of the drink, isn't he Doctor?'* What should Dr Linton do?

As has already been said, the GMC is clear that Dr Linton has a duty to act. However, the work of the GMC in regulating the profession does not reach the majority of practising doctors.[194] It remains likely that expressions of concern will be shared, initially and perhaps exclusively, with other clinicians and possibly managers. The discretion of first-line responders, such as Dr Linton, is considerable and the ways in which those initially approached, such as the senior partner in the case study, choose to interpret the problem and subsequently respond carries considerable moral and professional responsibility.

Whilst it is essential not to jump to conclusions, there does seem to be evidence of a change in Dr Prince's behaviour and performance which warrants attention. However, it is inevitably easier to agree, in the abstract, that Dr Linton has a duty to act than it is to determine what her response should be in practice. It is probable that Dr Linton will feel loyal to Dr Prince and reluctant to 'rock

---

[194] Kultgen, J. (1998) *Ethics and Professionalism*. Philadelphia: University of Pennsylvania Press; 1988; Stacey M. (1995) 'Medical Accountability' in Hunt, G. (ed.) *The Health Service: Accountability, Law and Professional Practice*. London: Edward Arnold; 1995.

the boat' in the surgery where she is both junior and dependent on senior colleagues for her training. Dr Linton may feel that she is merely 'passing through' (a sentiment I hear often from students and junior staff whose time with a particular firm or at a GP surgery is limited) and therefore she does not need to engage with the problem. However, there are no exemptions for trainees or those who are with a team for a defined period: the bottom line is that Dr Linton has observed, and heard of, concerns about Dr Prince's behaviour. Dr Linton must act carefully, she must act in accordance with proper processes and she must act cautiously and honestly, but act she must.

The first issue to consider is the way in which Dr Linton should respond to the patient. She cannot ignore what the patient has said but she should not be drawn into investigation or even gossip. For someone who is both relatively junior and new to the practice, the best course of action is likely to be to express a neutral acknowledgement of the patient's perception of Dr Prince such as *'I am sorry to hear you think that but I appreciate you telling me'*.

Secondly, what is the nature of the problem facing Dr Linton? It seems that Dr Prince's practice is potentially compromised. It is not clear what prompted the patient's remark to Dr Linton or what other evidence exists to support the claim that Dr Prince has been abusing alcohol aside from Dr Linton's own experience of thinking that she has smelled alcohol. It is easy, perhaps natural, to assume that the Dr Prince's competence is in question. However, that is not necessarily the case. Often in such cases, the problem is one of potential incompetence or increased risk of poor performance (although Dr Prince has made errors, all doctors make errors and there may not be a link between the mistakes and his changed behaviour). Irrespective of the actual effects, or otherwise, on Dr Prince's competence, there is an issue that needs to be addressed: doctors who behave in ways that may compromise their performance cannot be ignored. By way of illustration of the relative moral status of risk in medicine, most would accept that a surgeon conducting an operation may have 70% mortality rate, provided he has done all he can to ensure he is proficient at performing the operation, that he performs it to the best of his ability and that he reviews his practice to ensure that he remains acceptably proficient; but not if the same surgeon has a 70% mortality rate for an operation for which he is inadequately trained, that he conducts with a hangover or other impairment and that he chalks up to experience. Clinicians must put themselves in the best position to be competent notwithstanding the inherent risks of healthcare: the moral difference is between avoidable and unavoidable mistakes.[195] Impaired practice matters whether or not harm is likely or ensues: patients come to clinicians expecting a basic level of competence and care, and the relationship depends on trust. A surgery or hospital makes representations to patients that foster and maintain trust. Representations that a doctor is someone in whom a patient should place his trust inform the whole process of seeking care – from a plaque on the wall bearing a clinician's name, credentials and status to offering appointments with, and providing a consulting room or theatre for, individual practitioners. It is ethically unacceptable to disregard concerns about Dr Prince, irrespective of the risk of harm, because it indicates collective misrepresentation and dishonesty by the practice.

Having determined that Dr Linton cannot ignore the problem, she should be aware that other members of staff may respond variably. For example, there may be conflicts of interest: the partners and other staff at the surgery are likely to feel loyalty towards Dr Prince as a close colleague, and perhaps even a friend. It may be significant that it is a relative newcomer, ie Dr Linton, to whom the patient has expressed concerns about Dr Prince. It has been suggested that those who raise concerns about clinical performance are, like Dr Linton in the case study, most likely to be new to existing organisations and systems.[196] The ties that bind clinical teams, and perhaps particularly GPs in partnership[197], are considerable and perhaps more fundamental than is routinely acknowledged. However, using Ronald Dworkin's[198] terminology, the duty to patients is clear, overrides the duties to Dr Prince and the profession, and is reinforced by the GMC which states

---

[195] Rosenthal, M. *The Incompetent Doctor*. Buckingham: Open University Press, 1996, at pp. 14–19.

[196] Martin, J.P. *Hospitals in Trouble*. Oxford: Blackwell; 1985; Pilgrim, D. *'Explaining Abuse and Inadequate Care'* in Hunt, G. (ed.) *The Health Service: Accountability, Law and Professional Practice*. London: Edward Arnold, 1995.

[197] Rosenthal, M. *The Incompetent Doctor*. Buckingham: Open University Press, 1996.

[198] Although Dworkin uses the term 'trumping' in relation to rights; see Dworkin, R. *Taking Rights Seriously*. London: Gerald Duckworth, 1977.

unequivocally that doctors must *'must make the care of the patient your first concern'* and requires that *'where there are serious concerns about a colleague's performance, health or conduct, it is essential that steps are taken without delay to investigate the concerns to establish whether they are well-founded, and to protect patients'*.[199] These professional imperatives reflect the principle of respect for persons. Patients are not means to an income, professional advancement, security or self-worth, but ends in themselves. Patients are dependent upon clinicians for care and they do not come to the relationship with equal status or knowledge. Put simply, most patients trust their professional carers: they believe they are competent.

In addition to the personal loyalty to Dr Prince as a colleague, there may be financial conflicts of interest. GP surgeries are small businesses and the impact of disrupting the partnership is considerable. The impact of dissolving partnership is even greater. Inevitably these factors, while perhaps not articulated, will have a bearing on how other members of staff perceive and respond to concerns. In addition to the inconvenience and cost of losing Dr Prince's services either temporarily or permanently, there may be less quantifiable effects on the reputation of the practice; the relationship of the practice with external parties who may have an interest in Dr Prince's performance, for example the Primary Care Organisation; and the ways in which Dr Prince's difficulties reflect on those who appointed him as a partner and staff workload.

It is to be hoped that Dr Prince isn't also a patient of the practice where he is a partner[200], but he may be given that significant numbers of doctors don't register with a GP, self-medicate and/or find seeking help difficult[201]. Someone, such as the senior partner, should ensure that Dr Prince has access to advice and support outside the practice, for example, a GP, support organisations or an occupational health service. There are a number of excellent services that specialise in treating healthcare professionals including the

---

[199] *Good Medical Practice.* London: General Medical Council, 2006

[200] *Ethical Responsibilities in Treating Doctors who are Patients: Guidance from the Ethics Department.* London: British Medical Association, 2004.

[201] Chambers, R., Belcher, J. Self-Reported Healthcare over the Past Ten Years: A Survey of General Practitioners. *Br J GP* 1992; 42: 153–6; Thompson, W.T. *et al.* Challenge of Culture, Conscience and Contract to General Practitioners' Care of their Own Health: Qualitative Study. *BMJ* 2001; 323: 728–31.

Practitioner Health Programme[202] and Mednet.[203] The BMA also runs a confidential counselling and advice service.[204]

If, as seems likely, there is reason to be concerned about Dr Prince's health and fitness to practise, Dr Linton must ensure that the appropriate person or people are informed promptly both of her observations and the patient's comments about Dr Prince. In a general practice setting, that might mean talking to the senior partner or a GP trainer. It is likely that the next step will be for the appropriate senior member of staff to talk to Dr Prince directly. If Dr Prince accepts that there are problems, it may be possible to negotiate actions that will ameliorate the situation. If, as is perhaps more likely, Dr Prince does not accept there is a problem with his performance, how should the practice proceed? Again, the GMC is clear:

> *You must give an honest explanation of your concerns to an appropriate person from the employing authority ... If there are no appropriate local systems, or local systems cannot resolve the problem, and you remain concerned about the safety of patients, you should inform the relevant regulatory body.*

It is likely that the next stage for the surgery partners would be to contact the relevant contact at the primary care organisation. Another source of advice is the National Clinical Assessment Service which draws on its national and international expertise in performance problems while emphasising local resolution. Although both Dr Linton and those in whom she confides are ethically obliged to act, the emotional impact of discharging this obligation is considerable and there is notable ambivalence about the role of whistleblowers, beautifully encapsulated by Hunt, who describes them as *'a peculiar and fascinating hybrid ... half trouble-maker, half-hero'.*[205] Dr Linton and all those involved in handling

---

[202] www.php.nhs.uk/ [accessed 27 June 2011].

[203] For details of how *Mednet* works with the London Deanery to support doctors in difficulty, see www.londondeanery.ac.uk/var/supporting-professional-performance/mednet [accessed 27 June 2011].

[204] www.bma.org.uk/doctors_health/index.jsp [accessed 27 June 2011].

[205] Hunt, G. 'Introduction: Whistle-blowing and the Breakdown of Accountability' in Hunt, G. (ed.) *The Health Service: Accountability, Law and Professional Practice.* London: Edward Arnold, 1995.

concerns about Dr Prince may wish to identify a trusted mentor or third party with whom they can debrief.

Complaints and Negligence

Complaints and possible litigation are often brought by patients who feel aggrieved for reasons that may be unconnected with the clinical care that they have received. It is an old and untraceable adage that 'a doctor who is nice to his or her patients can get away with murder' but the spirit of this saying is true. When patients are asked about their decisions to complain or to sue doctors, it is common for poor communication, insensitivity, administrative errors and lack of responsiveness to be cited as motivation.

Openness is a valuable asset in medicine and particularly when something has gone wrong. The question of whether or not to apologise when something has gone wrong is sometimes considered to be a confusing area for doctors. The advice from the main defence organisations is that a prompt apology is an appropriate response to an adverse incident, as is an accurate account of the facts. Indeed, the GMC goes further and states that all doctors have a moral obligation to apologise and explain when medical errors and accidents occur. As a medical student and future doctor, you are not compromising your position by apologising. Indeed, you may be preventing further complaints, and/or future legal action by a courteous and appropriate apology.

The courts are neither concerned with best practice nor with unfeasibly high standards of care. It is not expected that doctors are 'super doctors' who always make perfect decisions, accurately identify rare conditions and never make a mistake. What is expected is that doctors behave in a way that accords with the practice of a reasonable doctor – and the reasonable doctor is not perfect. However, the law is not the best means to achieve justice for either claimants or defendants. Claimants generally feel aggrieved that the system is slow, costly, and alienating. Defendants, unsurprisingly, frequently feel persecuted and defensive. During the lengthy period that many legal actions take, both claimants and defendants will be expected to conduct some semblance of a normal life under conditions of enormous stress and anxiety. Furthermore, the legal process itself is an artificial one. Cases will often be decided on the basis of technical legal points such as causation and the admissibility of evidence rather than on the basis of substantive clinical merit.

Moreover, the most incompetent doctors will probably not end up in court at all because such cases are commonly indefensible and, will therefore be settled discreetly by the relevant defence organisation: a fact that somewhat undermines claims that legal regulation has significant effects on the practice of the medical profession at large. Thus the law is far from an ideal check, and regulation, of standards in the medical profession. However, perhaps some understanding of how the standards of care are judged and the cases decided makes it easier to protect oneself and avoid contact with the dreaded lawyer in future practice.

What then are the components of a negligence action? An action in negligence[206] comprises three elements, namely:

(i)   A duty of care between claimant and defendant;
(ii)   A breach, by an act or omission, that falls below the standard of care expected;
(iii)   Causation, ie the breach resulted in loss or damage to the claimant that was reasonably proximate

What is the clinical duty of care?

The first component of a negligence claim is to establish that the defendant owed a duty of care to the claimant. Usually, this is not difficult in cases of medical negligence, as all doctors are considered at common law to owe a duty of care to their patients. Indeed, in an emergency, the duty of care may extend beyond the patients on a doctor's list or in a hospital catchment area to anyone whom one may encounter. The technical difficulties lie in proving that the duty of care was breached in such a way as to fall below the standard of care that could reasonably be expected, and establishing that it was the breach that actually *caused* damage to the patient.

---

[206] As a civil action in the law of torts, claims have to be proven on the balance of probabilities.

What is the standard of care in medicine?

In the UK, the standard of care is common to all negligence claims. For many years, the courts considered whether a defendant had behaved in a way that accorded with a responsible body of professional opinion. It need not be a majority opinion, but it does need to be considered reasonable and not reflect a perverse or esoteric professional perspective. This way of determining the standards of care was known as the 'Bolam test' after the case in which it was first articulated.[207] In practice, for matters of clinical judgement, an expert or number of experts would advise the courts on the acceptability or otherwise of a defendant's conduct. Therefore, on the application of the *Bolam* test, if an expert witness stated that a clinician's actions (or omissions) were those of a reasonable practitioner, it was most unlikely that he or she would be found negligent. The *Bolam* test was criticised by those who believed that it invested the power to make determinative judgment in medical opinion (as represented by medically qualified expert witnesses).[208] The test was also perceived as flawed because it equated commonly accepted practice with acceptable practice.[209]

At the end of the twentieth century, the courts showed signs of dissatisfaction with the role of experts and its effect on standards of care. In 1997, in the case of *Bolitho v City and Hackney Health Authority*[210], the House of Lords introduced a new element to the assessment of standards of care. The Lords held that a court was not bound to accept that a doctor had not been negligent merely because expert opinion affirmed that a defendant's actions accorded with those of a responsible body of his peers. The House stated that, in order to be judged 'reasonable', a defendant's actions (and the expert's opinion of those actions) should be capable of withstanding logical analysis by the court. Thus, for the first time, there was a clear statement by the most senior members of the judiciary that courts should scrutinise medical opinion rather

---

[207] *Bolam v Friern Hospital Management Committee* (1957) 1 WLR 582.

[208] Stacey, M. 'Medical Accountability' in Hunt, G. (ed.) *Whistleblowing in the Health Service: Accountability, Law and Professional Practice*. London: Edward Arnold, 1995.

[209] Samanta, A., Samanta, J. Legal Standard of Care: a Shift from the Traditional *Bolam* Test. *Clin Med*. 2003; 3(5): 443–6.

[210] [1993] 4 Med LR 381.

than simply accept the assessments of expert witnesses. *Bolitho* is significant because it indicates that the interpretation of guidance on consent is not the preserve of experts but something on which the court can, and where appropriate, will comment. The decision generated much comment in professional and academic literature and was interpreted (and indeed welcomed) by many as marking the demise of the power of the medical profession to determine an appropriate standard of care.[211] However, in practice, only a negligible number of cases will produce expert opinions that are so unreasonable that they do not withstand logical analysis. It seems that the essence of the *Bolitho* amendment to the standard of care test is to introduce an element of objective risk/benefit analysis into the equation.

The use of guidelines and protocols in medicine has been steadily increasing. Along with the emergence of evidence-based medicine, there is more information available for anyone (including patients and lawyers) who wishes to explore standards of clinical care. Whilst guidelines can be valuable in assessing what standards are expected of clinicians in specific areas of practice, there are limitations. First, the validity and acceptability of guidelines are inextricably dependent upon the quality (or otherwise) of both the evidence on which the guidance is based and the skills of those interpreting the evidence. The critical appraisal skills of both practitioners and expert witnesses are subject to increasing scrutiny in negligence actions. Secondly, a false sense of security can result as a consequence of adhering to and relying on protocols and guidelines. Thus, there is a danger of believing that by following the protocol or guidelines one is immune from complaints or legal challenges. Even 'best practice' guidelines can be followed negligently.

So, what is the status of protocols and guidelines in law? Strictly speaking protocols and guidelines will not be recognised in law unless there is a mandate or a sanction that accompanies the protocol or guidelines. However, that is not to suggest that the

---

[211] Teff, H. The Standard of Care in Medical Negligence – Moving on from *Bolam*? *Oxford J Legal Studies.* 1998; 18(3): 473–84; Brazier, M. Miola, J. Bye-bye *Bolam*: A Medical Litigation Revolution? [2000] 8 *Med LR* 85–114; Khan, M. (2001) *Bolitho* – Claimant's Friend or Enemy? *Med Law.* 2001; 20(4): 483–91; McHale, J. Quality in Healthcare: A Role for the Law? *Qual Saf Health Care.* 2002; 11(1): 88–91.

courts disregard guidelines. Essentially, the court will seek to assess whether the guideline for that particular case is established ie do the guidelines reflect recognised practice that falls within the standards of care required by the cases of *Bolam* and *Bolitho*? The answer to this question is likely to come from an expert witness (or several) giving evidence; the guidelines will rarely substitute for that specialist testimony. Written guidelines cannot be subjected to cross-examination, and it would be contrary to legal process to find a clinician negligent (with all its concomitant consequences for careers, self-esteem and income) 'by default' simply because guidelines were not followed.

Notwithstanding the rise of evidence-based medicine and formal guidelines, the courts have traditionally recognised that medicine is an art and not a science. As yet, there is no legal authority to assume that deviation from guidelines will automatically be considered indicative of negligent practice. It remains that the court will examine whether the clinician's actions were reasonable, with reference to whether or not the defendant's actions were acceptable to a reasonable body of practitioners (who need not necessarily form the majority opinion), *in the particular circumstances of the case.* Perhaps the best advice is that, as in any area of medical practice, actions and decisions must be justifiable: for, should there be a court case, the clinician will surely be asked why the decision was made not to follow guidelines.

What is causation in clinical negligence?

Many medical negligence cases turn on this often complex and technical issue. In medicine, where illness, diagnosis, treatment and a therapeutic relationship evolve over time, it can be difficult to say when damage occurred and at what point a clinician was negligent. Many clinical negligence cases will fail on the basis of causation. The significance of causation was well illustrated by legal claims concerning the prescription of benzodiazepines. In many of those cases, the initial decision to prescribe a tranquillizing drug was appropriate, but the continued prescription of the drug without review was inappropriate once it was known that benzodiazepines are highly addictive. The claimants in these actions had to establish, on the balance of probabilities, exactly when they became addicted to the drug *and* whether addiction or dependence coincided with inappropriate prescribing.[212] An action would only succeed if the point at which the patient became addicted, the inappropriate prescribing and awareness of the risk of addiction coincided to cause damage to the patient.

Clinical risk

Many negligence actions in medical practice emanate from errors in communication and administration rather than from clinical and diagnostic errors. The legal implications are numerous and failure of the simplest processes can expose patients to harm. Most analyses of what constitutes good medical practice are not readily divided into clinical and the non-clinical. Rather, good practice is a package involving a wide range of administrative, communication, diagnostic and prescriptive skills. However, when asked about litigation and their fears, doctors will commonly mention clinical issues such as misdiagnosis and the failure to investigate and prescribe appropriately; rarely are the issues of communication and administration considered as medico-legal concerns. This section of the chapter discusses some of the principal areas where clinical risk should be considered and actively managed to avoid error, complaints and litigation.

Notes and records

The significance of good, accurate and contemporaneous notes cannot be overstated. As a medical student, you are likely to be invited to write in the notes at some stage in your clinical training. From the earliest days at medical school, it is worth taking the time to review the notes of others and to identify what constitutes an effective entry in the medical records. The effect of good record-keeping on diagnostic decisions and in any ensuing complaint or legal proceedings can be considerable. In negligence proceedings, the judge will sometimes state that the quality or otherwise of the notes has been a strongly persuasive factor in determining liability.[213]

---

[212] The appropriateness or otherwise of the prescribing will be assessed with reference to the standards of the time.

[213] For example, in anaesthetics, clear, accurate and meticulous notes detailing drug doses and vapour concentrations can help to defend cases in which allegations of awareness are made.

Medical notes and records have been said to be the single most important piece of evidence in a legal action. Furthermore, doctors who regularly give evidence in medical negligence litigation reveal that, whilst their involvement in clinical negligence actions has had an impact on their own practice of medicine, it is in the specific area of record- and note-keeping that the impact has been greatest. Many experts discuss the notes and medical records under a distinct heading in their medico-legal reports: a trend that is increasingly being encouraged by those with responsibility for advising on the compilation of such reports. Given the usual delay that occurs between the cause of action occurring and any ensuing proceedings, good notes are vital not only as formal evidence but also as a means of recalling the events accurately and consistently.

So, what constitutes 'good' record keeping? The box below describes the features of effective record-keeping.

Features of effective medical record-keeping

☑ If handwritten, the notes should be legible.

☑ The date and time of the consultation should be included.

☑ Notes should be signed by name and the signature should be accompanied by a printed name and description of role eg Dr James Bloggs, Specialist Trainee, General Medicine.

☑ Only approved and unambiguous abbreviations should be used in notes.

☑ An entry should never be altered nor an addition disguised. If an addition or amendment is required, it should be made in the form of a dated, signed addendum.

☑ Where electronic records are used there should be an audit trail.

☑ Insulting, humorous or personal comments should never be included in the notes.

☑ If notes/letters are dictated and typed up by someone else, the contents of the hard copy should be checked to ensure that it is an accurate representation of the dictated version.

☑ Reports should be seen, evaluated and initialled by a clinician before they are filed.

☑ Notes and records should not be thrown away.

☑ Access to records should be provided in accordance with the law eg the Data Protection Act 1998.

Co-operation with other health professionals

Referrals can be compromised by simple administrative errors eg letters that aren't written, letters that are not sent promptly or at all, and letters that are sent to the wrong recipient. Doctors must do what is reasonable to discharge their liability when referring patients and this includes the basic checks to ensure that the communication has been received by the correct person.

The importance of a coherent and complete referral letter is hard to overstate. As with all areas of medical law, the question of whether or not a letter complies with the standard of care expected is assessed in accordance with the *Bolam* principle as amended by *Bolitho* (discussed earlier in this chapter). The referral letter must be comprehensive ie it should provide as complete a picture as possible of the patient's condition and the degree of urgency with which the referral appointment is required. The recipient is, in turn, expected to prioritise according to the terms of the referral letter and to clarify any ambiguity in the referral letter. Although it is important to involve patients in decision-making and communicate openly, that does not mean it is reasonable to expect patients to be able to provide accurate details about their medical history and care. Clinical practice should never rely solely on patients remembering information and/or conveying it accurately between clinical teams. In addition to the difficulties that can occur in respect of referrals to different teams, problems can arise when patient care involves any multidisciplinary team handing over care between its members. Particular issues recur when doctors are covering for each other, and especially when locums and junior staff are involved. The significance of an effective handover on the quality of care provided is considerable.

A second area of potential risk is that of following-up patients. Where a patient is receiving long term therapy, eg the prescription of anti-coagulants, clear advice should be given about when to return for review, the importance of monitoring and what symptoms or signs may indicate adverse effects. In acute episodes, for example presenting in A&E, it is good practice to give the patient a clear idea of the possible effects of treatment, when some improvement may be expected and under what circumstances the patient should make contact again, be it with a GP or directly with the hospital.

Failure to follow up investigations is an increasing source of both complaints and claims. When an investigation of any kind is ordered, it is incumbent upon the doctor who requested the investigation to check that the result arrives, to review that result and to ensure that appropriate steps are taken to arrange such further investigation and treatment as may be necessary.

Writing prescriptions

Basic administrative errors occur when writing prescriptions and there are many junior doctors who have been saved from making an error by a sharp-eyed nurse or pharmacist picking up prescription mistakes. Before writing a prescription or making an entry on a drug chart, a doctor should consider why a particular medication is indicated and check for contraindications, interactions with other medication and/or allergies. On the prescription itself, both the patient and drug name must be correctly written and the dosage checked and transcribed to the prescription or drug chart accurately.[214] Finally, if appropriate, provision should be made for monitoring and follow-up, including advice about repeat prescriptions. It is particularly important for junior doctors to remember that even though a prescription may be written on the advice of a consultant or senior clinician, in law, it is the doctor who signs the prescription that bears legal responsibility.

Conclusion

This chapter has discussed competence, complaints and negligence in medical practice which are discomforting subjects for most medical students and doctors. It is important not to overstate the potential risks and to understand that as long as one adheres to the basic principles then it is possible to practise *defensible* rather than *defensive* medicine. The reassuring aspect of many of the issues discussed in this chapter is that much potential complaint and litigation is avoidable simply by developing and maintaining good standards of communication, organisation and administration; these good habits begin in medical school. In particular, effective communication is a potent weapon in preventing complaints and,

---

[214] Prescriptions involving calculations and decimal points are notoriously susceptible to human error.

ultimately, encounters with the legal system. In any contemporary medical student education, much emphasis will rightly be placed on the need for, and benefits of, effective communication.

Openness and accountability are the watchwords of medical practice in the twenty-first century. Mistakes will always occur whilst medicine is practised by fallible human beings (and tired, overstretched and sometimes inexperienced human beings at that). All doctors, like all people, are fallible. A minority of doctors will be unlucky. Incompetence remains the most difficult of all the concepts to define. Medical error is a multifactorial concept encompassing:

- Social psychology
- Risk management
- Systems failure
- Socio-economic factors
- Individual knowledge and skills (clinical, communication and administrative)
- Personal relationships
- Political agendas
- Legal definitions
- Professional codes of conduct
- Available resources and support mechanisms

As a student, try to be alert to how clinicians organise their practice and manage potential risks and conflict. You will have the opportunity to see doctors making and communicating decisions, handling disagreement, responding to mistakes and working with others – make the most of these opportunities, for learning to be a safe, reliable and effective doctor in a complex health system depends as much on developing skills in organisation and communication as it does on learning anatomy and physiology.

Looking after yourself as a medical student

Medical training and work are stressful and everyone will, at some point, be performing below their best. Medical training is also bonding – you are likely to make friends for life and the shared experience of exams, ward rounds and the early days of navigating an operating theatre give a sense of common purpose and an atmosphere of collegiality. Inevitably perhaps, a tribal trench spirit and camaraderie develops from the shared experiences of training to be a doctor. That common purpose and collegiality can be invaluable when times are tough, but it cannot be allowed to compromise patient care.

Fortunately, obvious unsuitability for medicine and abject incompetence are rare and medical education is improving at detecting and responding difficulties early. However, there may be times when you are concerned about a fellow student or colleague or when someone is concerned about you. Naturally, medical students worry about fitness to practise and there are many myths and misunderstandings about showing vulnerability and the implications for being 'fit to practise'. All medical schools are responsible for producing graduates that are fit to practise medicine. Questions about fitness to practise may be raised in response to concerns about a student's honesty, probity, ability to work effectively and professionally with others or their regard for the ethical rules that apply to good clinical practice. Although the subject of fitness to practise can be worrying for students, it is sensible to read the General Medical Council's guidance on student fitness to practise[215] and to understand how that guidance is interpreted and applied at your medical school.

Proceedings relating to a student's fitness to practise are rare. Often proceedings are preceded by a pattern of behaviour that has not responded to appropriate warnings, advice and remediation. Occasionally, a single episode is so concerning that it triggers an investigation and formal fitness to practise proceedings. There is a misapprehension that disclosing or showing any vulnerability, perhaps particularly in relation to mental health, might lead to fitness to practise proceedings. That misapprehension prevents many students from seeking and receiving the support they deserve. To be clear: fitness to practise is about a student's ability to do the job of being a doctor and judgements have to be based on evidence of past behaviour. Any diagnosis (of physical or mental illness) is relevant only so far as it has an effect on a student's behaviour. For the overwhelming majority the effect of an illness on their training and work as a future doctor is positive not negative: students

---

[215] *Medical Students: Professional Values and Fitness to Practise.* London: General Medical Council, 2009

understand what it is like to be a patient and are better able to empathise and support their own patients in turn.

Looking after yourself and seeking help or support makes you a better doctor. It does not indicate someone about whom there are questions of fitness to practise. There are many doctors practising medicine who have experienced painful personal circumstances. The obligation is to be sufficiently self-aware to realise when your personal difficulties might compromise your clinical care. Most medical schools have members of staff who are available to support students and who will want to help you. If you prefer to seek help outside the medical school faculty members, there are counselling and GP services, student-led support groups and specialist organisations that can help. Do not suffer alone and do not allow others to suffer alone.

Speaking out as a medical student

You will doubtless encounter a range of clinical practice in your training. Much of it will be admirable and inspiring but occasionally you will find yourself in a position where you have concerns. I sometimes ask medical students who have witnessed or participated in something that they know to be wrong what prevented them from speaking out. The commonest response is '*I am only a medical student*'. Some honest students explain that they want to fit in and depend on their seniors for teaching and being signed off at the end of their placement. I understand those responses: medicine is tribal and hierarchical. However, learning to stand up for yourself, and perhaps more importantly, your patients, is a crucial part of your training. You need not do so alone: I work hard to support and, where necessary, protect students who find themselves in a difficult position. However, you cannot escape the fact that at some stage, even if it is not until after qualification, you will have to make a choice about whether to remain silent or act in the face of sub-optimal care. The scenario below is an example of such a situation.[216]

---

[216] This scenario and the commentary are adapted from Bowman, D. Changing Places: Ethical Choices as a New Doctor. *The New Doctor* 2011; 4(1): 6–8. London: Medical Protection Society.

Scenario

Sadiq Haq was pleased to begin his final year medicine placement at a district general hospital located near to his medical school. He joined a busy medical firm and works most closely with Dr Hopkins, the FY1 doctor. Sadiq believes that the consultant, Dr Tan, is a skilled clinician but he has concerns about some of the interactions between her and patients, particularly on ward rounds where she rarely acknowledges or discusses care with the patient. One morning, Sadiq is part of a large ward round comprising a dozen people. Dr Tan reviews the care of a patient, Mr Yates, who was admitted for investigations following an unexplained 'collapse'. She proposes that the patient should have an echocardiogram, an exercise stress test and begin treatment for hypertension. Dr Tan does not explain her decision to the patient. Later, Dr Hopkins and Sadiq are asked by the nursing staff to see Mr Yates who is distressed and refusing to go down for investigations because he *'has no idea what is going on'*. Dr Hopkins and Sadiq go to see the patient but he insists that he will only *'talk to the woman in charge – the consultant'*. Dr Hills and Sadiq know that Dr Tan has an outpatient clinic followed by a research meeting off-site.

Sadiq and the Foundation Year doctor with whom he is working, Dr Hopkins, have encountered ethics in a context that is so common that it is considered by many not only to be the norm but a necessary medical tradition: the ward round. Sadiq and Dr Hopkins face a multifactorial ethical dilemma.

First, there is the immediate 'presenting ethical problem': a patient is refusing treatment that is in his best interests because he does not feel sufficiently informed to give valid consent. To proceed under such circumstances would not only be unethical, it would be an assault. Secondly, the therapeutic relationship and trust between the patient and the clinical team has been compromised. It is upon trust that effective care depends. The diminution of trust is a significant ethical challenge with potentially serious consequences for both the patient and the clinical team. Thirdly, both Sadiq and Dr Hopkins have competing personal and professional interests. Dr Hopkins is likely to want to impress Dr Tan. At the very least, Dr Hopkins will be concerned about irritating her while she is busy. Sadiq, in turn, will want to remain on good terms with Dr Hopkins and not alienate the Foundation Year doctor with whom he is likely to get the most experience. A patient has made a specific request to see Dr Tan but it is a natural human response for Dr Hopkins and Sadiq to consider the implications for them of contacting the consultant.

Many readers will already be taking a practical approach to this scenario. If Sadiq or Dr Hopkins can find the time to sit with the patient, perhaps they can rectify the situation by apologising for his distress, explaining what is happening and seeking his consent to proceed. Even if Sadiq and Dr Hopkins have the skills and sensitivity to manage the situation (and as a medical student Sadiq should not be expected to respond to a distressed and angry patient), it will still involve several ethical compromises. First, the patient has explicitly requested time with the consultant. It may be that time can be negotiated and that the patient will agree to seeing Dr Tan at a more convenient point, but there are strong signs that he is unhappy about the extent to which the consultant has involved him in his care. Moreover, it is likely, given Sadiq's and Dr Hopkins' existing concerns about the ways in which Dr Tan interacts, or rather doesn't interact, with patients that the issue is greater than just this particular patient's concerns. By seeking to manage the situation, Sadiq and Dr Hopkins are making a choice not to engage with an ethical issue that affects care within the team for which they are working and goes to the heart of the therapeutic relationship. There may be good reasons for Sadiq and Dr Hopkins not wishing to tackle the wider issue: they may each feel that they are too junior to speak out; they may be unsure whether their concerns are legitimate; they, particularly Dr Hopkins, may feel that they have responsibility but no power; or they may be keen to preserve relationships with their clinical seniors. Nonetheless, if Sadiq and Dr Hopkins choose not to do more than merely contain the crisis, they are making a significant ethical choice and one that has implications for patient care. Furthermore, this is an opportunity to practise something that is difficult and likely to recur in their careers, namely speaking out or disagreeing with a colleague. Just as it takes practice to hone skills in cannulation or lumbar punctures, so it takes practice to learn how to challenge, question and constructively disagree with someone whose approach is compromising patient care.

Why are standards of care compromised? It is not usually because clinicians are 'unethical', 'cruel' or 'indifferent'. Rather, it is because there is an enormous and significant gap between ethics in the abstract and its embodiment day after day in the provision of care.

To be ethical is easy in the abstract: ethical dilemmas in the lecture theatre and seminar room often appear to be deftly resolvable. Ethics is part of practice; it is a practical pursuit and it is the practice of ethics that is most difficult. The challenge of ethics in practice is not to provide logical, rigorous and intellectual analysis of moral problems but to live and embody ethics, values and virtues.

What is the difference between those who are able to enact and remain true to their ethical values, and those who remain silent and do not challenge others when they are ethically discomforted? It is unlikely to be a question of knowledge. Indeed, there is not much knowledge required of either Sadiq or Dr Hopkins in addressing the ethical dilemma in which they find themselves. It may be that Sadiq enjoyed his education in ethics and is skilled at analysing ethical problems. It may be that he tolerated or even disliked the ethics sessions that he has encountered in his training and has forgotten everything he ever learned. It does not matter: it does not take the conceptual frameworks of bioethics and familiarity with moral philosophy to recognise that he and Dr Hopkins should not collude with Dr Tan. Sadiq and Dr Hopkins are likely to know what they should do, but what will determine whether they actually do what they know they should? It is a question that has long occupied bioethicists, but it is the field of business that provides one of the more useful explanations for why putting ethics into practice can be so difficult. Professor Mary Gentile has spent her career as an academic in business education and leadership. Having observed the dissonance between professional ethics in theory and what individuals actually do in the workplace led her to develop the 'Giving Voice to Values' project.[217] Drawing on research published after the Second World War that explored why some individuals acted as rescuers to save those threatened by the Nazis[218], Gentile argues that the act of speaking out and being loyal

---

[217] Gentile, M.C. Turning Values into Action. *Stanford Social Innovation Review*, Fall 2010; Volume 8(4): 42–47; Gentile, M.C. *Giving Voice to Values: How to Speak Your Mind When You Know What's Right.* Yale, New Haven: Yale University Press, 2010.

[218] London, P. 'The Rescuers: Motivational Hypotheses about Christians who Saved Jews from the Nazis' in *Altruism and Helping Behaviour: Social Psychological Studies of Some Antecedents and Consequences.* New York: Academic Press, 1970; Huneke, D.H. *The Moses of Rovno: The Stirring Story of Fritz Graebe, A German Christian who Risked His Life to Lead Hundreds of Jews to Safety During the Holocaust.* New York: Dodd Mead, 1985.

to ethical precepts is a skill that requires practice like any other professional skill. Thus, those who have early experience of standing up for values and acting ethically in the face of pressure are more likely, Gentile argues, to find it possible to resist and even confront organisational pressure to behave unethically. Gentile suggests it is therefore possible to learn the skills that are required to avoid ethical erosion and remain true to one's values and those of one's profession. She has developed a skill-based model that draws on seven principles which are shown, with a brief explanation, in the box below.

Giving voice to values: seven principles (Mary C. Gentile)

1. Values: identifying and agreeing what is core and fundamental to one's work.
2. Choice: recognising that there are options and that everyone has experience of making difficult choices.
3. Normality: acknowledging that conflict about values is to be expected and avoiding demonising those with whom one disagrees.
4. Purpose: defining one's role and being explicit about aims.
5. Self-knowledge and Alignment: challenging one's perception or characterisation of self with reference to personal strengths and previous successes.
6. Voice: developing and practising 'scripts' that enable individuals to speak out and confront conflict about values or ethics.
7. Reasons and Rationalisation: anticipating the reaction of those with whom we disagree and developing effective and relevant responses.

If Sadiq and Dr Hopkins remind themselves of their values; draw on previous occasions (in both their personal and professional lives) where they have addressed a difficult situation; neither vilify nor defer to Dr Tan; focuses on the patient, Mr Yates, and his care as their purpose; and plan explicitly what they could say to Dr Tan and anticipate her response, they are more likely to find it possible, even essential, to question Dr Tan. It is not a matter of knowledge, reasoning or intellectual debate: it is a practical exercise that depends on skills that are rarely taught formally and yet are an essential part of being 'an ethical practitioner'.

Ethical practice requires us to grapple with taboos: the person whom we dislike, the boredom of daily responsibilities, personal ambition, competitiveness and professional rivalries are just some examples of context that inevitably shapes practice but is not often discussed at all, let alone with reference to ethics. For most junior doctors, ethical questions do not relate to the life and death crises that often dominate ethics teaching. The issues are more mundane. Yet, it is that very ordinariness that makes those challenges fundamental to, and at the heart of, what it means to be an ethical doctor.

Clinical ethics necessarily extends well beyond that which can be learned in lectures and tutorials. The practice of ethics is reinterpreted according to speciality, personalities and the culture of the working environment. Even the 'core' concepts that most students master early in their training become nuanced and contestable in practice, where much of what has been learned has to be revisited. Whilst there are concepts within bioethics that warrant reinterpretation when in a particular clinical environment, there are also rules to which no exception should be made. Honesty, respect, fairness and kindness are non-negotiable and easy to support in the abstract, yet it can be a struggle to remain true to that support when one is overburdened, irritable, intimidated, tired or fed up. The reality of health and social care is that many, if not all, will be challenged to 'make an exception' and compromise personal and professional values at some stage. It is on those occasions that we learn that meaningful ethics is an integral part of practice which depends on practising skills that are rarely addressed by formal teaching sessions in ethics. It is those occasions that make the difference.

 ## Core Concepts: Competence, Whistleblowing, Negligence and Clinical Risk

---

Traditionally many doctors have been reluctant to act on concerns about a colleague.

Following a series of medical 'scandals' in the 1990s, medical accountability and professionalism have been in the spotlight, leading to a number of new agencies and organisations charged with reviewing quality and performance in healthcare.

> The GMC requires doctors to act if they have concerns about a colleague and believe patients are at risk.

> All NHS Trusts are required to have whistle-blowing policies and The Public Interest Disclosure Act 1998 exists to protect those who express concern appropriately.

> Good communication is an effective prophylactic against complaints and litigation.

> Negligence comprises three elements, namely (i) a duty of care between claimant and defendant; (ii) a breach, by an act or omission, that falls below the standard of care expected; and (iii) causation, ie the breach resulted in loss or damage to the claimant that was reasonably proximate.

> The standard of care expected of doctors is that of acting in accordance with a responsible body of medical opinion (the *Bolam* test), and in a way that withstands logical analysis (the *Bolitho* amendment).

> There are particular areas of clinical risk involving administrative and organisational aspects of clinical care of which students should be aware, including record-keeping, referrals, following up investigations, communication with other healthcare professionals and prescribing medication.

 # Assessments: Competence, Whistleblowing, Negligence and Clinical Risk

1. Health, competence and colleagues

Sample SAQ

Dr John Rees is a GP Principal in a four-partner practice. Over the last few months, his partners have been concerned because of the deterioration in the quality of care he is delivering to his patients. One of his partners, Dr Evans, is aware that he has had problems with alcohol abuse in the past and she suspects that he has relapsed.

(a) Describe the duty imposed by the General Medical Council in respect of colleagues who abuse alcohol and/or drugs. How should Dr Evans discharge this duty? (5 marks)

(b)   It has been estimated that approximately 10% of doctors have a dependency problem at any one time. List three UK-based services that exist specifically to help doctors, like Dr Rees, who become dependent on drugs or alcohol. Suggest one advantage and one disadvantage of these services run specifically for doctors.   (4 marks)

Guidance notes

Part (a)   The GMC states in *Good Medical Practice* that all doctors have a duty to protect patients when they believe that a colleague's health, conduct or performance poses a risk to patient care. The GMC advises that the appropriate way in which Dr Evans should discharge this duty is:

- Try to find out the facts (eg talk to Dr Rees and/or the other partners).
- Follow employer's procedures – this is less easy in general practice where GPs have the status of self-employed contractors as opposed to the employed status of doctors working in secondary care. However, there may be a practice policy on ill health, which Dr Evans should investigate. If there is not practice policy, a discussion with the other partners would be a logical next step if Dr Rees refuses to acknowledge that there is a problem.
- Seek advice from an appropriate person eg the PCT lead.
- Comments made by Dr Evans about Dr Rees must be honest.
- Ultimately, the GMC states that 'the safety of patients must come first at all times'

Part (b)   Organisations that exist specifically to support doctors include:

- Mednet (at the Tavistock and Portman NHS Trust)
- National Counselling Service for Sick Doctors
- The Practitioner Health Programme

Chapter 11

- The Sick Doctors Trust
- The BMA 24-hour Counselling Service
- Doctors' Support Network
- British Doctors and Dentists Section of the Medical Council on Alcoholism
- Local NHS Occupational Health Services

The potential advantages of such specialised services include that they are:
- Anonymous
- Easier to access for many doctors who might not be registered with a GP, or are reluctant to consult GP.
- Familiar with the particular pressures of being a doctor
- A source of peer group support

The potential disadvantages of such specialised services include:
- They could prevent doctor from seeking advice of GP
- They are not as proactive as a GP could be with an 'ordinary' patient with dependency problems
- The help provided depends on doctor recognising problem in first instance
- The public perception of the 'closed shop' effect of such support groups

2. Negligence and clinical risk

Sample SAQ

Dr Paros intends to take advice from the local diabetic clinic regarding appropriate therapy for one of his patients, Mr Henry, because he is unsure whether insulin should be started straight away. Mr Henry has renal impairment. Dr Paros asks Mr Henry to return in a few days. Mr Henry is increasingly anxious about his condition and attends his usual doctor, Dr Dawson, for a second opinion. Dr Dawson does not usually manage the diabetic patients within the practice and is not up to date in this area. He starts him on Metformin, which is contraindicated in renal impairment.

> (a) What standard of care is used to determine whether Dr Dawson's error constitutes negligence? (3 marks)
> (b) Suggest five areas of potential risk in clinical practice that can lead to errors and/or give rise to negligence claims.
> (5 marks)

Guidance notes

Part (a)   The standard of care is the *Bolam* test subject to the *Bolitho* amendment, ie did Dr Dawson act as a body of reasonable practitioners would have acted and do his actions or omissions withstand logical analysis by the court?

Part (b)   Areas of potential clinical risk that may given rise to errors and/or negligence claims include:

- Note-keeping – incomplete, illegible, non-contemporaneous
- Prescribing – second common cause of negligence actions (failure to meet four-fold duty as set out by defence organisations)
- Follow-up – administrative error, duty of care to meet administrative responsibilities as part of follow-up eg to send letters, communicate with other professionals etc
- Confidentiality – data sharing, DPA and access to medical records and information
- Communication between primary and secondary care
- Monitoring in chronic illness eg international normalised ratio (INR) for patients on Warfarin, blood pressure measurement for patients on oral contraception etc.
- Consent – insufficient information, seeking invalid consent eg from relatives/next of kin
- Capacity – determination without regard to the Mental Capacity Act 2005
- Interaction with other professional groups and agencies eg radiographs mislabelled, referrals to and from social services etc.
- Implementation of guidelines and protocols

Chapter 12

Publish or Perish: Research and Publication Ethics

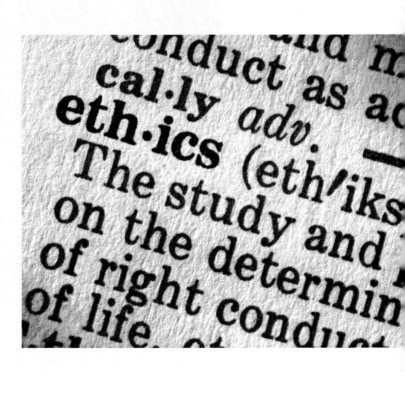

Publish or Perish: Research and Publication Ethics

Introduction

Whether or not you, as a medical student, are involved in research (and increasing numbers of students are participating in research projects as part of their education and training), you will be working with treatments that have been developed by research, often involving both animal and human subjects. This chapter discusses the ethico-legal framework for research involving both animals and people and considers its relevance for medical students.

Research with human subjects

Since the Nuremberg trials and the promulgation of the Nuremberg Code, research on human subjects has been regulated. The key source of regulatory information on biomedical research on human subjects is found in the Declaration of Helsinki[219] (which is revised and updated regularly). In the United Kingdom, the regulation of research on human subjects that involves NHS staff, patients or premises falls within the remit of the National Research Ethics Service (NRES)[220] which is currently part of the National Patient Safety Agency.[221] NRES oversees the framework for research governance. It provides an Integrated Research Application Service for those wishing to undertake research in the fields of health, social and community care.

One of the first and most fundamental ethico-legal questions to be considered is whether a proposed project is research at all. If a project is not research, it will not be required to undergo the same ethical review that applies to proposed research. The line between research, service evaluation and clinical audit can be confusing, especially for medical students who may be new to the field. The National Research Ethics Service issues guidance on how

---

[219] www.wma.net/en/30publications/10policies/b3/ [accessed 27 June 2011].

[220] www.nres.npsa.nhs.uk/ [accessed 27 June 2011].

[221] At the time of writing, the National Patient Safety Agency was to be disbanded following the Coalition Government's review of Arms Length Bodies; see *Liberating the NHS – Report of the Arms-Length Bodies Review*. London: Department of Health, July 2010.

to distinguish between research, audit and service evaluation[222]. That guidance suggests that if the following four conditions apply, the project is likely to be research: (i) the intention of the project is to generate generalisable and new information; (ii) it involves providing a treatment or service; (iii) a protocol is used to allocate services or treatment; and (iv) participants are randomised.

For all research, including that conducted by medical students[223] and pilot studies which involves NHS staff, patients or premises, an application for ethical review should be made prior to any work being conducted. The application will be considered by a NHS Research Ethics Committee (REC). All RECs are subject to the Governance Arrangements for NHS Research Ethics Committees (GAfREC). Membership of Research Ethics Committees is intended to be balanced and to include lay members. The intention is to achieve a range of perspectives on research and its ethics. The materials reviewed by the REC include the research protocol, any participant recruitment or information material, the consent form and the research expertise and experience of the investigators. Applicants are encouraged to attend the REC meeting where their application is being considered but are not required to do so.

For research that does not fall within the remit of NRES and the NHS REC system, for example educational research or inquiry in the social sciences that does not involve health, social or community care, there is a requirement to have the proposal reviewed by an institutional or organisational ethics committee eg a university or charity ethics committee. It is the obligation of the researcher to submit an appropriate application and to follow the governance requirements that apply to his or her particular project.

Whether research is reviewed by a NHS REC or another institutional committee, there are ethical dimensions to all research that should be considered. It may be helpful to think about the ethical dimensions of research as comprising four elements, namely: (i) the validity and rigour of the proposed research; (ii) the balance of potential risks and benefits arising from the research; (iii) how

---

[222] *Defining Research*. London: National Research Ethics Service, December 2009
[223] All student research that is below doctoral level must have a named supervisor who acts as the Chief Investigator for the purposes of the application for ethical review.

to provide information such as to facilitate valid consent; and (iv) the processes involved in carrying out the research itself. In short and in the words of Grbich, conducting research in an ethical way requires the researcher to take *'demonstrable responsibility for the issues of power, negotiation and transformation'* at all stages.[224]

The validity and rigour of research

Validity and rigour are fundamental ethical requirements of research. Any research will entail some degree of inconvenience and/or risk for the participants. As such, the potential benefits and quality of the proposed research must be considered and scrutinised. The research must be designed to ask an important question with appropriate and adequate methodology, so that an answer can be obtained within a reasonable period of time. Whilst the scientific paradigm will apply when considering the validity of many proposals reviewed by NHS Research Ethics Committees, there is an increasing (and welcome) emphasis on qualitative inquiry in health and social care and the requirements for methodological rigour may differ from the focus on randomisation and statistical power that is relevant to traditional quantitative studies. Research that is poorly designed, inadequately rigorous or unduly repetitive of earlier work can be said to be *prima facie* 'unethical' because it necessarily compromises the balance of benefits and harms, although the terms 'poorly designed', 'inadequately rigorous' and 'unduly repetitive' are themselves statements of judgement and value. The concept of what research is worthwhile is itself socially constructed, and frequently reflects the dominance of positivistic enquiry conducted by the disinterested investigator and quantitative paradigms of generalisability and causation. Methodological preferences and choices of method depend on the aims of the research; the methodological approach should be that which allows the researcher to address the question(s) he or she poses.

Imagine, for instance, that you are a researcher embarking on an interview study in which you wish to find out about medical students' perceptions of stress. If you are interested in perception,

---

[224] Grbich, C. *Qualitative Research in Health: An Introduction.* London: Sage, 1999 at p. 77.

it is likely that talking to people directly and in person is going to produce the richest accounts. The nuances and silent cues of nonverbal communication are too important to be eliminated by telephone interviews or written questionnaires. Given the potentially sensitive subject of the research, focus groups or other collective interviews would probably not be suitable. Although the interaction and stimulation of a focus group is sometimes appealing, group dynamics might adversely affect and inhibit participation and the method does not lend itself to in depth discussion of personal experience like a one-to-one interview. For a student or novice researcher, whether you are planning qualitative or quantitative research, it is essential that you have the support of an experienced supervisor who is familiar with, and skilled in, the type of research that you wish to pursue.

The fact that a proposed study has validity and rigour does not necessarily mean that the research is justifiable. Thus, questions will be asked about the relevance of the research (in the context of existing knowledge and likely benefits). In short, all researchers should ask themselves the 'so what?' question when proposing a particular project or study. What is it that this particular proposal has to offer the body of knowledge? What would happen if this research were *not* to take place? However, in evaluating the potential value of a research proposal it must be remembered that research is a process of continued development and unexpected evolution. A single experiment or study may not in itself be immediately beneficial or significant, but it may build on and develop the ideas and findings of earlier research and raise relevant questions to be asked in future experiments. Is it appropriate only to think of benefits from research in terms of the micro effect for an individual participant of a single experiment or study? Or is it more appropriate to think of benefits in terms of the macro effect for communities of patients (present or future) of a series of experiments or studies within an institution, a country or even globally? How far removed from the experimental process does the 'benefit' need to be before it can be considered significant? There is a history of serendipitous discoveries in biomedical research ranging from the discovery of penicillin to the role of insulin in diabetes; luck and chance can lead to positive but unexpected discoveries that were not even conceived of as possibilities by a researcher investigating something else entirely. Ethical reviews of research have to be sufficiently flexible to allow for serendipity, the slow pace of many biomedical advances, and creativity, whilst protecting those who participate in the research and ensuring it remains rigorous.

Balancing risks and benefits in research

Once a project has been determined to be valid, rigorous and methodologically appropriate, the relative risks and benefits must be considered. Essentially, as with clinical work, the researcher must seek to balance her obligations to do good (although see the discussion above for the challenges inherent in determining 'good' in biomedical research) which may be both for her own patients and the wider interests of those with a particular condition, and to prevent harm to her individual participants (benevolence and non-maleficence).

Before thinking about the balance of risks and benefits in practice and in relation to different types of research, it is worth taking time to think a little more deeply about what constitutes a 'risk' in research. Often there will be obvious risks: the potential side-effects of a new drug, the discomfort of a procedure or the inconvenience of an admission for the research to be conducted under supervision. However, there are also subtler and more nuanced ways of thinking about 'risk' in research that tend to be underconsidered. To return to our imaginary interview study in which you wish to talk to medical students about the stress that they encounter in their practice, what might a broader approach to risks and benefits require?

First, the researcher should be alert and sensitive to his or her place in developing the interview, engaging with potential participants, conducting interviews, hearing the participants' voices, interpreting narratives, analysing and eventually presenting the data.

The question is whether the researcher is sufficiently reflective about the possible influence of status as presented and perceived in the project. In other words, status is relevant because the researcher must remain sensitive and alert to the mutual and dynamic interaction of the interviews. Whether you choose to interview students who are known to you, or those from another institution where you are unknown, there will be different issues to consider but nonetheless you do need to reflect on the effect of your relationship with your interviewees (as a peer or stranger). As a medical student yourself, you are likely to have your own experiences of and views about stress. You must think about your own perceptions and how those have informed your research. The use of interviews as a research tool has similar potential for the transference and counter-transference more familiar in the fields of psychiatry, psychotherapy and psychoanalysis. Age, gender, accent, ethnicity, dress, perceived attractiveness and demeanour all contribute to how we are perceived and perceive others. All interviewers and interviewees are engaged in what psychologists call 'impression management'. The ways in which 'self' is perceived by others in interview-based research is particularly important given the closeness, sociability, active participation and intimacy inherent in an interview. Both interviewer and interviewee will be engaged in 'interview work' and their respective roles, perceptions and responses contribute to this interview work. It is in this context that information is shared, presented, received and interpreted and why the researcher's status influences the interaction he or she has with the interviewees.

Feminist methodologists have written extensively about the shared enterprise of research in which the power imbalance between researcher and subject is deliberately acknowledged and addressed. A research partnership, rather than a research hierarchy[225] is likely to be both more effective and more ethical. It is important to allow the interviewees time and space to respond as they wished, to acknowledge and respond humanely to visible distress. Although this project involves interviewing members of a high status and articulate group, there is no reason to reject the feminist model of interviews in which equality, compassionate and mutual exchange are prioritised.

Other ethical issues relate to the subject matter and what participants might disclose in the interviews about stress and its effects on clinical practice. It has been suggested that unpredictability is a defining methodological criterion in qualitative research but can

---

[225] Sprague, J., Zimmerman, M.K. 'Overcoming Dualisms: A Feminist Agenda for Sociological Methodology' in Hesse-Biber, S. N., Leavy, P. (eds.) *Approaches to Qualitative Research: A Reader on Theory and Practice.* Oxford: Oxford University Press, 2004.

render consent a particular challenge.[226] Asking students about stress might be unsettling and even distressing for interviewees. A researcher must not underestimate the privilege of hearing such personal stories. The interview should be designed with emotional pace in mind. If consent is to be not merely informed but continuing, the researcher has to respond to distress, encourage participants to take their time, offer to stop the interview, and remind them only to discuss what felt comfortable. The question of the boundaries and extent of a researcher's duty of care is particularly difficult in the context of psychological symptoms and emotional distress,[227] and it can be helpful to have a list of sources of support or advice to hand to share should it be appropriate.

It is easy for a researcher to be so focused on the project in hand that they forget that the participants are people who have given up their time and, sometimes, shared personal details with them. Small, but important acknowledgements of the value of an individual's participation can be invaluable. In our imaginary project, it might be that when the interview is complete, participants receive a letter or email of thanks. Some researchers, in the spirit of a true research partnership, offer to share transcripts, data, results and any subsequent publication.

What happens if one encounters information during research that is alarming? Although it is unlikely, it is another potential ethical dilemma that researchers should consider when planning their projects. Much, perhaps most, research offers confidentiality and anonymisation of data. Before doing so, however, one has to be clear that such promises about confidentiality and anonymisation can be met. As a researcher working with participants with whom one has no contractual or professional connection, the question of whether there were any circumstances under which confidentiality might be breached is complex, but nonetheless cannot be disregarded. Traditionally, researchers have defended the confidentiality of their

---

[226] Eisner, E. W. *The Enlightened Eye*. New York: Macmillan, 1991.

[227] Eccleston, C. Commentary on Ethical and Research Dilemmas Arising from a Questionnaire Study of Psychological Morbidity among General Practice Managers. *British Journal of General Practice* 2001; 51:34; Dickson-Swift, V., James, E. L., Kippen, S. and Liamputtong, K. P. Blurring Boundaries in Qualitative Health Research on Sensitive Topics. *Qual Health Res* 2006; 16(6): 853–871.

data completely, even to the point of going to prison.[228] However, for most researchers there are limits to confidentiality, particularly in relation to serious harm. These limits are embodied in ethical codes. As a medical student, you too are working within an ethico-legal framework where there are limits to the confidentiality that you can offer. When medical students qualify as doctors, the guidance from the General Medical Council on confidentiality and its relationship to research sets the boundaries for the confidentiality that can be offered. A related point with respect to confidentiality is how data are handled, protected and subsequently anonymised. Inclusion of detail can inadvertently result in easy identification and therefore constitute a breach of confidentiality. You should consider how you will anonymise your data and include the details of anonymisation in the information for participants. It is essential to work out the extent to which any information shared with you in research is confidential and to include an honest account of confidentiality and anonymisation to all prospective participants. You might also, if you are conducting an interview-based study or have the opportunity to speak to prospective participants, explicitly invite questions about confidentiality and anonymisation to ensure that it has been properly understood and allow an opportunity for discussion.

Valid consent in research

As in clinical practice, in research, valid consent is essential and the validity of consent depends on the same four elements (discussed in Chapter 3) as applied in clinical practice, namely (i) capacity; (ii) information; (iii) voluntariness; and (iv) ongoing permission. Consent matters because not only does it demonstrate that someone has evaluated the risks and benefits and freely chosen to take part in the research, but also because it demonstrates that participants in research are moral agents in their own right and not simply 'a means to an end'. Again like clinical practice, the consent form is an acknowledgement that consent has been sought from the patient, and is not a substitute for a discussion in which the proposed research is fully explained (in non-technical language) and the patient's questions and concerns addressed. In research, such discussion

---

[228] Kvale, S. *Interviews: An Introduction to Qualitative Research Interviewing*. London: Sage, 1996.

is usually reinforced by written information, partly because the details of the study or project are often complex and it is helpful to give people something to read and consider before they agree to participate and partly because NHS Research Ethics Committees expect to see patient information and a written consent form.

All prospective participants who are approached about participating in research must be assured that a refusal to participate in research will not affect their clinical care in any way. In some cases it may be more appropriate for an independent third party to seek consent from possible participants; there is already a power imbalance between doctors and patients and the desire to 'please' or 'thank' the doctor may lead to a sense of obligation in some people, which is avoided when a third party, unknown to the patient from their routine clinical care, seeks consent to participate in research. Indeed, it has been argued that no matter how fairly the invitation to participate in research is expressed, recipients of the approach will feel in some way indebted or obliged to agree.[229] Ways to ensure patients are not pressured into participating might include the use of a formal letter sent by post as the initial contact (rather than an email), a telephone call or even opportunistic meeting, to allow recipients time to deliberate and reflect on whether they wish to participate in research. If potential participants are encountered in the clinical setting or elsewhere after a formal letter of invitation has been sent, it is wise to avoid mentioning the research and letter if the individual does not refer to it, and to avoid sending reminders to those who do not respond to the letter. Payments are a vexed area in research. If a payment is too great, it is an inducement and invalidates consent. However, it is usual for expenses to be reimbursed, and sometimes for inconvenience to be recompensed. All participants should be aware that they can withdraw from the research at any stage and that their decision to withdraw from the research will not affect their clinical care in any way. However research teams seek to address the issue of voluntariness, it is essential that deliberate attention is paid to maximising the freedom to choose.

Information is central to consent. Prospective participants should have sufficient information to enable them to make a choice. The

---

[229] Sapsford, R., Abbott, P. *Research Methods for Nurses and Caring Professionals.* Buckingham: Open University Press, 1992.

provision of information is not a one-way conversation in which the expert researcher transmits information to a passive patient. Rather, information should be shared. Information should not just include an account of the research project. Prospective participants should understand the practical implications of taking part. Patients should be encouraged to ask questions, explain how he or she feels about what has been said and convey his or her own priorities. At different stages of a research project, participants might be reminded of the aims of the research, invited to ask questions and offered the opportunity to receive updates on the progress of the research. The ethical review process will look closely at both the information that is provided to prospective participants, and the opportunities to discuss that information in a way that is timely and responsive.

Particular ethical questions arise in respect of vulnerable participants eg unconscious and cognitively impaired patients and children. An absolutist perspective suggests that vulnerable patients should never be able to participate in research. However, the repercussions of such a position for research would be huge. Therefore, it is more usual for ethics committees to adopt a risk assessment approach to vulnerable participants: the greater the likely risk[230] to the patient ,the less justification there is likely to be for the proposed research. Where a person does not have the capacity (as determined by the Mental Capacity Act 2005; see Chapter 3) to make a choice about participating in research, guidance suggests that assent should be sought. Assent demonstrates a commitment to seeking the agreement of those who have a sense of the incapacitous patient's best interests and wishes. In paediatrics, assent might be sought from the child[231] and/or person with parental responsibility (see Chapter 6). In the ICU, assent may be sought from a patient's partner, spouse or adult child. The Mental Capacity Act 2005[232] emphasises the need to consult someone who can represent the incapacitated person's wishes and interests. That consultation does not equate to legal or proxy consent but is, instead, an opportunity to find out more

---

[230] Risk should include not only physical risks, but also inconvenience, discomfort, embarrassment and invasion of privacy.

[231] For a thoughtful account of assent in paediatrics, see Wendler, D.S. Assent in Paediatric Research: Theoretical and Practical Considerations. *J Med Ethics* 2006; 32: 229–234.

[232] See Section 32 of the Act and Chapter 11 of the Code of Practice.

about the incapacitated person's values, preferences and priorities to inform any decision about participation in research.

Therapeutic and non-therapeutic research

Research ethics guidance has traditionally distinguished between therapeutic and non-therapeutic research for the purposes of evaluating risks and benefits. Therapeutic research is that which has the potential to produce a benefit to participants; non-therapeutic research is that which may generate knowledge that benefits groups of patients in the future, but that is unlikely to benefit the participants in the research.

In therapeutic research the key principle is that, without the research, there can be no certainty as to which of the treatments or interventions being tested will be of benefit, thereby justifying the random allocation of therapies, interventions or treatments to patients. If it becomes clear during the course of a study that one particular treatment or intervention is more effective than another, then the research must cease. Concomitant risks that arise during the research must be minimised wherever possible and safety of the participants is the primary concern. In non-therapeutic research, the rights of the participants are central. Many patients will agree to participate in such research (where there is no benefit to them) for altruistic reasons.

Although the distinction between therapeutic and non-therapeutic research continues to appear in guidelines, the distinction can be inconsistently drawn or difficult to delineate consistently. Furthermore, participants who act as controls in therapeutic research are in the same position as participants in non-therapeutics research in that no benefit is likely to accrue to them. It may be more meaningful to think about the ethical aspects of research with reference to the principles described in this chapter, irrespective of the type of research being considered.

Research raises particular ethico-legal issues regarding confidentiality and access to, and the management of, data. The most important piece of law with which researchers should be familiar is the Data Protection Act 1998. The Data Protection Act 1998 (DPA) is an immensely complex piece of legislation and only the basic principles of the statute are discussed in this paper. A useful starting point for specific queries is the Information Commissioner's website which can be found at www.ico.gov.uk

The DPA 1998 came fully into force in 1999. However, there are provisions to allow for the development of transitional mechanisms eg for data held before 24 October 1998, the data controller has three years (longer in the case of some manual data) to conform to the requirements of the DPA 1998. The DPA 1984 is repealed by the 1998 Act. The 1998 Act contains eight principles of data protection. The definition of 'data' within the 1998 Act would seem likely to incorporate information that might be held by either a Primary Care Trust (PCT) or a Health Authority, such information being *'recorded as part of a relevant filing system'* and forming *'part of an accessible record'* (DPA 1998, section 1(1)). Note no distinction is drawn between manual and electronic data. The emphasis is on the thematic 'setting' or structuring of information rather than the physical filing systems used. The Data Commissioner recommends that organisations undertake an audit of existing data to evaluate how well the storage of that data complies with the DPA 1998. Such an audit would be a large undertaking for PCTs and Health Authorities but should be considered.

'Personal data' is information by which an individual can be identified and includes statements of opinion (as well as fact) and indications of any intentions of the data controller in respect of the named individual. Thus, in terms of performance assessments and information about potentially poorly performing doctors, it is not only the factual information which falls within the DPA 1998, but also expressions of opinion about an individual doctor and recommendations or proposals that affect that doctor.

The DPA 1998 significantly broadens the definition of data 'processing' to incorporate the obtaining, holding and disclosing of information. This is clearly at the heart of the issues surrounding the communication of information about potentially poorly performing doctors.

Data controllers, ie those responsible for managing data, should seek consent from those about whom they are holding data. In general, the more ambiguous and implied the consent on which the data controller relies, the more likely the Data Commissioner is to question its validity. This has relevance when considering how doctors should be advised that personal data may be held and processed by PCTs and/or health authorities.

Data should be accurate and the onus is on the data controller to take all reasonable steps to verify the accuracy of the data, rather than simply rely on the word of third parties. Thus, careful documentation of how information (about potentially poorly performing doctors) is evaluated by the relevant data controller will be important to the work of the PCTs and Health Authorities in investigating and managing potential poor performance in primary care.

Individuals are entitled to be told by data controllers whether data is being processed about them by or on behalf of an organisation. If the latter, individuals can seek a description of (i) the data held; (ii) the purposes for which data are being processed; and (iii) persons/third parties to whom data may be disclosed. Individuals can ask for a copy of the data (which must be in an accessible and intelligible form). Requests must be made in writing and the data controller can charge a fee.

If decisions are likely to be made solely on the basis of the data, the individual is entitled to be told of the logic and reasoning behind such decision-making. There is a further important reason why all decision-making must be well reasoned and clearly documented, which is to prevent the potential challenges that could be made via judicial review. Where an individual discovers that data are inaccurate, he can apply to have the data corrected, blocked, erased or destroyed. This might be a particular issue in data describing a doctor's performance.

Activities: Research with human subjects

Consider the principles discussed in so far in this chapter with reference to the following scenarios.

Scenario

Mrs Woolf presents to her GP, Dr Leonard, for a routine cervical smear. As she lies on the examination couch, the Dr Leonard tells Mrs Woolf that *'the teaching hospital is doing a study on chlamydia, would you mind if I take a swab while you're here for that study?'*

(i) What do you think of Dr Leonard's approach?
(ii) What information would you require if you were Mrs Woolf?
(iii) If Mrs Woolf agreed to take part and was found to have chlamydia, who should be responsible for informing Mrs Woolf?
(iv) What criteria should have been included in the study protocol to ensure that Mrs Woolf was properly informed and able to give adequate consent?

Scenario

You are working with Professor Ridley, a Professor of Haemotology, on a research project. One morning, Professor Ridley asks you to contact the lecturer in clinical skills because *'the students are practising cannulation this morning, and we should be able to take the blood samples to use in the lab'.*

(i) Is Professor Ridley's request ethical?

Guinea pigs as guinea pigs: the ethics of using animals in biomedical research

Research on animals has been regulated since the Cruelty to Animals Act 1876. The current law is found in the Animals (Scientific Procedures) Act 1986. The Declaration of Helsinki states that any health research involving human participants *'should be based on adequately performed laboratory and animal experimentation'*. However, to examine only the regulation of experimentation on animals is to presume that the use of animals in scientific research is *a priori* ethical. This section will consider the main ethical arguments for and against the use of animals, and the UK regulatory framework for the use of animals, in biomedical research.

The ethics of research involving animals

One of the most prominent ethicists to write extensively about the use of animals in biomedical research is Peter Singer.[233] Singer suggests that the key to understanding the debate about the use of animals is not equality of treatment but equality of *consideration*. He argues that once we have considered how animals should be treated we might well conclude that the logical thing is that they should be subject to different treatment and different entitlements. However, Singer argues, we have not yet reached a position where we have afforded equal consideration to animals and are therefore not yet in a position to justify different treatment. 'Speciesism' is the term used by Singer to describe discrimination against non-humans. Singer argues that if we do not discriminate against our fellow human beings because they are less intelligent than us, then we cannot sustain a moral argument for treating animals differently simply because they are apparently 'less intelligent' than us. Singer suggests it is sentience, not intelligence, that is the criterion for the right to equal consideration (note, not necessarily treatment). Indeed, Singer has suggested that mature cats, dogs and mice are more aware of what is happening to them than human infants. Does sentience entitle animals to the same consideration as non-animals? Or does the argument lead to equal rights for animals? If it is the latter, Singer argues that the protection offered to animals should be the same as that given to humans who are incapable of giving consent.

What can be said in response to the point that benefits (to humans, other animals, or both) have followed from animal experimentation? The way in which the 'benefit' argument is addressed depends upon the way in which distinctions are drawn between human beings and animals. If we adopt Singer's test of sentience, why could experiments with obvious and proven benefits not be performed on humans for the same benefit? Benefit alone may not be enough to justify experimentation on animals unless we can distinguish

---

[233] Singer, P. *Animal Liberation*. New York: Random House. 1975. The title was revised and a second edition published in 1995.

animals from humans in an intellectually convincing and morally significant way. As discussed, Singer, of course, believes that intelligence is not the way to do this but sentience which results in there being parity and equality between the species. Moreover, if Singer's sentience criterion is used, the question has to be whether it is sentience of pain or simply an awareness of surroundings that might also be significant, since experiments may be painless.

If sentience is not the means by which to attempt to distinguish humans from animals, what alternative arguments have been made? The basic principle to which philosophers most often return is that human life is intrinsically more valuable than animal life. What is it that makes so many commentators convinced of the increased value of human life? Can human beings be distinguished on the grounds of their unique capability for moral agency? Only humans have the capacity to make moral distinctions and to constrain their behaviour as appropriate. Yet there are people who do not have the capacity for moral agency eg babies or severely cognitively impaired adults. How might we protect those human beings if we determine that the capacity for moral agency is the distinguishing feature of humans as compared with animals? Campbell *et al.*[234] suggest these examples are distinguishable because of the capacity of babies to develop into moral agents as adults, and because of the unique relationship mentally impaired adults have with their fellow humans. Our obligations to both children and mentally impaired adults must exceed our obligations to animals, argue Campbell *et al.*

Some argue that it is the capacity for spiritual or religious experience that demarcates humans from animals. Others cite the more complex constitution of the human as the rationale for the belief in the greater value of human life. It is the fact that we enjoy a wider range of relationships, occupations and purpose than animals. Our lives are more valuable because, in the words of the philosopher, Frey, *'of the many more possibilities for enrichment they contain'*.[235] However,

---

[234] Campbell, A., Charlesworth, M., Gillett, G. and Jones, G. *The Use of Animals in Medical Research* in *Medical Ethics* (2nd ed.) Oxford: Oxford University Press, 1997 at p. 179.
[235] Frey, R. G. 'Vivisection, Morals and Medicine' in Kuhse, H., Singer, P. *Bioethics: An Anthology*. Oxford: Blackwell, 1999 at pp. 471 ff.

such an argument may not help us with human beings whose quality of life is poor (although we should be aware of the perils of making such moral judgments eg how do we know whether the quality of life of someone with cognitive impairment is poor?). To adopt such a position one needs to be convinced that the quality of all human life is inherently richer and more valuable than that of any animal. Frey[236] is unable to identify human life as inherently richer, and thus concludes that experiments should be performed on human subjects (with appropriate precautions). Paton[237] counters Frey's conclusions by suggesting that the examination of extreme examples, such as the comparison of an anencephalic foetus with a highly trained, intelligent and valuable sheep dog, does not give us any workable principles or criteria for evaluating 'quality of life', but simply invites emotional comment on a hard case. Paton argues that it is human achievement that distinguishes human life (and that this is not contingent upon contribution to the future). It is the continuum of human progress that distinguishes human beings from animals.

This section has outlined some of the main moral arguments for and against the use of animals in research. There are many variations and subtleties in the debate, which are not discussed due to the constraints of space. However, before moving on to discuss the regulation of animal experiments in the UK, it should be asked whose moral problem is the question of animal experimentation? Is it the preserve of researchers, drug companies, scientific institutions, regulatory agencies and the law or society at large? If as a society we are to believe in the value of science and to overcome some of the latent suspicion of science and scientists, there must be a culture of moral accountability, democracy and openness. There cannot be dogma without discussion and discussion must be informed, consistent and intelligent.

---

[236] Frey, R. G. 'Vivisection, Morals and Medicine' in Kuhse, H., Singer, P. *Bioethics: An Anthology*. Oxford: Blackwell, 1999.

[237] Paton W. 'Commentary from a Vivisecting Professor of Pharmacology' in Kuhse, H., and Singer, P. *Bioethics: An Anthology*. Oxford: Blackwell, 1999 at pp. 476–8.

The regulatory framework for the use of animals in research

Under the Animals (Scientific Procedures) Act 1986, the Home Office, advised by the Animal Procedures Inspectorate[238], is responsible for the use of animals in experiments. The statute applies to all protected animals ie all living vertebrates and one invertebrate, the common octopus. The Home Office's policy on the regulation of animal experiments is often described as 'The Three Rs' and prioritises:

- **Replacement**: non-animal methods should be used wherever possible eg researchers should consider the use of computer simulators or tissue samples rather than animals;
- **Reduction**: the numbers of animals used in experiments should be the minimum needed to give clear experimental results; and
- **Refinement**: the smallest degree of pain and distress should be inflicted and for a justifiable purpose.

Replacement may be possible in some circumstances by the use of computers that simulate body systems, cell culture and isolated tissues and organs. However, these alternatives are not always available. In addition to serving as a direct replacement for animals in research, computers may also contribute to an overall reduction in the number of experiments because literature searches may result in more thorough and better designed studies. Refinement requires that, as a minimum requirement, researchers are trained in the use of anaesthesia, caring for animals, analgesia and post-operative care. Premises licensed to conduct research involving animals are regularly inspected by teams of specialists employed by the Animal Procedures Inspectorate. The inspection teams will often arrive unannounced. At a local level, all institutions carrying out research on animals must have an animal ethics committee and a remit to establish ways in which 'The Three Rs' can be practicably implemented. The committees are responsible (within the Home Office and statutory framework) for reviewing and monitoring all research proposed or taking place within an institution.

---

[238] The Animal Procedures Inspectorate composition includes scientists, animal welfare experts and lawyers.

Three licences are required for any scientific work controlled by the Act, namely (i) a certificate of designation for the research site; (ii) a personal licence for the researcher(s); and (iii) a project licence. For the project licence, it must be shown that the experiments are well designed and are to be performed for justifiable reasons – the so-called 'cost-benefit assessment'. The higher the levels of potential distress, and the more invasive an experiment is, the more the project will be scrutinised. An individual researcher may only perform animal experiments if she is personally licensed to do so. Before a licence is granted, it must be shown (in both a written and a practical assessment) that the individual has been trained on an accredited course. Any applicant for a licence must show:

- An understanding and awareness of the ethical debate about animal experiments;
- A working knowledge of the law on animal experiments;
- An understanding of the health, safety and wellbeing of the animals;
- An understanding of minor and common surgical procedures, anaesthesia, analgesia and euthanasia
- A practical understanding of restraint and handling of animals in a laboratory.

When a licence is first issued to an individual they will have to work under the supervision of an experienced licence holder. The licence allows the holder to do only that which has been agreed as being within the terms of her licence. The aims of the research must be shown to be in the interests of the advancement of medical or scientific knowledge and the experiments should be designed to cause minimum distress to the animal.

Even if you never participate in research involving animals, as a medical student and future doctor the treatment you offer and the evidence on which you base your clinical practice will be derived from research with animals. As such, it is valuable to think about the moral dimensions to that work and become familiar with the regulation of the research that will inform so much of what you do in your career.

Publication Ethics

The ethico-legal questions relating to research do not end once a study is complete. There is increasing attention to, and interest in, the ethico-legal issues that arise in relation to the publication of research. Medicine and the biosciences have led the way on publication ethics. The Committee on Publication Ethics (COPE)[239] began life in 1997 as a result of the commitment of a small group of editors of medical and scientific journals. Since its early days, COPE has facilitated discussion of ethical issues involved in publishing and produced guidance, including a Code of Practice for journal editors. So what sorts of ethical questions can arise in relation to publishing research?

Authors and Contributors

It may surprise some readers, but the question of whether someone is an author, a contributor or neither in relation to research can be a vexed and morally complex matter. Unfortunately, there is a long and ignoble tradition of 'gift authorship' in academic research. Gift authorship refers to naming someone who has not made a meaningful contribution as an author. Sometimes the 'gift' is expected, sometimes it is bestowed unsolicited. Whatever the circumstances, it is not acceptable.

Fortunately, there are criteria available that define what is required to be considered an author. The International Committee of Medical Journal Editors require anyone claiming to be an author to be involved in all three of the following stages of preparing research for publication:

- Conception and design of the study and/or data collection and/or the analysis and interpretation of the data;
- Drafting/revising article critically for important intellectual content;
- Final approval of version to be published.

If a person does not meet the criteria above, he or she should be considered a contributor and a statement to that effect included in the acknowledgements at the end of the submitted manuscript.

---

[239] www.publicationethics.org

Research and 'salami slicing'

The slightly curious term 'salami slicing' refers to the practice of dividing up data/research to produce more papers, often at the expense of quality. The practice can result in difficulties in understanding the context in which the research has been conducted, and duplicate or dual publication which can lead to double-counting of the same data in subsequent aggregate studies. Authors are asked to declare that the work they are submitting is original and has neither been submitted for consideration nor published elsewhere.

Conflicts of interest

All researchers have to interact with a range of people and there will be conflicts of interests/agendas. It may be that the funding organisation has a particular interest in the research findings. The hierarchies within a research team can lead to pressures and tensions. The duties owed to the research participants can collide with a desire to contribute to the professional and academic communities. An awareness of the potential for conflicts of interest is vital for all researchers. Awareness means being sensitive to the potential for others to perceive a conflict of interest, not merely reaching one's own conclusion about whether you believe there is, in fact, a conflict of interest. Consideration of possible conflicts of interest should happen at all stages of the research process: collaborations, citations, data analysis, peer review and choice of journal can all be influenced unduly by conflicts arising from loyalties and hierarchical relationships, financial interests, professional ambition and academic rivalries.

Conclusion

All research, whether with human subjects or animals, involves consideration of how the interests of diverse parties can be protected. Research in healthcare is essential to improve the quality of care available for all. Therefore the ethico-legal issues in biomedical research are relevant to all who work in the healthcare professions. Whilst there are established governance and regulatory frameworks for both research involving people and that involving animals, history is littered with examples of researchers who have found themselves in ethical hot water. From outright fraud to plagiarism and from authorship disputes to undisclosed conflicts of interest, the range of offences committed (often by the most senior people in the field) suggests that many are prepared to take an 'ethical shortcut'. Whatever the perceived pressures that lead to a disregard for the ethical standards required in all research, ultimately medical science is the loser. Insufficient attention to ethical aspects of developing evidence base may not only result in skewed 'evidence' but irrevocably damage the relationship between scientists, doctors, patients and society.

Research and publication ethics and medical students

One of the most noticeable changes I have observed in my career is the eagerness of medical students to publish work. Many students now seek opportunities to participate in existing research projects or to develop their own studies with a view to publication. It is easy to see why. Medicine has always been competitive and publication has become a way of standing out, be it in the Foundation School application process or later in one's career. Unfortunately, the pressure to publish can lead to poor ethical decisions. This section considers some of the common pitfalls that students encounter when seeking to produce some publishable research.

The first issue is a lack of awareness of the processes for ethical governance. Often this is not the student's fault – unfortunately, some supervisors are less assiduous than they might be about seeking ethical review and students, understandably, assume that their supervisors are correct. However, if you put your name to a research project, it is your responsibility to ensure that you have followed the proper governance procedures. In a similar vein, sometimes supervisors will suggest that a questionnaire study is a 'survey' and does not require ethical review. Regrettably, I hear from students who, on submitting their work to a journal, are surprised to be asked for evidence of ethical review and approval. If you are unsure, seek advice from someone who has expertise in research ethics and seek it early.

The second issue relates to ideas for research that are not covered by the National Research Ethics Service because it falls outside its remit. For example, many students are keen to participate in research overseas or other non-NHS settings. In such cases, the local Research Ethics Committee will not be able to review your project or give ethical approval. That does not mean however that you can disregard the ethical aspects of your work. Many universities and third sector organisations have their own ethical governance procedures including ethics committees. Your medical school is likely to want assurance that you have considered the ethical issues arising from your project (and these may be significant if you wish to work with vulnerable or marginalised populations in resource-poor countries) and obtained appropriate permission or approval. It can be a complicated and lengthy procedure obtaining valid ethical review for such projects, so begin early and again, seek advice promptly.

Plagiarism is, unfortunately, a common problem in all academic writing. It is essential that you are aware of the definition of plagiarism that is used by your institution and are scrupulous about referencing. If you are unsure about how to reference, seek help and guidance. Most universities incorporate education about plagiarism into their courses and also often supplementary guidance in course handbooks or from libraries. The use of plagiarism detection software is increasingly common and members of academic staff are trained to detect plagiarism. As a student who is training for a career in which the highest standards of probity and integrity are expected, allegations of plagiarism can raise questions about fitness to practise and seriously affect your career. Simply put: protect yourself against plagiarism by understanding what it is and how to avoid it.

Issues that arise in relation to publication can be particularly problematic for students. The criteria from the International Committee of Medical Journal Editors can be invaluable in deciding whether a supervisor or tutor qualifies for authorship or is a contributor who should be acknowledged. If your tutor or supervisor is an author on the paper, consideration of conflicts of interest should include his or her interests, which are likely to be more complex than yours as a student. It goes without saying that you must follow all the procedures required of authors when submitting your paper; this will include obtaining original signatures from all involved in the project, so allow time to chase people.

Core Concepts: Research and Publication Ethics

Since the Nuremberg trials and the promulgation of the Nuremberg Code, research on human subjects has been regulated. The key source of regulatory information on biomedical research on human subjects is found in the Declaration of Helsinki.

Research involving NHS staff, patients or sites is subject to ethical review by NHS Research Ethics Committees.

The process of ethical review of research in the NHS is co-ordinated by the National Research Ethics Service.

It is important to distinguish between research, audit and service evaluation. If the intent is to generate new knowledge by providing an intervention, it is likely that what is proposed is research.

NHS Research Ethics Committees have a wide membership including clinicians, scientists, lawyers, statisticians and lay members.

Broadly speaking, ethical review of research with human subjects will consider (a) the validity and methodological rigour of the proposal; (b) the balance of risks and benefits; (c) the provision of information and consent process; and (d) the ethical conduct of the project.

Particular ethical questions arise in respect of vulnerable participants eg unconscious and cognitively impaired patients and children. In such cases consultation of those who can represent the patient's best interests takes place and assent is sought.

Some ethical guidance distinguishes between therapeutic and non-therapeutic research, but it may be more helpful to consider each research project with reference to basic ethical principles, irrespective of the type of research.

The ethical issues relating to research on animals have been long debated. Peter Singer argues for equality of consideration on the basis of sentience.

For some, there is a relationship to philosophical arguments about personhood which seek to distinguish human beings by reference to variables, including: the capacity for relationships, the potential for moral reasoning, the nature of human progress and faith-based beliefs about the intrinsic value of human life.

Research on protected animals (vertebrates and one invertebrate, the common octopus) is regulated by the Animal (Scientific Procedures) Act 1986

Regulation is overseen by the Animal Procedures Inspectorate which regularly visits sites where research involving animals is conducted.
The policy regarding research in animal research is often described as 'The Three Rs': replacement, reduction and refinement.
Three types of licence are required to conduct research with animals: a designating certificate for the site, a personal and a project licence.
Publication ethics refers to the ethical issues that can arise in respect of preparing research for publication. In recent years, the Commission on Publication Ethics has led the way in facilitating discussion and issuing guidance on publication ethics.
There are criteria for authorship which should be followed when preparing papers for publication. Gift authorship is unacceptable.
'Salami slicing' refers to splitting a single research project or study into multiple papers to maximise publication. It can skew the literature and lead to distortion of knowledge. Authors are expected to declare if work has been submitted or published elsewhere.
All researchers should consider conflicts of interest in their work. A conflict of interest is what might be perceived by others as influencing the research.

Assessments: Research and Publication Ethics

1.   Animals in biomedical research

Sample OSCE station

You are a student who has just begun work on Dr Carter's firm. Dr Carter is a physician who carries out research on animals. Dr Carter is very keen to ensure that students understand the legislative provisions relating to research on animal subjects, and have considered ethical and moral arguments about such research in order that he can allocate tasks appropriately. Dr Carter does not want those who object to research on animals to be asked to work in the laboratory, and he wishes to ensure that those who do not object to research on animals are aware of the law relevant to such work. Dr Carter routinely sees each student who is new to his firm to discuss the issue of research on animals.

You have been invited to meet Dr Carter to discuss (i) what you know about how research on animals is regulated; and (ii) your personal position on the ethics of using animals in biomedical research.

Guidance notes

- The principal aim of this slightly unusual station is to assess your understanding of the law relating to medical research on animals, and your ability to discuss the main moral arguments relevant to such research.
- You are not being marked on your views, but on your capacity to demonstrate that you are familiar with the law that regulates such research and have thought about the ethical issues sufficiently to substantiate your personal position.
- You should explain that in the UK there is statutory regulation of research on animals in the form of the Animals (Scientific Procedures) Act 1986. Under that law, the Animals Procedure Inspectorate conducts inspections of premises on visits that are often unannounced.
- There are three types of licence of which you should be aware: (i) the certificate of designation for the site; (ii) the project licence; and (iii) the personal licence. There are particular requirements for the training and skills of those holding personal licences.
- The policy in the UK is often described as 'The Three Rs': (i) replacement; (ii) reduction; and (iii) refinement.
- After describing the legal position you should try to explain the ethical issues. Essentially, you should be considering perspectives on whether animals are different from humans and in what way(s). There are several ways of looking at this question, but you might want to consider: sentience, the capacity of human beings for loving relationships and moral choice, human progress, faith-based positions and equality of consideration.
- As the station draws to a close, explain your own view about animals in biomedical research and why you hold that view.

2. **Research ethics**

Sample SAQ

You are attached to an oncology team and have been looking after Mr Harris who has leukaemia. Mr Harris has not responded to treatment. He is expected to live for between six months and a year. The consultant is carrying out research into a new drug that has shown promising results in animal models. He asks you to approach Mr Harris to seek his consent for participation in a trial of the new drug.

(a)   How is research on animals regulated in the UK?
                                                            (4 marks)
(b)   How is research involving NHS staff and patients regulated in the UK?   (4 marks)
(c)   Suggest four points that a Research Ethics Committee considers as part of its ethical review of research involving human subjects.   (4 marks)

Guidance notes

Part (a)   How is research on animals regulated in the UK?

- Research on animals is regulated by the Animals Scientific Procedures Act 1986. The policy in the UK is often described as 'The Three Rs': (i) replacement; (ii) reduction; and (iii) refinement. Under that law, the Animals Procedure Inspectorate conducts inspections of premises on visits that are often unannounced. There are three types of licence for research involving animals, namely: (i) the certificate of designation for the site; (ii) the project licence; and (iii) the personal licence. There are particular requirements for the training and skills of those holding personal licences.

Part (b)   How is research involving NHS staff and patients regulated in the UK?
            The regulation of research on human subjects involving NHS premises, staff and/or patients is overseen by the National Research Ethics Service (NRES). Local Research Ethics Committees review project proposals and the oversight of NRES enhances efficiency and consistency. Membership of Research Ethics Committees is by application and includes statisticians, scientists, clinicians, lawyers, ethicists and lay members.

Part (c)   Suggest four points that a Research Ethics Committee considers as part of its ethical review of research involving human subjects.

            A Research Ethics Committee will consider a range of ethical issues; the more interventionist the proposed research, the greater the scrutiny. Ethical review is likely to include:
            •   Considering the validity and rigour of the proposed project, with particular attention to methodology and methods which should be appropriate to the research question(s).
            •   Weighing the ratio of risks and potential benefits to explore how the burden of research weighs against the potential benefits for both the participants and society at large. Sometimes a distinction is drawn between therapeutic and non-therapeutic research. However, although it is possible that there is greater potential for immediate benefit in therapeutic research, the preferred way to assess the ethical acceptability of the research is to consider first principles, rather than rely on the somewhat artificial distinction between therapeutic and non-therapeutic research.
            •   The provision of information and seeking of consent is vital to ethical research. Information leaflets in non-technical

language should be provided and potential participants invited to discuss the study and ask questions. The consent form is written evidence that a proper discussion has taken place and it is not a substitute for that discussion.

- Scrutiny of the procedures for managing research, including how the team will respond to adverse or unexpected events and the provision for protecting the wellbeing of the participants throughout the project.

Chapter 13

It's Another World: Healthcare Policy, Resource Allocation and Ethics

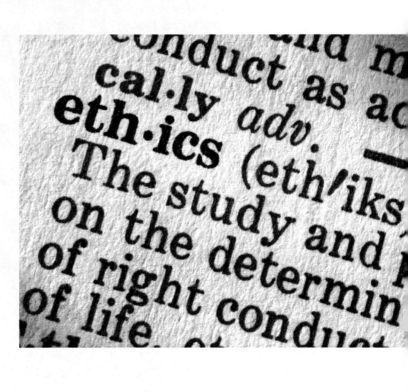

It's Another World: Healthcare Policy, Resource Allocation and Ethics

Introduction

Health policy is often a somewhat neglected subject in medical education. In a crammed curriculum, it is often not seen as something of which medical students need much more than a rudimentary grasp. Yet healthcare policy is what shapes the world of medical students and doctors. If a student remains in clinical practice, he or she may experience the effects of health policy for over 40 years. From the number of places available to prospective students to study medicine to the system for applying for training to posts, and from the resources available in clinical practice to the organisations of clinics, wards and surgeries, you will be living and working in a policy framework throughout your medical education, training and practice.

What is the relationship between ethics and policy? The governance and practice of healthcare is an ethical matter. The values that underpin the organisation and delivery of healthcare are unavoidable and moral in character. Professionals and patients don't interact in a vacuum but in the complex machinery of the NHS as envisaged by its political masters. Yet healthcare and its ethics often seek and claim a position of moral neutrality. The convention for a disinterested (note, not 'uninterested') perspective begins early. In some situations, this is desirable: the therapeutic relationship would likely be compromised by stridently and inappropriately expressed personal opinions. However, the daily work that doctors, dentists and other clinicians do is an inherently political business in that the provision of healthcare is the enactment of policy. And that policy has a moral dimension: it is predicated on particular values and it has far-reaching effects on the practice of millions.

Many medical students and practising clinicians, even the avowedly apolitical, have fantasised about the ways in which the NHS could be improved. Many more have probably groaned as successive Secretaries of State seek to impose their reforming vision on healthcare. Those fantasies and groans may seem at first glance to be nothing more than a healthy reflex to political meddling, but they warrant closer attention. For such responses demonstrate two ethical points: first, the vast majority of healthcare professionals care about how healthcare is provided; secondly, there is a relationship between how individuals aspire to serve patients and how policy influences their daily work. In other words, medical students and clinicians can be politically disinterested but never uninterested.

What then is the ethical significance of health policy? Political reform has a moral dimension and it is always worth reflecting on the ethical assumptions embedded in policy. What does a particular policy or proposal for reform assume about fairness, equitable access, the role of the clinician and distributive justice? Having identified the moral foundations on which a policy is built, it is time to return to ethical basics. How will a particular policy inform that which is the daily bread of clinical practice? What are the implications of a particular proposal for the therapeutic relationship? Will the virtuous medical student or doctor differ in the newly envisaged NHS or are the virtues of altruism, service and inclusivity secure? How will conflicts of interest be conceptualised and understood in a world of commissioning and multiple providers of healthcare? What skills and competencies should medical and healthcare education develop in those new to the clinical professions and are they unaltered by the changing policy landscape?

This chapter explores the moral dimension and effects of health policy in relation to one of the recurring themes within the NHS: the allocation of resources. Politicians, the law, professional organisations, policy makers, patients and clinicians have all had to grapple with the difficulties of providing care that is fairly allocated, accessible, justly distributed and appropriately resourced. In a healthcare system that is unable to meet demand, how should decisions be made about who should be treated and what are the ethical assumptions, preferences and challenges embedded in resource allocation decisions?

Resource allocation: the challenges

Resources are inevitably constrained in the NHS. 'Resources' comprise budgets and financial provision, but also staff, time, facilities, estates and administrative or systemic assets. An ageing population, a growing number of people with chronic diseases, expensive medical advances and novel treatments all contribute to financial pressures that are indicative of a context in which economic constraint is creating difficulties for all public services. Yet the NHS was created on the basis that it should offer free healthcare for all on the basis of need. The question therefore is what is meant by 'need', and how easy are needs to distinguish from 'wants' or desirable outcomes? The distinction may sound seductively neat, but it is inevitably a judgement made by human beings, albeit those with 'authority' to make these decisions and human beings are partial, value-driven creatures with biases and preferences. For example, is screening a want or a need? Is pain relief in labour a want or a need? Is the prescription of Zyban to a dependent smoker a want or a need? Is the side effect profile of a drug relevant to meeting patient needs or wants? These are the judgements that have to be made and are not made uniformly.

If it is accepted that there are few absolute 'needs', how can a limited budget best be managed to achieve maximum advantage to the maximum number of patients when faced with myriad conflicting demands? The complexity of allocating resources is often focused on managing the relative value of competing needs in a way that is logical, reasonable and consistent.

One way of thinking about resource allocation, and its relationship to healthcare policy, is to categorise the decision-making process into three types of questions shown in the box below.

Macro Questions	These are questions that are considered at a national level, eg how should we allocate resources within the NHS? What proportion of the NHS budget should be allocated to particular services? What systems should we use to make national resource allocation decisions?
Midi Questions	These are questions for consideration at a regional level eg which services should be given priority within a particular area, group of healthcare providers or Primary Care Trust? How should the public be engaged in resource allocation decisions?
Micro Questions	These are the questions that occupy the minds of individual practitioners or clinical teams eg how can I be an advocate for my patient? How do resource constraints inhibit my ability to act in my patient's best interests? Can I reconcile the competing and conflicting demands on my practice?

Although these categories of decision-making can be presented as distinct, they are necessarily interrelated. For instance, national policy on resources for the National Health Service affects how much money a health authority or NHS Trust has available which, in turn, will determine clinical practice locally.

Ethical approaches to resource allocation

Any publicly funded, resource-limited system will struggle to reconcile demand and available facilities and there are different ways of approaching the resource question. Many discussions about resources assume a utilitarian position: crudely put, the NHS exists to serve the greatest number of people in the best, most efficient way possible. Such utilitarian-based positions often seek ways of evaluating the value or worth of healthcare to particular groups of people. One of the best known and most controversial of the methods used to weigh the benefit of a particular intervention or treatment is Quality Adjusted Life Years or QALYs.

Quality Adjusted Life Years weigh a patient's life and the effect of an intervention eg a year of healthy life expectancy is worth +1, a year of life compromised by ill health is worth -1, etc. Healthcare interventions are measured according to the likely extension of years of life and improvement in quality of life. If all interventions are given an agreed QALYs value, they can then be ranked against each other. However, QALYs assume that quality of life can and should be measured objectively. They could be said to be ageist in that quantity of life expectancy is important in making the calculation – so the older one is, the less time one has to live and therefore that can be counted in the life expectancy part of the QALY calculation. In practice this means those who are older have a shorter life expectancy for the purpose of calculating QALYs; many interventions do not have an agreed QALY value and the act of determining a particular intervention's QALY is problematic and morally contestable in itself. QALYs work at a population rather than individual level and therefore generalise about patients, diseases and interventions. Pre-existing disabilities will influence the assessment of QALY, leading to 'double jeopardy' for those who are already vulnerable and should be advocated within the health service. Finally, QALYs inevitably focus on outcome rather than need: those who are most likely to benefit are treated instead of those who most need treatment. Patients may neither have long to live nor enjoy good health by objective standards, but nonetheless will value extra time albeit in pain or discomfort because they want to see a grandchild born, celebrate a graduation or attend a special event.

A similar, consequentialist approach focuses on the goals, perceived benefits and outcomes of healthcare as a means of deciding what sorts of services should be prioritised. Such an approach is seductive, particularly in a discipline such as medicine which is naturally outcome-focused. Yet, there are difficulties. Identifying the goals of treatment does not necessarily make it any easier to determine which interventions should be funded and which should not. In the face of competing approaches to reaching the same clinical goal, is it morally acceptable to oblige a clinician to take the least resource-draining option? A second difficulty is the inherent uncertainty in defining and predicting the effectiveness and benefits of treatment. For example, a patient may prefer a more expensive drug with fewer side effects. Should his or her doctor include the side effect profile of a drug as part of its 'benefits'? Is it a goal of treatment to minimise side effects? And who should decide?

Other ethical approaches to resource allocation focus on need, with the aim of promoting and protecting the interests of the weakest irrespective of resource or likely benefit. Since the days of Aristotle, philosophers have thought and written about inequality and the distribution of social resources. Aristotle's formal principle of equality essentially asserts that the equal in society should be treated equally whilst the response to inequalities should be proportionate according to the degree of inequality. As such, when thinking about resource allocation in healthcare, we need to consider what criteria make someone equal or not eg health needs, individual vulnerability, socio-economic status, etc. Unlike the QALYs approach, the focus is on treating people according to their needs and interests rather than the benefits that might ensue as a result of treatment. It also has the potential to recognise and respond to health inequalities allowing, or even demanding, that more resources are given to those groups who bear a disproportionate burden of disease, poor health and disadvantage in society.

A further alternative to the Utilitarian approaches can be found in the work of the lawyer and political philosopher John Rawls. In his seminal work *A Theory of Justice*[240], Rawls proposed a thought experiment to facilitate thinking about fairness and equity in society as a counter to Utilitarian thinking. In his thought experiment, Rawls asks what version of justice would be selected by people who were behind a 'veil of ignorance' which precluded them from knowing what sort of person they were or represented in society. In other words, if you were contributing to a society in which no one knew about their relative social status, wealth, talents and ability, health, intelligence or ethnicity, what sort of just society would emerge? It is a thought experiment that Rawls analyses with meticulous detail in over 600 densely-argued pages and he concludes that a just society would comprise two principles. The first principle provides for equality of basic rights and liberties. The second principle is in two parts and requires social inequalities to be arranged for the benefit of the least advantaged and for there to be equality of opportunity in society. Whilst Rawls was using his thought experiment to facilitate theorising about social justice, it is a thought provoking stimulus for discussion of what a just healthcare system might be like if it were devised behind a veil of ignorance.

Some ethical debate focuses on the processes by which resource allocation decisions are made, often arguing for transparent, inclusive and accountable systems in which society is engaged in determining how scarce healthcare resources should be spent. In short, not only should the allocation of resources be equitable, it must also be seen to be equitable. A well-known example of public engagement and transparency in the resource allocation decision-making is the Oregon Experiment.[241] As is so often the case in resource allocation debates, it was a particular patient who led to the Oregon Experiment: a child with leukaemia who had not received a publicly-funded bone marrow transplant. The case highlighted the number of people who did not have access to healthcare and the need to establish a cost-effective way to

---

[240] Rawls, J. *A Theory of Justice.* Cambridge, MA: Belknap Press, 1971. Rawls revised, clarified and updated his ideas in a later work, Rawls, J., Kelly, E. (eds.) *Justice as Fairness: A Restatement.* Cambridge, MA: Belknap Press, 2001.

[241] For an excellent discussion of the Oregon Experiment, see Haas, M., Hall, J. *The Oregon Experiment in the Provision of Universal Healthcare.* Centre for Health Economics Research and Evaluation: Discussion Paper 4, University of Sydney, 1992.

provide healthcare. The idea was that the equitable and democratic way to prioritise healthcare services was to ask members of the public to rank healthcare treatments for particular conditions. From the outset, the need to allocate services on the basis of cost-effectiveness was explicit. In practice, there were difficulties with the experiment. It was difficult to determine the costs and benefits of particular treatments. The focus on particular diseases and treatment meant that some individuals were more disadvantaged than before eg due to disability. Unfortunately, efforts to engage the public widely were not as successful as had been hoped. There were some surprises too. Many had feared that public opinion might lead to some so-called 'Cinderella' services being neglected; in the event, that seemed not to happen. For example, addictive disorders were ranked immediately behind the treatment of a closed hip fracture.

There is ethical value in processes, particularly in resource allocation decision-making, and the creation of a transparent and clear process, even if it has imperfect results, could be argued to be as important as the decisions eventually reached. There is greater moral legitimacy in decisions taken by public, acceptable and well-understood processes, rather than in secrecy or opacity.

The law and resource allocation

The law does not require the NHS to provide treatment. Essentially, legal challenge comes about when a person or group of people claims that a decision about how to allocate resources has been made improperly or irrationally. In such a situation, an action for judicial review may be heard by a court. Most of the case law involves judicial reviews of health authorities and NHS Trusts that are seeking to limit available but expensive treatment, the benefits of which are contestable.

One of the most notable cases involving the allocation of resources involved the refusal of the Cambridgeshire Area Health Authority to fund further treatment for Jaymee Bowen[242], a ten-year-old girl

---

[242] *R v Cambridge HA, ex parte B (No 2)* [1996] 1 FLR 375.

who had leukaemia.[243] The court stated that there whilst there was no duty to prescribe or give expensive treatment, refusal to offer treatment must not be motivated *'solely or exclusively by financial considerations'*.[244] However, the question of resource allocation was overshadowed by concern expressed by the court in response to clinical evidence that the treatment sought by Jaymee Bowen's family was experimental, had a slight chance of success[245] and was likely to have significant and debilitating side effects which could not be in the child's best interests.

A later notable case involved an action by a patient with breast cancer, Ann Marie Rogers, against Swindon Health Authority which refused to fund treatment with the drug Herceptin.[246] Mrs Rogers succeeded on appeal albeit for reasons that were somewhat different from those portrayed in media accounts of the case. The court held that Swindon Primary Care Trust had been irrational and arbitrary in refusing to prescribe on the basis that their policy was flawed. In its policy on prescribing, the PCT specifically excluded cost as a consideration. Therefore if cost was not the reason for not funding Herceptin, it appeared to be an inexplicable decision by the PCT, given the available evidence for the drug and the clinical need of Mrs Rogers. By saying that cost was not a factor in their decision, the PCT could not justify the decision to deny treatment on rational grounds. The appeal therefore succeeded on a narrow legal basis, rather because of any 'treatment as of right' which was how the case was reported in many publications. The case confirmed that costs could legitimately be *part* of an exercise in weighing access to treatments. The court also noted that different NHS Trusts might adopt contrasting approaches to resource allocation.

The legal emphasis then is on decisions about resources that are rational within context. That context includes the biomedical

---

[243] For a thoughtful and thought-provoking account of Jaymee Bowen's case, including interviews with those clinicians who were involved in caring for Jaymee, see Ham, C., Pickard, S. *Tragic Cases in Health Care: The Case of Child B.* London: The King's Fund, 1998.

[244] Per Lord Bingham.

[245] Estimated at between 10 and 20 per cent; see 'The Provision of Hospital Care' in Kennedy, I., and Grubb, A., (eds.) *Principles of Medical Law*. Oxford: Oxford University Press, 1998.

[246] *Rogers v Swindon Primary Care NHS Trust and the Secretary of State* [2006] EWCA Civ 392.

evidence, clinical judgement and financial constraints. Context is to be judged in its entirety. Where, as in the Jaymee Bowen case, an expensive treatment is not considered to be in a patient's best interests clinically, that is a rational justification for not funding the treatment. Conversely, as in the case of Ann-Marie Rogers, where a healthcare organisation claims that a treatment that is clinically indicated is not being provided but not for reasons of financial constraint, the court may conclude that the decision is irrational as there is no reasonable explanation for the decision to withhold treatment.

How then is 'rational' policy created?

Resource allocation and health policy

The establishment of the National Institute for Health and Clinical Excellence (NICE)[247] in 1999 was intended to establish a formal, centralised and independent process of reviewing the clinical and cost-effectiveness of particular medicines. It was a bold attempt to end 'postcode lotteries'. To return to the idea of an ethical process for making difficult resource decisions, there may be moral value in collective and accountable decision-making. In doing so though, we may be acknowledging that the determination of wants and needs is inherently imperfect. NICE publishes guidance on therapies, interventions and treatments, the clinical management of particular diseases or conditions and health promotion. Guidance is based on both clinical efficacy and cost effectiveness and informed by expert opinion, computer-based economic modelling, the available evidence-base and public consultation. Issuing such guidance could be said implicitly to be making a judgement about whether a treatment is a want or a need. An example of a treatment that NICE has rejected on the basis of cost-effectiveness include expensive drugs, for the treatment of cancer, such as Avastin. However, there have been examples of NICE changing its guidance on particular treatments, for example the prescription of Aricept for those showing early signs and mild symptoms of dementia.

The ethical basis for NICE's work is utilitarian. It uses QALYs to make calculations about the value of therapies and treatments which,

---

[247] Originally, it was known as the National Institute for Clinical Excellence. It was renamed in 2005, but the acronym 'NICE' remained.

as has already been discussed, is a controversial method that does not allow for consideration of individual circumstances, priorities and need. The determination of the value of a particular treatment is also problematic. For example, are 'core' cancer services the priority given the prevalence of cancer in the UK or the so-called 'last chance' drugs like Avastin? NICE has been criticised for the economic models that it uses in evaluating the worth of a treatment or intervention. NICE decisions have also been the subject of legal challenge in the form of judicial review.[248] The guidance that is issued by NICE informs the decisions that are made at regional and local level about prescribing. Sometimes, local healthcare providers may sometimes want to wait until a particular medicine has been reviewed by NICE before approving it for general use on patients, even though the drug has a licence.

The fact that NICE has not recommended a particular drug or therapy for use in the NHS does not prevent individuals from obtaining that treatment but, and it is a significant 'but', it would have to be either entirely or in part privately funded. There is also provision for NHS Trusts to provide drugs in exceptional cases, but what makes an exceptional case? It is a difficult question to answer because the nature of special cases is that they are individual assessments of particular situations rather than generalised determinations. The advocacy and opinion of clinical staff is likely to be relevant and, in practice, such cases will be considered on an individual basis by a sub-group of the NHS Trust or Health Authority. One difficulty is that provision for exceptional cases creates potential for the campaigning or articulate patient who achieves access to healthcare via media coverage or threatened legal action, whilst those who are less able to advocate themselves, engage the media or navigate the system find it harder to claim that they are an 'exceptional case'.

The existence of NICE has not prevented high profile interventions from lobbyists, pharmaceutical companies and politicians. For example, in 2005 when there were a number of highly publicised cases of women who were seeking treatment of breast cancer with the drug Herceptin, the then Secretary of State for Health, Patricia

---

[248] *R (Eisai Ltd) (Alzheimer's Society & Shire Ltd, Interested Parties) v the National Institute for Health and Clinical Excellence* [2007] EWHC 1941 (Admin).

Hewitt, announced that Herceptin should be fast-tracked for use within the NHS.[249] Such intervention can be interpreted in different ways. It could be seen as advocacy for, and on behalf of, patients. However, it might also be argued that politicians and pharmaceutical companies are exploiting patients who will understandably try anything, even at great cost, to treat their disease. Drug pricing is high and patients are desperate, therefore companies stand to profit and politicians to win votes by championing specific patients or diseases over others. The implications of high profile political intervention may be unforeseen and unacknowledged. However well intentioned a public statement[250] made by a politician in response to a sympathetic patient, it is difficult to see that it can be congruent to the declared principle of the NHS ie fair access based on clinical need. It is also difficult to accept that a remote politician has sufficient knowledge of individual cases to make an assessment on the provision of care, particularly in respect of novel treatments that may be unlicensed for the proposed use, as Herceptin was when Patricia Hewitt intervened.

Political attention may be better focused on the pharmaceutical industry and its relationship with the health service. For example, Avastin was priced at a level that is commonly reserved for rare conditions affecting only small numbers, yet its potential market is a large group of patients. Market forces may not be desirable in healthcare. There is also the knock on effect of contagious pricing ie other companies will price their drugs accordingly. Who should contain the pharmaceutical industry? Is that part of an ethical health policy?

Resource allocation in clinical practice

How does health policy on resource allocation affect the daily practice of clinicians? The dominant model in medicine has been dyadic, emphasising the duty of care to each individual patient, but resource constraints are inevitable background noise. Is the individual clinician's duty to provide the best available care for each

---

[249] 'Hewitt Steps In as Trust Refuses Herceptin to Cancer Patient'. *The Guardian*, 9 November 2005.

[250] Although Patricia Hewitt's intervention was subsequently judged to be 'for guidance' only to PCTs in the Rogers case, that fine legal detail was somewhat lost in the media reporting of her statements.

patient without reference to any duty of 'stewardship' of collective resources? Or is such an individual approach fundamentally selfish and unacceptable?

A key factor in considering these questions is the imbalance between the information available to the doctor and the patient about resources. It may be that it is this imbalance in information that makes prioritisation decisions inequitable. Resource allocation may be more ethically acceptable if there is openness about the available evidence and the reasoning behind the recommendations made by national and local guidance on the allocation of resources. In which case, an individual doctor may have an important role in explaining the function of NICE and other policy-making bodies in determining the care that is available locally to patients.

A further question arises in relation to personal responsibility in an environment of scarce medical resources. As the burden of chronic diseases that are linked to, or exacerbated by, lifestyle grows, how can health professionals strike a balance between friendly support and making morally inappropriate judgements on autonomous adults? In the 1980s, some individual clinicians and some NHS organisations did limit the availability of coronary artery bypass graft procedures to patients who were smokers. Such an approach was challenged legally and held to be an unacceptable way of excluding large sections of the population from access to essential healthcare services.

From both an ethical and legal perspective, moral judgement about people that results in discrimination is unacceptable. Clinicians are expected to allocate scarce resources according to patients' comparative needs and taking account of the time at which they sought treatment eg a waiting list for non-urgent cases. Clinical practice is built on the principle of equality of access and treatment according to the patient's needs and without reference to other variables. A system of triage is a practical example of how need and time of presentation are combined to provide fair access to healthcare.

Whilst lifestyle undoubtedly has an effect on health and illness and it is a doctor's duty to provide health promotion advice, no one should be denied potentially beneficial treatments on the basis of his or her lifestyle. Such decisions usually tend towards the prejudicial. For example, why single out smokers or the obese for blame as opposed to those who engage in dangerous sports (and who often crowd busy A&E departments on a Saturday afternoon)? People do not have equal opportunities to lead healthy lives and to make wise healthcare choices. Education, wealth, social pressures, personal confidence and access to support all contribute to, and determine, health.

Conclusion

This chapter has taken resource allocation as an example of how health policy that is developed at national level shapes the daily work of doctors and their patients. Whatever you believe to be the best, or at least better, model of allocating resources, it will be an issue, along with many policy issues, that affects you every day of your practising life. Taking time to think about the resources that are being used to provide care to patients you meet on the wards and in clinics will be time well spent, and provides an invaluable opportunity to think for yourself about the values, priorities, assumptions and implicit choices that are embedded in each and every treatment decision in the NHS.

Healthcare policy and medical students

Medical school is a time to think about, and develop into, the sort of doctor you want to be. Part of that development involves thinking about the system(s) in which you will be working throughout your career and understanding the ways in which the policies of that system will inform your practice. Whilst finding out about health policy may seem less pertinent than learning anatomy, practising clinical skills and observing theatre, it is at the heart of what you are doing and will be doing for the rest of your life.

If you take the time to talk to doctors, patients and your peers about different aspects of health policy, you will encounter widely variable responses. That does not matter. Indeed, a range of response and divergence of opinion are usually beneficial for the quality of ethical debate. The point is that these are questions for everyone studying to be a doctor or working as a healthcare professional to consider. Whether you are excited by a particular aspect of healthcare policy or uneasy about its effects on clinical practice, time spent reflecting on the reasons for your position is worthwhile and taking time to consider the underlying ethical dimension to policy change is instructive. Whatever your response to health policy, it reveals something about your moral compass and the ways in which you believe healthcare should be practised. It is via the medium of policy that fundamental ethical questions are raised. These questions matter because they are not often explicitly considered yet they shape every moment of a future clinician's professional life: what we believe the aims of healthcare to be, how the clinician-patient relationship should be, what it means to serve the public sector, the ways in which limited resources are distributed and ultimately what makes a 'good' doctor.

Core Concepts: Healthcare Policy

Healthcare policy informs everything that medical students and doctors do in their education, training and practice. It is underpinned by moral assumptions and engaging with policy reveals much about not only the healthcare system, but also one's own values and ideals in relation to healthcare and the practice of medicine.

Resource allocation is an example of health policy that prompts myriad ethical questions. When resources are limited, and the burden on the NHS continues to grow, attention must be paid to the ethico-legal framework in which resources are allocated.

Resource allocation takes place at a macro (national or even international), midi (regional) and micro (within the clinical consultation) level.

Quality Adjusted Life Years (QALYs) are a way of evaluating the cost-effectiveness or benefit of a particular treatment, using an equation that gives an intervention a value and considers it in relation to expected duration of healthy or impaired life.

QALYs can be problematic in the emphasis they place on populations and disease rather than individuals and personal experience and the difficulties in attributing a value to all interventions.

Other ethical approaches emphasise fairness and justice. Aristotle's theory of distributive justice and Rawls' theory that justice depends on equity, fairness and protection of the most vulnerable are two examples of such approaches.

Some ethicists focus on the system for allocating scarce resources arguing that such systems must be accepted, inclusive, accountable and transparent in its decision-making.

The Oregon Experiment was one of the most notable attempts to involve the public in making decisions about prioritising healthcare according to perceived need in order to maximise access to healthcare resources.

The law is concerned with ensuring that decisions about healthcare resources are made in a reasonable way. Cases pivot on whether a decision to withhold treatment was made irrationally. Two examples are the cases of Jaymee Bowen and Ann Marie Rogers.

Individual clinicians have to make decisions in the best interests of their patients with regard to the stewardship of resources without making inappropriate moral judgements about lifestyle.

Medical students and doctors should take time to engage with health policy and to understand how it will shape their careers and the care that is provided to their patients.

 # Assessments: Healthcare Policy

1. A request for expensive cancer treatment

Sample OSCE station

You are a student at the oncology outpatient clinic. The consultant, Dr Beauchamp, invited you to observe her consultation with Mr Cheever who consents to you being present. Mr Cheever is 46 years old and he has metastatic colorectal cancer. He has become aware that Bevacizumab ('Avastin') has improved survival time in patients with metastatic colorectal disease. He asks Dr Beauchamp why he is *'not receiving Avastin if it has proven benefits. It might help me live long enough to see my daughter's eighteenth birthday. Surely that's got to make it worth a try?'*

After Mr Cheever leaves, Dr Beauchamp asks you what your views are about the availability of Avastin for Mr Cheever.

Guidance notes

- Questions of resource allocation are common and increasingly vexed as newer, more expensive drugs are licensed and the population served by the NHS increases. Although Mr Cheever is a cancer patient, few, if any, areas of medicine are exempt from decisions which could be seen to have been taken on fiscal rather than clinical grounds. The National Institute for Health and Clinical Excellence was established to offer a transparent process in which diverse interests could be considered and best evidence would inform the availability of treatment. NICE to uses evidence and efficacy to inform decisions about equitable access.

- Patients, such as Mr Cheever, may not have long to live nor enjoy good health by objective standards, but nonetheless will value extra time (albeit in pain or discomfort) because they want to see a grandchild born, celebrate a graduation, attend an assembly, etc. You may wish to discuss the difficult distinction between 'wants' and 'needs' and the contestable nature of a 'benefit' in making treatment decisions. Is Mr Cheever's desire to receive Avastin and potentially prolong his life a need or a wish? Is it essential that Mr Cheever lives as long as possible? Or even simply long enough to see his children grow up? Or is the extension of Mr Cheever's life and his presence at his daughter's eighteenth birthday merely a so-called 'desirable outcome'?

- From the perspective of the clinician, there is often considerable discretionary power to shape, if not determine, resource decisions. The opinion of clinical staff is likely to be sought when difficult decisions about healthcare resources are being made. If Mr Cheever were to pursue his wish to receive Avastin, the local prescribing committee would probably ask whether his clinical team believe that he should receive the drug. Discretion may be part of the determination of resource allocation decisions which, taken with other factors such as efficacy and clinical evidence, combine to provide the rationale for choices made about healthcare on a case by case basis.

- The difficulties surrounding the ethically and legally defensible allocation of resources are further exacerbated by the potential impact of the HRA, particularly Article 14. If a particular group of patients can show that decisions about available treatments are based on criteria that could be considered discriminatory eg age, gender, sexuality, marital status etc. it is possible that they could bring an action on the grounds of discrimination. In the case of Mr Cheever, it does not appear that there is any question of discrimination, but it is always a variable that should be considered in the context of resource allocation to ensure that particular groups are not discriminated against, either directly or indirectly.

- Mr Cheever is a cancer patient and it is the field of oncology that there has been discussion of mixing public and private provision. What would the position be if Mr Cheever asked to combine standard NHS and publicly-funded treatment, such as chemotherapy and radiotherapy, with private treatment such as the prescription of Avastin? Although much of the recent debate about combining public and private healthcare provision has suggested that it is a new issue in healthcare, there are already examples of mixed provision eg a NHS consultation may result in a private prescription. However, the general principle of the NHS is one of universal equality. As originally conceived, the NHS was intended to provide that all patients receive the same treatment irrespective of their social or economic status. This is a familiar ethical precept and is based on the notion that equality and fairness require us to protect the weakest as a society. An alternative perspective on mixing public and private provision is what might be called a 'libertarian' position in which individuals are free to supplement their care in a system that provides basic provision. This view would argue that for the hospital management to refuse any request from Mr Cheever to combine NHS treatment with the private prescription of Avastin would be to infringe his autonomy. In one account of mixing NHS and private healthcare for patient on an NHS ward, nursing staff reported significant difficulties in providing differential care.[251]

- What about the duty a doctor owes to a patient such as Mr Cheever? Doctors have traditionally been the advocate of the individual patient. The relationship has been constructed as a dyadic one with little attention to broader notions of resource management, even though the NHS is a fundamentally utilitarian system. Thus, the ethical preference has been to represent both the area in which one works and particular patients *in extremis* ie in this situation, oncology and Mr Cheever. Doctors have made representations to funding committees and such representations have been seen as part of the role of a doctor. However, increasingly there is a responsibility on everyone in the NHS, including doctors, to make resource decisions. The GMC requires doctors to make the patient their first concern but also to be aware of scarce resources – these may be difficult duties to reconcile eg how are sick patients to have therapeutic relationships with those who are apparently 'denying' them treatment?

- As well as the advocacy role, there are interesting issues raised by cases like Mr Cheever's for the doctor-patient relationship. First, if the patient is able to request and fund treatment, is the doctor relegated to the role of technician and does this matter? Secondly, how can individual doctors ensure informed consent in the context of 'wonder drugs'? There may be a paucity of data with limited follow-up and unclear information about side effects which may be significant eg cardiac toxicity in relation to Herceptin. The information available can be difficult to assess critically, even for the medical community; see for example Richard Horton's critique of the Herceptin trials in *The Lancet*[252] when the same trials were praised as 'revolutionary' by oncologists writing in the *New England Journal of*

---

[251] Richards, C., Dingwall, R. and Watson, A. Should NHS Patients be Allowed to Contribute Extra Money to their NHS Care? *BMJ* 2001; 323: 563–565.

[252] Horton, R. Herceptin and Early Breast Cancer: A Moment for Caution. *Lancet* 2005; 366: 1673.

Medicine three weeks earlier.[253] For some patients, including Mr Cheever perhaps, the drug that appears to offer benefit may harm. In any event, there remains considerable uncertainty surrounding the effect(s) of Avastin, making consent a difficult concept. And medicine is sadly familiar with drugs that are initially hailed as a revolution and later revealed to have serious adverse effects eg Thalidomide, Vioxx, etc. Yet the cautionary notes sounded are far harder to hear than the 'miracle drug' stories, especially when patients, such as Mr Cheever, are vulnerable and desperate.

- Individual doctors have to make individual choices about the extent to which they are cognisant of the less familiar and perhaps less appealing role of allocating resources. Centralisation and committees notwithstanding, there remains local discretion, although many would argue it is diminishing. Furthermore, in the unlikely event that doctors have all their discretion removed in relation to treatment decisions, this does not equate to removing responsibility to consider these vexed questions and contribute to the debate. Ideally, this 'representation' is as inclusive as possible, and has an eye on the silent patient who has healthcare needs but perhaps has a diagnosis that is not well-known or 'appealing' eg care of the elderly, mental health, and individuals who are less able to engage the powerful (media, politicians and even doctors themselves) in his or her cause.

2.   Resource allocation

Sample SAQ

Mrs Trapido is 56 years old. She has been diagnosed as having the early signs and symptoms of Alzheimer's disease. She has read about the drug Aricept in the newspaper and understands that the NICE reversed the decision regarding the availability of

---

[253] Romond, E.H., Perez, E.A., Bryant, J., *et al.* Trastuzumab plus Adjuvant Chemotherapy for Operable HER2-positive Breast Cancer. *N Engl J Med* 2005; 353: 1673–1684; Piccart-Gebhart M.J., Procter M., Leyland-Jones B., *et al.* Trastuzumab after Adjuvant Chemotherapy in HER2-positive Breast Cancer. *N Engl J Med* 2005; 353: 1659–1672.

the drug on the NHS. Mrs Trapido approaches her GP, Dr Byatt, and asks him to prescribe Aricept for her.

(a) What is the role of NICE in determining whether drugs, like Aricept, should be available? (2 marks)

(b) NICE uses QALYs to make its decisions about particular therapies and treatments, explain what QALYs are (3 marks)

(c) There are criticisms that can be made of QALYs. Suggest three such criticisms. (3 marks)

(d) If Dr Byatt did not prescribe Aricept for Mrs Trapido, on what basis might she be able to challenge the decision legally? (2 marks)

Guidance notes

Part (a) The role of NICE is to provide a centralised and accountable system for evaluating treatments and therapies for clinical and cost-effectiveness. To do so, NICE consults widely and uses information gathered in that consultation process to analyse the evidence and efficiency of a particular treatment, eventually leading to guidance that is disseminated throughout the NHS.

Part (b) QALYs or Quality Adjusted Life Years weigh a patient's life and the effect of an intervention eg a year of healthy life expectancy is worth +1, a year of life compromised by ill health is worth -1. Healthcare interventions are measured according to the likely extension of years of life and improvement in quality of life. If all interventions are given an agreed QALY value, they can then be ranked against each other.

Part (c) Criticisms of QALYs include:
- The assumption that quality of life can and should be measured objectively.
- QALYs could be said to be ageist in that quantity of life expectancy is important in making the calculation so the older one is, the less time one has to live and therefore

that can be counted in the life expectancy part of the QALY calculation;

- Many interventions do not have an agreed QALY value
- The act of determining a particular intervention's QALY is problematic and morally contestable in itself;
- QALYs work at a population rather than individual level and therefore generalise about patients, diseases and interventions;
- Pre-existing disabilities will influence the assessment of QALYs, leading to 'double jeopardy' for those who are already vulnerable and should be advocated within the health service; and
- Finally, QALYs inevitably focus on outcome rather than need: those who are most likely to benefit are treated instead of those who most need treatment.

Part (d)   Mrs Trapido would only be able to challenge any decision legally if she were able to show, via judicial review, that the decision to withhold Aricept from her had been made in a way that was demonstrably irrational or unreasonable.

Chapter 14

Putting it Together: Concluding Thoughts

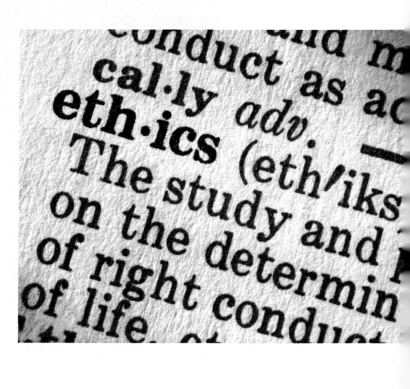

Putting it Together: Concluding Thoughts

The act of writing a book is always an opportunity to pause and reflect on the subject. This book is no exception. Whilst it began life as a resource for students to help their learning, it has become a rich and welcome opportunity for someone who has spent her life thinking about the ethico-legal dimensions of medicine and healthcare to consider what it is we try to do when we teach ethics to medical students, trainees and practising clinicians.

For many medical students and doctors, it is the place of ethics and law in assessments and examinations that prompts attention. Sometimes that attention is reluctant and partial, but I hope that the legacy of learning ethics and law for undergraduate and postgraduate exams lingers even in the most ambivalent student or junior doctor. Yet, preparing for exams is a very particular and partial version of ethics education. It is necessary perhaps, but not sufficient for those who want to become good doctors. The real business of ethics does not take place in the examination room but on the wards, in clinics and in the community and that is where students must be able to thrive.

Ethics is a practical subject. It requires practice and it is the enactment of ethical choices and decisions in the clinical setting that is regrettably overlooked by many curricula in ethics and law. It is a failing of education if we produce students who are able to recite the four principles, describe the legal position of euthanasia and proffer an opinion about cloning, but are unable to step in when a consultant fails to introduce students in clinic, or, who unquestioningly accede to requests to conduct intimate examinations on anaesthetised patients from whom consent has not been sought. Developing the moral awareness of medical students and junior doctors is as integral to medical education and training as sharing knowledge, diagnostic and clinical skills. If ethical education raises moral awareness (as it should), it must also give students the facility to respond to that moral awareness and act with integrity in the face of challenge or pressure. Students have to learn how to respond to questions about the difference between learning from or on patients, the dissonance between 'classroom ethics' and observed behaviour in the clinical setting, and the effects of professional hierarchy, competition and insecurity on remaining true to ethical ideals. The practical skills involved in becoming and remaining an ethical practitioner are not learned by osmosis in medical school; they have to be made explicit, modelled and practised. From such practice comes confidence and control – you can become the doctor you want to be, and the doctor that your patients have a right to expect.

Ethics education should not be the preserve of the 'expert': it must be owned, shared and developed by the widest and most inclusive group possible and, as a student, you can begin to play your part from the earliest days. In particular, clinicians who provide an integrated approach to ethics as part of good patient care are powerful role models, with the potential to reach students more effectively than many ethics specialists who may sometimes be charged with teaching in something of an academic vacuum. Teaching ethics in the clinical setting allows for a rich and responsive approach in which generic principles or virtues can be demonstrated 'in action' while modelling best practice in seeking consent for patient participation; remaining alert to, and respectful of, patient dignity; and encouraging learners to participate in care rather than remain passive recipients of 'teaching'. As students qualify, and sometimes even before graduation, they become role models themselves. Remember that role modelling is unlike other forms of education in that one does not 'do it' intermittently in a pre-determined format, as is the case with lectures or bedside teaching. Role modelling occurs constantly, whenever the learner is able to observe. Doctors and academic staff are role models to their students and juniors irrespective of whether they are interacting and whether the teacher realises he or she is being observed. If you can make a simple commitment to discuss ideas with others, to seek out those who disagree, and think differently from oneself and to listen carefully when an opposing or challenging argument is presented, you will retain the value of multiple perspectives.

Ethics, both in education and in clinical practice, can be an emotional business. Notwithstanding the historical emphasis that ethics has placed upon rationality, in teaching and learning ethics everyone has to be aware of the significance of emotion and its effects. The feelings that arise between teacher and learner may not be explicitly acknowledged or considered, but nonetheless exist and can powerfully influence the effectiveness of the education. Such emotional responses and different experiences of 'teaching', particularly perhaps in a subject such as ethics where the focus is commonly on multiple perspectives and diverse ways of understanding a problem, are inevitable. Awareness of emotion reveals values, differences and hierarchy of priorities.

Rather than being an 'irrational', undesirable or obfuscatory response, emotion is significant to both the learning and practice of ethics because it indicates one is making a judgement about an important issue; suggests that the issue is complex, uncertain and yet, in some way, intrinsic to being 'a good clinician'; and reveals the nature of ethical decision-making to be related to values, discretion and multilayered responses rather than a purportedly 'neutral' endeavour.

Those invited to teach ethics and facilitate the ethical development of future clinicians bear both educational privilege and power. To teach ethics is to learn ethics. Ethics teaching and learning extends well beyond the boundaries of a 'core curriculum'. Everyone, including you, has the power to show and to foster a culture of caring professionalism, moral imagination and ethical courage in medicine. This book is aimed at the worried student. However, at the end of the volume, the conclusion is perhaps that a little, appropriately contained worry is desirable because it denotes engagement, interest, a commitment to doing well and insight that ethical questions are multifaceted and not susceptible to easy resolution. If you can accept that residual worry, use the skills and knowledge you have developed, find supportive mentors and practise ethics throughout your career, you and your patients will thrive.

Appendix

A Literary Potpourri: Recommended Resources and Further Reading

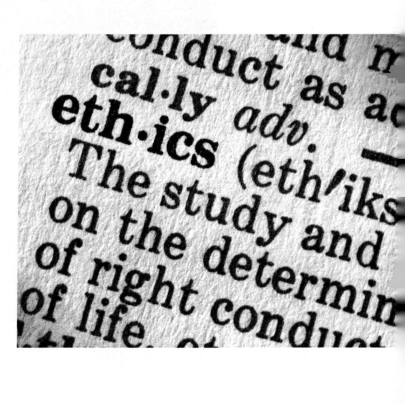

A Literary Potpourri: Recommended Resources and Further Reading

This section contains an eclectic and highly personal selection of books, papers and resources that have been important to me and to which I return regularly. I have included titles from a wide range of academic disciplines, novels, poetry, plays, biographies and memoirs; all have something to say about humanity, health, disease, morality and the practice of medicine in its broadest sense. The titles are grouped according to the theme of each chapter in this volume. I hope you enjoy selecting from this literary potpourri of medically-related texts.

1. Entering the Medical Moral Maze

Atkinson, P. *Medical Talk and Medical Work* (London: Sage, 1995)

Azzone, G. F. *Medicine: From Art to Science* (Amsterdam: IOS Press, 1998)

Balint, M. *The Doctor, the Patient and the Illness* (Edinburgh: Churchill Livingstone, 1957)

Bamforth, I. (ed.) *The Body in the Library: A Literary History of Modern Medicine* (London: Verso Books, 2003)

Berger, J. *A Fortunate Man: The Story of a Country Doctor* (London: Random House, 1997)

Brennan, T. *Just Doctoring: Medical Ethics in the Liberal State.* (Berkeley: University of California Press, 1991)

Bulgakov, M. A Country Doctor's Notebook. (London: Harvill Press, 1995)

Cassell, E. J. *The Healer's Art: A New Approach to the Doctor-Patient Relationship* (Boston, Mass: Massachusetts Institute of Technology Press, 1985)

Cassell, E. J. *The Nature of Suffering and the Goals of Medicine* (Oxford: Clarendon Press, 1991)

Cavel, H. *Illness (Art of Living)* (Durham: Acumen Publishing, 2008)

Charon, R., Montello, M. *Stories Matter: The Role of Narrative in Bioethics* (New York: Routledge US, 2002)

Clement, G. *Care, Autonomy and Justice: Feminism and the Ethic of Care* (Boulder, Colorado: Westview Press, 1998)

Conley, F. K. *Walking out on the Boys* (New York: Farrar, Straus and Giroux, 1998)

Crellin, J. K. *Public Expectations and Physicians' Responsibilities: Voices of the Medical Humanities* (Oxford: Radcliffe Medical Press, 2005)

Dally, A. *The Trouble with Doctors: Fashions, Motives and Mistakes* (London: Robson Books, 2003)

Downie, R. S. *The Healing Arts: An Illustrated Anthology* (Oxford: Oxford University Press, 2002)

Drane, J. F. *Becoming a Good Doctor: Place of Virtue and Character in Medical Ethics* (Lanham MD: Sheed and Ward US, 1988)

Elliott, C., Lantos, J. (eds.) *Walker Percy and the Moral Life of Medicine* (Durham: Duke University Press, 1999)

Frank, A. W. *The Wounded Storyteller: Body, Illness and Ethics* (Chicago: The University of Chicago Press, 1995)

Frank, A. W. *The Renewal of Generosity: Illness, Medicine and How to Live* (Chicago: University of Chicago Press, 2004)

Gawande, A. *Complications: A Surgeon's Notes on an Imperfect Science* (New York: Metropolitan Books, Henry Holt and Company, 2002)

Good Medical Practice (London: General Medical Council, 2006)

Golub, E. S. *The Limits of Medicine: How Science Shapes our Hope for the Cure* (Chicago: University of Chicago Press , 1997)

Glover, J. *Causing Death and Saving Lives* (London: Penguin, 1990)

Groopman, J. *Second Opinions: Stories of Intuition and Choice in the Changing World of Medicine* (New York: Viking, 2000)

Illich, I. *Limits to Medicine: Medical Nemesis – The Expropriation of Our Health* (New York: Pantheon, 1976)

Irvine, D. *The Doctor's Tale: Professionalism and Public Trust* (Oxford: Radcliffe Medical Press, 2003)

Kapp, M. B. *Our Hands Are Tied: Legal Tensions and Medical Ethics* (Connecticut: Greenwood Press, 1998)

Kennedy, I. *The Unmasking of Medicine* (London: Allen & Unwin, 1981)

Klass, P. *Love and Modern Medicine* (Houghton Mifflin, 2001)

Le Fanu, J. *The Rise and Fall of Modern Medicine* (London: Little Brown and Company, 1999)

Lindemann Nelson, H., Lindemann Nelson, J. *The Patient in the Family* (New York: Routledge US, 1995)

Massad, S. *Doctors and Other Casualties* (Lincoln: iUniverse.com Inc, 1993)

Mercurio, J. *Bodies* (London: Jonathan Cape, 2002)

Misselbrook, D. *Thinking about Patients* (Newbury: Petroc Press, 2001)

Pellegrino, E. D., Veatch, R. M., Langan, J. P. (eds.) *Ethics, Trust and the Professions: Philosophical and Cultural Aspects* (Washington DC: Georgetown University Press, 1991)

Pellegrino, E. D., Thomasma, D. C. *The Virtues in Medical Practice* (New York: Oxford University Press, USA, 1993)

Petit-Zeman, S. *Doctor, What's Wrong? Making the NHS Human Again* (London: Routledge, 2005)

Porter, R. *Blood and Guts: A Short History of Medicine* (London: Penguin Books, 2003)

Sanderson, M. *Wrong Rooms: A Memoir* (Roseburg, OR: Scribner, 2002)

Seglow, J. (ed.) *The Ethics of Altruism* (Southgate: Frank Cass Publishers, 2004)

Shaw, G. B. *The Doctor's Dilemma: A Tragedy* (London: Penguin, 1911)

Sontag, S. *Illness as Metaphor and AIDS and its Metaphors* (Penguin Classics, 2009)

Tallis, R. *Hippocratic Oaths: Medicine and its Discontents* (London: Atlantic Books, 2004)

Vickers, S. *The Other Side of You* (London: Fourth Estate, 2006)

Weatherill, D. *Science and the Quiet Art* (Oxford: Oxford University Press, 1993)

Wiltshire, J. *Samuel Johnson in the Medical World: The Doctor and the Patient* (Cambridge: Cambridge University Press, 1991)

Winterson, J. *Written on the Body* (London: Vintage, 2001)

Woolf, V. *On Being Ill* (Minnesota: Consortium, 2002)

Wootton, D. *Bad Medicine: Doctors Making Mistakes since Hippocrates* (Oxford: Oxford University Press, 2006)

2. Morality Tales: Ethics and Medical Education

Albanese, M. The Decline and Fall of Humanism in Medical Education. *Medical Education* 2000; 34: 596–597

Becker, H. S., Geer, B., Hughes, E. C. and Strauss, A. L. *Boys in White: Student Culture in Medical School* (Chicago: University of Chicago Press, 1961)

Bowman, D. The Challenges of an Ethical Education in Europe. *Die Psychiatrie* 2005; 2: 158–164

Broadhead, R. S. *The Private Lives and Professional Identity of Medical Students* (New Brunswick: Transaction Books, 1983)

Brody, H. *The Future of Bioethics* (Oxford: Oxford University Press, 2009)

Cooke, L., Halford, S., Leonard, P. *Racism in the Medical Profession: The Experience of UK Graduates* (London: British Medical Association, 2003)

DasGupta, S. *Her Own Medicine: A Woman's Journey from Student to Doctor* (New York: Ballantine Books, 1999)

Eckenfels, E. J. Learning about Ethics: The Cardinal Rule of Clinical Experience. *Med Educ* 2001; 35: 716–7

Gillon, R. White Coat Ceremonies for New Medical Students. *J Med Ethics* 2000; 26(2): 83–84

Hafferty, F. W. *Into the Valley: Death and the Socialization of Medical Students* (New Haven: Yale University Press, 1991)

Hafferty, H. W. Beyond Curriculum Reform: Confronting Medicine's Hidden Curriculum. *Acad Med* 1998; 73: 403–407

Halpern, J. *From Detached Concern to Empathy: Humanising Medical Practice* (Oxford: Oxford University Press, 2001)

Hunter, K. "Don't Think Zebras": Uncertainty, Interpretation and the Place of Paradox in Clinical Education. *Theoretical Medicine and Bioethics* 1996; 17(3): 225–241

Klass, P. *A Not Entirely Benign Procedure* (New York: Plume Books, 1994)

Konner, M. *Becoming a Doctor: A Journey of Initiation in Medical School* (New York: Viking, 1987)

Kushner, T. C., Thomasma, D. C. (eds.) *Ward Ethics: Dilemmas for Medical Students and Doctors in Training* (Cambridge: Cambridge University Press, 2001)

LeBaron, C. *Gentle Vengeance: An Account of the First Year at Harvard Medical School* (New York: Penguin, 1981)

Lindemann Nelson, H. (ed.) *Stories and their Limits: Narrative Approaches to Bioethics* (New York: Routledge USA, 1998)

Marion, R. *Learning to Play God: The Coming of Age of a Young Doctor* (New York: Fawcett Books, 2000)

Maudsley, G., Strivens, J. Promoting Professional Knowledge, Experiential Learning and Critical Thinking for Medical Students. *Med Educ* 2000; 34: 535–544

Noddings, N. *Caring: A Feminine Approach to Ethics and Moral Education* (2nd ed.) (Berkeley: University of California Press, 2003)

Raine, N. *Tiger Country* (London: Faber and Faber, 2011)

Reilly, P. *To Do No Harm: A Journey Through Medical School* (Dover MA: Auburn House, 1987)

Rennie, S. C., Crosby, J. R. Students' Perceptions of Whistle Blowing: Implications for Self-Regulation. A Questionnaire and Focus Group Survey. *Med Educ* 2002; 36: 173–179

Richardson, R. A Necessary Inhumanity? *J Med Ethics* 2001; 26(2): 104–106

Rothman, D. J. *Strangers at the Bedside: A History of How Law and Ethics Transformed Medical Decision-Making* (New York: Basic Books, 1991)

Schon, D. A. *The Reflective Practitioner: How Professionals Think in Action* (Aldershot: Arena, 1983)

Schon, D. A. *Educating the Reflective Practitioner* (San Francisco: Jossey-Bass, 1987)

Selzer, R. *Doctor Stories* (US: Picador, 1999)

Sinclair, S. *Making Doctors: An Institutional Apprenticeship* (Oxford: Berg, 1997)

Thistlethwaite, J., Spencer, J. *Professionalism in Medicine* (Oxford: Radcliffe Publishing, 2008)

Wear, D. and Bickel, J. (eds.) *Educating for Professionalism* (Iowa: University of Iowa Press, 2003)

3. It's My Life: Capacity and Consent

Bowman, D., Spicer, J., Iqbal, R. *Informed Consent: A Primer* (Cambridge: Cambridge University Press, 2011)

Donnelly M and Coulter C (eds.) *Consent and Medical Decision-Making: Bridging the Gap between Doctor and Patient* (Cork: University of Cork Press, 2002)

Foster, C. *Choosing Life, Choosing Death: The Tyranny of Autonomy in Medical Ethics and Law* (Oxford: Hart Publishing, 2009)

Gunn, T. *The Man with Night Sweats* (US: Farrar Straus & Giroux, 1992)

LEARNING MEDIA

Maclean, A. *Autonomy, Informed Consent and Medical Law: A Relational Challenge* (Cambridge: Cambridge University Press, 2009)

O'Neill, O., Manson, N. C. *Rethinking Informed Consent in Bioethics* (Cambridge: Cambridge University Press, 2007)

Noll, P. In the Face of Death. (translated by Nolls, H.) (London: Penguin Books, 1990)

Shapcott, J. *Of Mutability* (London: Faber and Faber, 2011)

4. Trust Me, I'm a Medical Student: Confidentiality

Jackson, J. *Truth Trust and Medicine* (London: Routledge, 2000)

O'Neill, O. *A Question of Trust: The BBC Reith Lectures 2002* (Cambridge: Cambridge University Press, 2002)

Walton, M. M. *The Trouble with Medicine: Preserving the Trust between Patients and Doctors* (St Leonards, NSW: Allen and Unwin, 1999)

5. New Beginnings: Reproductive Ethics

Desai, K. *Witness the Night* (London: Beautiful Books, 2010)

Jensen, L. *Egg Dancing* (London: Bloomsbury Publishing, 2006)

McCracken, E. *An Exact Replica of My Imagination* (New York: Little Brown and Company, 2008)

Patchett, A. *State of Wonder* (London: Bloomsbury Publishing, 2011)

Scully, D. *Men Who Control Women's Health: The Miseducation of Obstetrician-Gynaecologists* (New York: Teachers College Press, 1994)

Shapiro, D. *Delivering Doctor Amelia: The Story of a Gifted Young Obstetrician's Error and the Psychologist Who Helped Her* (New York: Vintage Books USA, 2004)

6. Minor Morality: Children and Adolescents

Anspach, R. *Deciding who Lives: Fateful Decisions in the Intensive Care Nursery* (Berkley CA: University of California Press, 1993)

Batmanghelidjh, C. *Shattered Lives: Children Who Live with Courage and Dignity* (London: Jessica Kingsley Publishers, 2006)

Christensen, R. *Ask Me Why I Hurt* (New York: Broadway Books, 2011)

Fadiman, A. *The Spirit Catches You and Then You Fall Down: A Hmong Child, Her American Doctors and the Collision of Two Cultures* (Farrar Straus & Giroux, 1998)

Lantos, J. *The Lazarus Case: Life and Death Issues in Neonatal Intensive Care* (Baltimore, MD: The Johns Hopkins University Press, 2007)

Lantos, J. *Neonatal Bioethics: The Moral Challenges of Medical Innovation* (Baltimore MD: Johns Hopkins University Press, 2008)

Mardell, D. *Danny's Challenge: Learning to Love My Son* (Short Books Ltd, 2005)

McCarthy, C. *Everyone's Children* (New York: Scribner, 1998)

Nichols, P. *A Day in the Death of Joe Egg* (London: Faber and Faber, 2001)

Wakenshaw, M. *This Child of Mine* (Richmond, VA: Harbinger Press, 2001)

7. A Meeting of Minds: Mental Health Ethics and Law

Allen, S. *Wish I Could Be There: Notes from a Phobic Life* (Viking Penguin, 2007)

Cockburn, P, Cockburn, H. *Henry's Demons: Living with Schizophrenia, a Father and Son's Story* (London: Simon and Schuster Ltd, 2011)

Eysenck, H. J. *The Decline and Fall of the Freudian Empire* (London: Penguin, 1985)

Fallon, P., Katzman, M. A. , Wooley, S. C. (eds.) *Feminist Perspectives on Eating Disorders* (New York: The Guildford Press, 1994)

Foucault, M. *Madness and Civilisation* (London: Routledge, 1967)

Green, H. I Never Promised You a Rose Garden (Pan Books, 1967)

Healy, D. *The Anti-Depressant Era* (Cambridge MA: Harvard University Press, 1997)

Healy, D. *The Creation of Psychopharmacology* (Cambridge MA: Harvard University Press, 2002)

Healy, D. *Let Them Eat Prozac: The Unhealthy Relationship between the Pharmaceutical Industry and Depression* (New York: New York University Press, 2004)

Hyland, M. J. *How the Light Gets In* (Canongate, 2004)

O' Donoghue, J. *Sectioned: A Life Interrupted* (London: John Murray Publishers, 2009)

Peay, J. *Decisions and Dilemmas: Working with Mental Health Law* (Oxford: Hart Publishing, 2003)

Penhall, J. *Blue Orange* (London: Methuen Drama, 2000)

Redfield-Jamison, K. *An Unquiet Mind* (Vintage, 1995)

Stout, C. E. *From the Other Side of the Couch: Candid Conversations with Psychiatrists and Psychologists* (Wesport CT: Greenwood, 1993)

Winter, S. *Freud and the Institution of Psychoanalytic Knowledge* (Stanford CA: Stanford University Press, 1999)

8. I Blame My Parents: Genethics

Bosk, C. L. *All God's Mistakes: Genetic Counselling in a Paediatric Hospital* (Chicago: University of Chicago Press, 1995)

Churchill, C. *A Number* (London: Nick Hearn Books, 2002)

Glover, J. *What Sort of People Should There Be?* (London: Pelican Books, 1984)

Ishiguro, K. *Never Let Me Go* (London: Faber and Faber, 2010)

9. Death, Distress and Decisions: End of Life

Diamond, J. C. *Because Cowards Get Cancer Too* (Vermillion, 1999)

Gordon, M. *Bea* (Oberon, 2010)

Picardie, R. *Before I Say Goodbye* (Penguin, 1998)

Tolstoy, L. *Death of Ivan Ilyich and Other Stories (Wordsworth Classics)* (London: Wordsworth Editions, 2004)

Verghese, A. *The Tennis Partner* (HarperCollins, 1998)

Warnock, M., Macdonald, E. *Easeful Death: Is There a Case for Assisted Dying?* (Oxford: Oxford University Press, 2006)

10. Rights and Wrongs: Human Rights and Global Ethics

Atwood, M. *Oryx and Crake* (London: Virago Press, 2006)

Dworkin R (1997) *Taking Rights Seriously* (Cambridge MA: Harvard University Press)

Galgut, D. *The Good Doctor* (New York: Atlantic Books, 2004)

Glover, J. *Humanity: A Moral History of the 20th Century* (London: Jonathan Cape, 1999)

Horton, R *Second Opinion: Doctors and Diseases – Wretched Arguments at the Sickbed* (London: Granta Books, 2003)

Verghese, A. *Cutting for Stone* (Vintage, 2009)

Wynne-Jones, R. *Something is Going to Fall Like Rain* (London: Reportage Press, 2009)

11. Fallibility, Being Human and Making Mistakes

Banja, J. *Disclosure of Medical Error and Medical Narcissism* (New York: Jones and Bartlett Publishers, 2005)

Berlinger, N. Broken Stories: Patients, Families and Clinicians after Medical Error. *Literature and Medicine* Fall 2003; 22(2): 230–240

Berlinger, N. *After Harm: Medical Error and the Ethics of Forgiveness* (Baltimore MA: Johns Hopkins University Press, 2005)

Bogner, M. S. *Misadventures in Health Care: Inside Stories* (New York: Lawrence Erlbaum Associates Inc, 2003)

Bosk, C. L. *Forgive and Remember: Managing Medical Failure* (Chicago: University of Chicago Press, 1979)

Cox, J., King, J., Hutchinson, A. and McAvoy, P. (eds.) *Understanding Doctors' Performance* (Oxford: Radcliffe Medical Press, 2005)

Fadon, V. A., Sharpe, A. L. *Medical Harm: Historical, Conceptual and Ethical Dimensions of Iatrogenic Illness* (Cambridge: Cambridge University Press, 1998)

Glynne, J., Gomez, D. *Fitness to Practise: Healthcare Regulatory Law, Principle and Process* (London: Thomason, Sweet and Maxwell, 2005)

Mulcahy, L. *Disputing Doctors: The Socio-legal Dynamics of Complaints about Doctors* (Buckingham: Open University Press, 2003)

Paget, M. *The Unity of Mistakes: A Phenomenological Interpretation of Medical Work* (Philadelphia: Temple University Press, 1998)

Rosenthal, M. *The Incompetent Doctor: Behind Closed Doors* (Buckingham: Open University Press, 1995)

Rosenthal, M., Mulcahy, L., Lloyd-Bostock, S. (eds.) *Medical Mishaps: Pieces of the Puzzle* (Buckingham: Open University Press, 1999)

Rubin, S. B., Zoloth, L. (eds.) *Margin of Error: The Ethics of Mistakes in the Practice of Medicine* (Hagerstown MD: University Publishing Group, 2000)

12. Publish or Perish: Research and Publication Ethics

Becker, H. S. *Tricks of the Trade: How to Think about Your Research While You're Doing It* (Chicago: University of Chicago Press, 1999)

Lee, R. M. *Doing Research on Sensitive Topics* (London: Sage, 1993)

Merton, R. K. *On the Shoulders of Giants: A Shandean Postscript – The Post-Italianate Edition* (Chicago: University of Chicago Press, 1993)

Oakley, A. *Experiments in Knowing: Gender and Method in the Social Sciences* (Cambridge: Polity Press, 2000)

Skloot, R. *The Immortal Life of Henrietta Lacks* (London: Random House, 2010)

Slater, L. *Opening Skinner's Box: Great Psychological Experiments of the Twentieth Century* (London: Bloomsbury, 2005)

13. It's Another World: Healthcare Policy, Resource Allocation and Ethics

Castro, A. *Unhealthy Health Policy: A Critical Anthropological Examination* (Lanham MD: Alta Mira Press, 2004)

Elliott, C. *White Coat, Black Hat: Adventures on the Dark Side of Medicine* (Boston, MA: Beacon Press, 2010)

Fitzpatrick, M. *The Tyranny of Health: Doctors and the Regulation of Lifestyle* (London: Routledge, 2001)

Ham, C. *Health Policy in Britain* (6th ed.) (Basingstoke: Palgrave Macmillan, 2009)

Klein, R. The New Politics of the NHS: From Creation to Reinvention (6th ed.) (Oxford: Radcliffe Publishing Ltd, 2010)

Phillips, A. *Equals* (London: Faber and Faber, 2002)

Pollock, A. *NHS Plc: The Privatisation of Our Healthcare* (London: Verso Books, 2005)

Shriver, L. *So Much for That* (London: HarperCollins, 2011)

Talbot-Smith, A., Pollock, A. M. *The New NHS: A Guide* (London: Routledge, 2006)

14. Putting It Together: Concluding Thoughts

Brody, H. *Stories of Sickness*. (2nd ed.) (Oxford: Oxford University Press, 2003)

Cassell, J. *Expected Miracles: Surgeons at Work* (Philadelphia PA: Temple University Press, 1991)

Cassell, J. *The Woman in the Surgeon's Body* (Cambridge MA: Harvard University Press, 1998)

Gawande, A. *Better: A Surgeon's Notes on Performance* (New York: Profile Books, 2008)

Gentile, M. *Giving Voice to Values* (New Haven, CT: Yale University Press, 2010)

Groopman, J. *How Doctors Think* (New York: Mariner Books, 2008)

Marion, R. *The Intern Blues* (New York: Harper Collins, 2001)

Montgomery, K. *How Doctors Think: Clinical Judgment and the Practice of Medicine* (Oxford: Oxford University Press, 2006)

Murray, J. F. *Intensive Care: A Doctor's Journal* (Berkeley: University of California Press, 2000)

Ofri, D. *Medicine in Translation: Journeys with My Patients* (Boston, MA: Beacon Press, 2010)

Peschel R E (1992) *When a Doctor Hates a Patient, and Other Chapters in a Young Physician's Life* (Berkley: University of California Press)

Sachs, D. (ed.) *Emergency Room* (New York: Little Brown and Company, 1996)

Stead, E. A., Haynes, B. F. (eds.) *A Way of Thinking: A Primer on the Art of Being a Doctor* (Durham NC: Carolina Academic Press, 1995)

Weston, G. *Direct Red: A Surgeon's Story* (Vintage, 2010)

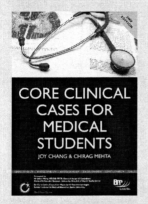
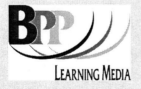

Medical Leadership: A Practical Guide for Trainees & Tutors

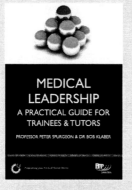

MEDICAL LEADERSHIP
A PRACTICAL GUIDE FOR TRAINEES & TUTORS
PROFESSOR PETER SPURGEON & DR BOB KLABER

£19.99
November 2011
Paperback
978-1-445379-57-9

Are you a doctor or medical student who wishes to acquire and develop your leadership and management skills? Do you recognize the role and influence of strong leadership and management in modern medicine?

Clinical leadership is something in which all doctors should have an important role in terms of driving forward high quality care for their patients. In this up-to-date guide Peter Spurgeon and Robert Klaber take you through the latest leadership and management thinking, and how this links in with the Medical Leadership Competency Framework. As well as influencing undergraduate curricula and some of the concepts underpinning revalidation, this framework forms the basis of the leadership component of the curricula for all medical specialties, so a prac-tical knowledge of it is essential for all doctors in training.

Using case studies and practical exercises to provide a strong work-based emphasis, this practical guide will en-able you to build on your existing experiences to develop your leadership and management skills, and to develop strategies and approaches to improving care for your patients.

This book addresses:

- Why strong leadership and management are crucial to delivering high quality care

- The theory and evidence behind the Medical Leadership Competency Framework

- The practical aspects of leadership learning in a wide range of clinical environments (e.g. handover, EM, ward etc)

- How Consultants and trainers can best facilitate leadership learning for their trainees and students within the clinical work-place

Whether you are a medical student just starting out on your career, or an established doctor wishing to develop yourself as a clinical leader, this practical, easy-to-use guide will give you the techniques and knowledge you require to excel.

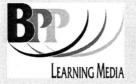

LEARNING MEDIA

More titles in the Progressing your Medical Career Series

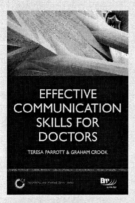

EFFECTIVE
COMMUNICATION
SKILLS FOR
DOCTORS

TERESA PARROTT & GRAHAM CROOK

£19.99
September 2011
Paperback
978-1-445379-56-2

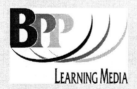

LEARNING MEDIA

Would you like to know how to improve your communication skills? Are you looking for a clearly written book which explores all aspects of effective medical communication?

There is an urgent need to improve doctors' communication skills. Research has shown that poor communication can contribute to patient dissatisfaction, lack of compliance and increased medico-legal problems. Improved communication skills will impact positively on all of these areas.

The last fifteen years have seen unprecedented changes in medicine and the role of doctors. Effective communication skills are vital to these new roles. But communication is not just related to personality. Skills can be learned which can make your communication more effective, and help you to improve your relationships with patients, their families and fellow doctors.

This book shows how to learn those skills and outlines why we all need to communicate more effectively. Healthcare is increasingly a partnership. Change is happening at all levels, from government directives to patient expectations. Communication is a bridge between the wisdom of the past and the vision of the future.

Readers of this book can also gain free access to an online module which upon successful completion can download a certificate for their portfolio of learning/Revalidation/CPD records.

This easy-to-read guide will help medical students and doctors at all stages of their careers improve their communication within a hospital environment.

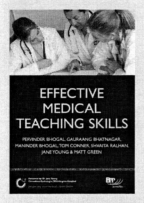
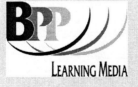

More titles in the Essential Clinical Handbook Series

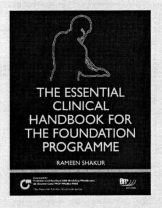

THE ESSENTIAL CLINICAL HANDBOOK FOR THE FOUNDATION PROGRAMME

RAMEEN SHAKUR

£24.99

October 2011

Paperback

978-1-445381-63-3

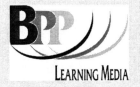

LEARNING MEDIA

Unsure of what clinical competencies you must gain to successfully complete the Foundation Programme? Unclear on how to ensure your ePortfolio is complete to enable your progression to ST training?

This up-to-date clinical handbook is aimed at current foundation doctors and clinical medical students and provides a comprehensive companion to help you in the day-to-day management of patients on the ward. Together with this it is the first handbook to also outline clearly how to gain the core clinical competencies required for successful completion of the Foundation Programme. Written by doctors for doctors this comprehensive handbook explains how to successfully manage all of the common cases you will face during the Foundation Programme and:

- Introduces the Foundation Programme and what is expected of a new doctor especially with the introduction of Modernising Medical Careers

- Illustrates clearly the best way to manage, step-by-step, over 150 commonly encountered clinical diseases, including NICE guidelines to ensure a gold standard of clinical care is achieved.

- Describes how to successfully gain the core clinical competencies within Medicine and Surgery including an extensive list of differentials and conditions explained

- Explores the various radiology images you will encounter and how to interpret them

- Tells you how to succeed in the assessment methods used including DOP's, Mini-CEX's and CBD's.

- Has step by step diagrammatic guide to doing common clinical procedures competently and safely.

- Outlines how to ensure your ePortfolio is maintained properly to ensure successful completion of the Foundation Programme.

- Provides tips and advice on how to start preparing now to ensure you are fully prepared and have the competitive edge for your CMT/ST application.

The introduction of the e-Portfolio as part of the Foundation Programme has paved the way for foundation doctors to take charge of their own learning and portfolio. Through following the expert guidance laid down in this handbook you will give yourself the best possible chance of progressing successfully through to CMT/ST training.

www.bpp.com/health

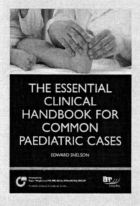
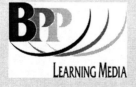

More titles in the Progressing your Medical Career Series

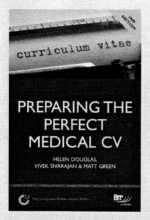

PREPARING THE PERFECT MEDICAL CV

HELEN DOUGLAS,
VIVEK SIVARAJAN & MATT GREEN

£19.99

October 2011

Paperback

978-1-445381-62-6

Are you unsure of how to structure your Medical CV? Would you like to know how to ensure you stand out from the crowd?

With competition for medical posts at an all time high it is vital that your Medical CV stands out over your fellow applicants. This comprehensive, unique and easy-to-read guide has been written with this in mind to help prospective medical students, current medical students and doctors of all grades prepare a Medical CV of the highest quality. Whether you are applying to medical school, currently completing your medical degree or a doctor progressing through your career (foundation doctor, specialty trainee in general practice, surgery or medicine, GP career grade or Consultant) this guide includes specific guidance for applicants at every level.

This time-saving and detailed guide:

- Explains what selection panels are looking for when reviewing applications at all levels.

- Discusses how to structure your Medical CV to ensure you stand out for the right reasons.

- Explores what information to include (and not to include) in your CV.

- Covers what to consider when maintaining a portfolio at every step of your career, including, for revalidation and relicensing purposes.

- Provides examples of high quality CVs to illustrate the above.

This unique guide will show you how to prepare your CV for every step of your medical career from pre-Medical School right through to Consultant level and should be a constant companion to ensure you secure your first choice post every time.

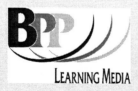

LEARNING MEDIA